Case Files™
Pharmacology

Second Edition

EUGENE C. TOY, MD
The John S. Dunn Senior Academic Chief and Program
 Director
Obstetrics and Gynecology Residency Program
The Methodist Hospital, Houston
Clerkship Director and Clinical Associate Professor
Department of Obstetrics and Gynecology
University of Texas Medical School at Houston
Houston, Texas

GARY C. ROSENFELD, PHD
Professor
Department of Integrative Biology and Pharmacology
Assistant Dean for Educational Programs
University of Texas Medical School at Houston
Houston, Texas

DAVID S. LOOSE, PHD
Associate Professor
Department of Integrative Biology and Pharmacology
University of Texas Medical School at Houston
Houston, Texas

DONALD BRISCOE, MD
Program Director
Family Medicine Residency
The Methodist Hospital, Houston
Medical Director
Houston Community Health Centers, Inc.
Denver Harbor Clinic
Houston, Texas

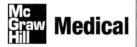

New York   Chicago San Francisco
Lisbon London Madrid Mexico City
Milan New Delhi San Juan Seoul
Singapore Sydney Toronto

Case Files™: Pharmacology, Second Edition

1 2 3 4 5 6 7 8 9 0   DOC/DOC   0 9 8

ISBN 978-0-07-148858-7
MHID 0-07-148858-8

Notice

Medicine is an ever-changing science. As new research and clinical experience broaden our knowledge, changes in treatment and drug therapy are required. The authors and the publisher of this work have checked with sources believed to be reliable in their efforts to provide information that is complete and generally in accord with the standard accepted at the time of publication. However, in view of the possibility of human error or changes in medical sciences, neither the editors nor the publisher nor any other party who has been involved in the preparation or publication of this work warrants that the information contained herein is in every respect accurate or complete, and they disclaim all responsibility for any errors or omissions or for the results obtained from use of the information contained in this work. Readers are encouraged to confirm the information contained herein with other sources. For example and in particular, readers are advised to check the product information sheet included in the package of each drug they plan to administer to be certain that the information contained in this work is accurate and that changes have not been made in the recommended dose or in the contraindications for administration. This recommendation is of particular importance in connection with new or infrequently used drugs.

This book was set in Times Roman by International Typesetting and Composition.
The editor was Catherine A. Johnson.
The production supervisor was Catherine Saggese.
Project management was provided by Gita Raman, International Typesetting and Composition.
The cover designer was Aimee Nordin.
RR Donnelley was printer and binder.

This book is printed on acid-free paper.

Library of Congress Cataloging-in-Publication Data

Case files. Pharmacology / Eugene C. Toy ... [et al.].—2nd ed.
    p. ; cm.
  Includes bibliographical references and index.
  ISBN-13: 978-0-07-148858-7 (pbk. : alk. paper)
  ISBN-10: 0-07-148858-8
    1. Clinical pharmacology—Case studies.   I. Toy, Eugene C.   II. Title: Pharmacology.
  [DNLM: 1. Pharmaceutical Preparations—Case Reports.   2. Pharmaceutical
  Preparations—Examination Questions.   QV 18.2 C337 2008]
  RM301.28.C37 2008
  615'.1—dc22

                                                                    2007038254

*To Dr. Larry C. Gilstrap III, whose encouragement is largely responsible for
my writing this series of books. He has been a personal inspiration, mentor,
and role model of an outstanding physician, teacher, and leader;
and to Dr. Edward Yeomans who has been a dear friend and
gleaming light of brilliance in obstetrics.*

—ECT

*To Dr. George Stancel who encouraged my passion for education;
to the medical students of the University of Texas, Medical School at Houston
who have consistently and constructively challenged me to be the
best teacher that I can be;
and to my special children and grandchildren,
Sydney, Stephanie, and Jacob.*

—GCR

*To the medical and graduate students of the
University of Texas Health Science Center in Houston who continually challenge
and make both teaching and research far more interesting;
and to William and Jane
for their patience and encouragement during the writing
and editing of the manuscript.*

—DSL

*To the dedicated staff, residents and faculty of the
Methodist Hospital Family Medicine Residency and Denver Harbor Clinic,
with whom I am privileged to work.*

—DB

❖ CONTENTS

❖ CONTRIBUTORS

Jeané Simmons Holmes, MD, FACOG
Assistant Clinical Professor
Obstetrics and Gynecology Residency Program
The Methodist Hospital, Houston
Houston, Texas
Polycystic Ovarian Syndrome

Lacy Kessler
Medical Student
Class of 2008
The University of Texas Medical School at Houston
Houston, Texas
Ergot Akyloids
Eicosanoids

Priti P. Schachel, MD
Assistant Professor
Department of Obstetrics and Gynecology
Weill Medical College of Cornell University
The Methodist Hospital, Houston
Houston, Texas
Polycystic Ovarian Syndrome

❖ ACKNOWLEDGMENTS

The inspiration for this basic science series occurred at an educational retreat led by Dr. L. Maximilian Buja, who at the time was the dean of the medical school. It has been such a joy to work together with Drs. Gary Rosenfeld and David Loose, who are both accomplished scientists and teachers. It has been rewarding to collaborate with Dr. Donald Briscoe, a scholar and an excellent teacher. I would like to thank McGraw-Hill for believing in the concept of teaching by clinical cases. I owe a great debt to Catherine Johnson, who has been a fantastically encouraging and enthusiastic editor.

At the University of Texas Medical School at Houston, we would like to recognize the bright and enthusiastic medical students who have inspired us to find better ways to teach. At The Methodist Hospital, I appreciate the support from Dr. Mark Boom, Dr. Karin Larsen Pollock, Mr. Reggie Abraham, Mr. John Lyle, and our fabulous Department Chair, Dr. Alan Kaplan. At St. Joseph Medical Center, I would like to recognize some of the finest administrators I have encountered: Phil Robinson, Pat Mathews, Laura Fortin, Dori Upton, Cecile Reynolds, John Bertini, MD, and Thomas V. Taylor, MD. I appreciate Marla Buffington's excellent advice and assistance. Without the help from my colleague and friend, Dr. John C. McBride, this book could not have been written. Most importantly, I am humbled by the love, affection, and encouragement from my lovely wife, Terri, and our four children, Andy, Michael, Allison, and Christina.

Eugene C. Toy

❖ INTRODUCTION

Often, the medical student will cringe at the "drudgery" of the basic science courses and see little connection between a field such as pharmacology and clinical problems. Clinicians, however, often wish they knew more about the basic sciences, because it is through the science that we can begin to understand the complexities of the human body and thus have rational methods of diagnosis and treatment.

Mastering the knowledge in a discipline such as pharmacology is a formidable task. It is even more difficult to retain this information and to recall it when the clinical setting is encountered. To accomplish this synthesis, pharmacology is optimally taught in the context of medical situations, and this is reinforced later during the clinical rotations. The gulf between the basic sciences and the patient arena is wide. Perhaps one way to bridge this gulf is with carefully constructed clinical cases that ask basic science-oriented questions. In an attempt to achieve this goal, we have designed a collection of patient cases to teach pharmacology-related points. More importantly, the explanations for these cases emphasize the underlying mechanisms and relate the clinical setting to the basic science data. The principles are explored rather than overemphasizing rote memorization.

This book is organized for versatility: to allow the student "in a rush" to go quickly through the scenarios and check the corresponding answers and to provide more detailed information for the student who wants thought-provoking explanations. The answers are arranged from simple to complex: a summary of the pertinent points, the bare answers, a clinical correlation, an approach to the pharmacology topic, a comprehension test at the end for reinforcement or emphasis, and a list of references for further reading. The clinical cases are arranged by system to better reflect the organization within the basic science. Finally, to encourage thinking about mechanisms and relationships, we used open-ended questions in the clinical cases. Nevertheless, several multiple-choice questions are included at the end of each scenario to reinforce concepts or introduce related topics.

HOW TO GET THE MOST OUT OF THIS BOOK

Each case is designed to introduce a clinically related issue and includes open-ended questions usually asking a basic science question, but at times, to break up the monotony, there will be a clinical question. The answers are organized into four different parts:

PART I

1. **Summary**
2. **A straightforward answer** is given for each open-ended question.
3. **Clinical Correlation**—A discussion of the relevant points relating the basic science to the clinical manifestations, and perhaps introducing the student to issues such as diagnosis and treatment.

PART II

An **approach to the basic science concept** consisting of three parts:

1. **Objectives**—A listing of the two to four main knowledge objectives that are critical for understanding the underlying pharmacology to answer the question and relate to the clinical situation.
2. **Definitions of basic terminology.**
3. **Discussion of the specific class of agents.**

PART III

Comprehension Questions—Each case includes several multiple-choice questions that reinforce the material or introduces new and related concepts. Questions about the material not found in the text are explained in the answers.

PART IV

Pharmacology Pearls—A listing of several important points, many clinically relevant, reiterated as a summation of the text and to allow for easy review, such as before an examination.

Applying the Basic Sciences to Clinical Medicine

PART 1. APPROACH TO LEARNING PHARMACOLOGY

Pharmacology is best learned by a systematic approach, understanding the physiology of the body, recognizing that **every medication has desirable and undesirable effects,** and being aware that the biochemical and pharmacologic properties of a drug affects its characteristics such as duration of action, volume of distribution, passage through the blood-brain barrier, mechanism of elimination, and route of administration. Rather than memorizing the characteristics of a medication, the student should strive to learn the underlying rationale such as, "Second-generation antihistamine agents are less lipid soluble than first-generation antihistamines and therefore do not cross the blood-brain barrier as readily; thus, second-generation antihistamines are not as sedating. Because they both bind the histamine H_1 receptor, the efficacy is the same."

KEY TERMS

Pharmacology: The study of substances that interact with living systems through biochemical processes.

Drug: A substance used in the prevention, diagnosis, or treatment of disease.

Toxicology: A branch of pharmacology that studies the undesirable effects of chemicals on living organisms.

Food and Drug Administration (FDA): The federal agency responsible for the safety and efficacy of all drugs in the United States, as well as food and cosmetics.

Adverse effect: Also known as side effect; all unintended actions of a drug that result from the lack of specificity of drug action. All drugs are capable of producing adverse effects.

Pharmacodynamics: The actions of a drug on a living organism, including mechanisms of action and receptor interaction.

Pharmacokinetics: The actions of the living organism on the drug, including absorption, distribution, and elimination.

Volume of distribution (V_d): The size of the "compartment" into which a drug is distributed following absorption and is determined by the equation:

$$V_d = \text{Dose (mg) drug administered/Initial plasma concentration (mg/L)}$$

Potency of drug: Relative amount of drug needed to produce a given response, determined largely by the amount of drug that reaches the site of action and by the affinity of the drug for the receptor.

Efficacy: Drug effect as the maximum response it is able to produce and is determined by the number of drug-receptor complexes and the ability of the receptor to be activated once bound. **EC-50** refers to the drug concentration that produces 50 percent of the maximal response, whereas **ED-50** refers to the drug dose that is pharmacologically effective in 50 percent of the population.

Absorption: The movement of a drug from the administration site into the blood stream usually requiring the crossing of one or more biologic membranes. Important parameters include lipid solubility, ionization, size of the molecule, and presence of a transport mechanism.

Elimination: Process by which a drug is removed from the body, generally by either metabolism or excretion. Elimination follows various kinetic models. For example, **first-order kinetics** describes most circumstances, and means that the rate of drug elimination depends on the concentration of the drug in the plasma as described by the equation:

Rate of elimination from body = Constant × Drug concentration

Zero-order kinetics: It is less common and means that the rate of elimination is constant and does not depend on the plasma drug concentration. This may be a consequence of a circumstance such as saturation of liver enzymes or saturation of the kidney transport mechanisms.

Bioavailability: The percentage of an ingested drug that is actually absorbed into the bloodstream.

Route of administration: Drug may be delivered **intravenously** (IV or iv) for delivery directly into the bloodstream, **intramuscularly** (IM), and **subcutaneously** (SC). The medication may be depot and slow release, **inhalant** for rapid absorption and delivery to the bronchi and lungs, **sublingual** to bypass the first-pass effect, **intrathecal** for agents that penetrate the blood-brain barrier poorly, **rectal** to avoid hepatic first-pass effect and for nausea, and **topical** administration when local effect is desired such as dermatologic or ophthalmic agents.

PART 2. APPROACH TO DISEASE

Physicians usually tackle clinical situations by taking a history (asking questions), performing a physical examination, obtaining selective laboratory and imaging tests, and then formulating a diagnosis. The synthesis of the history, physical examination, and imaging or laboratory tests is called the **clinical database.** After reaching a diagnosis, a treatment plan is usually initiated, and the patient is followed for a clinical response. Rational understanding of disease and plans for treatment are best acquired by learning about the normal human processes on a basic science level; likewise, being aware of how disease alters the normal physiologic processes is also best understood on a basic science level. Pharmacology and therapeutics require also the ability to tailor the correct medication to the patient's situation and awareness of the medication's adverse effect profile. Sometimes, the patient has an adverse reaction to a medication as the chief complaint, and the physician must be able to identify the medication as the culprit. An understanding of the underlying basic science allows for more rational analysis and medication choices.

PART 3. APPROACH TO READING

There are seven key questions that help to stimulate the application of basic science information to the clinical setting. These are:

1. **Which of the available medications is most likely to achieve the desired therapeutic effect and/or is responsible for the described symptoms or signs?**
2. **What is the likely mechanism for the clinical effect(s) and adverse effect(s) of the medication?**
3. **What is the basic pharmacologic profile (e.g., absorption, elimination) for medications in a certain class, and what are the differences among the agents within the class?**
4. **Given basic pharmacologic definitions such as therapeutic index (TI) or certain safety factor (TD_1/ED_{99}), or median lethal dose (LD_{50}), how do medications compare in their safety profile?**
5. **Given a particular clinical situation with described unique patient characteristics, which medication is most appropriate?**
6. **What is the best treatment for the toxic effect of a medication?**
7. **What are the drug-drug interactions to be cautious about regarding a particular medication?**

1. **Which of the following medications is most likely to be responsible for the described symptoms or signs?**
    The student must be aware of the various effects, both desirable and undesirable, produced by particular medications. Knowledge of desirable therapeutic effects is essential in selecting the appropriate drug for the particular clinical application; likewise, an awareness of its adverse effects is necessary, because patients may come into the physician's office with a complaint caused by a drug effect unaware that their symptoms are because of a prescribed medication. It is only by being aware of the common and dangerous effects that the clinician can arrive at the correct diagnosis. The student is encouraged not to merely memorize the comparative adverse effect profiles of the drugs, but rather to understand the underlying mechanisms.
2. **What is the likely mechanism for the clinical effect(s) and adverse effect(s) of the medication?**
    As noted above, the student should strive to learn the underlying physiologic, biochemical, or cellular explanation for the described drug effect. This understanding allows for the rational choice of an alternative agent or the reasonable choice of an agent to alleviate the symptoms or explanatory advice to the patient regarding behavioral changes to diminish any adverse affects. For example, if a 60-year-old woman who takes medications for osteoporosis complains of severe "heartburn," one may be suspicious, knowing that the bisphosphonate

medication alendronate can cause esophagitis. Instruction to the patient to take the medication while sitting upright and remaining upright for at least 30 minutes would be the proper course of action, because gravity will assist in keeping the alendronate in the stomach rather than allowing regurgitation into the distal esophagus.

3. **What is the basic pharmacologic profile (absorption, elimination, volume of distribution) for medications in a certain class, and what are differences among the agents within the class?**

Understanding the pharmacologic profile of medications allows for rational therapeutics. However, instead of memorizing the separate profiles for every medication, grouping the drugs together into classes allows for more efficient learning and better comprehension. An excellent starting point for the student of pharmacology would be to study how a **prototype drug** within a drug class organized by structure or mechanism of action may be used to treat a condition (such as hypertension). Then within each category of agents, the student should try to identify important subclasses or drug differences. For example, hypertensive agents can be categorized as diuretic agents, β-adrenergic-blocking agents, calcium-channel-blocking agents, and renin-angiotensin system inhibitors. Within the subclassification of renin-angiotensin system inhibitors, the angiotensin-converting enzyme inhibitors can cause the side effect of a dry cough caused by the increase in bradykinin brought about by the enzyme blockade; instead, the angiotensin-1 receptor blockers do not affect the bradykinin levels and so do not cause the cough as often.

4. **Given basic pharmacologic definitions such as therapeutic index (TI) or certain safety factor (TD_1/ED_{99}), or median lethal dose (LD_{50}), how do medications compare in their safety profile?**

Therapeutic index (TI): Defined as the TD_{50}/ED_{50} (the ratio of the dose that produces a toxic effect in half the population to the dose that produces the desired effect in half the population).

Certain safety factor (TD_1/ED_{99}): Defined as the ratio of the dose that produces the toxic effect in 1 percent of the population to the dose that produces the desired effect in 99 percent of the population; also known as **standard safety measure.**

Median lethal dose (LD_{50}): Defined as the median lethal dose, the dose that will kill half the population.

Based on these definitions, a desirable medication would have a high therapeutic index (toxic dose is many times that of the efficacious dose), high certain safety factor, and high median lethal dose (much higher than therapeutic dose). Likewise, medications such as digoxin that have a low therapeutic index require careful monitoring of levels and vigilance for side effects.

5. **Given a particular clinical situation with described unique patient characteristics, which medication is most appropriate?**

The student must weigh various advantages and disadvantages, as well as different patient attributes. Some of those may include compliance with medications, allergies to medications, liver or renal insufficiency, age, coexisting medical disorders, and other medications. The student must be able to sift through the medication profile and identify the most dangerous adverse effects. For example, if a patient is already taking a monoamine-oxidase-inhibiting agent for depression, then adding a serotonin reuptake inhibitor would be potentially fatal, because serotonin syndrome may ensue (hyperthermia, muscle rigidity, death).

6. **What is the best treatment for the toxic effect of a medication?**

If complications of drug therapy are present, the student should know the proper treatment. This is best learned by understanding the drug mechanism of action. For example, a patient who has taken excessive opioids may develop respiratory depression, caused by either a heroin overdose or pain medication, which may be fatal. The treatment of an opioid overdose includes the ABCs (airway, breathing, circulation) and the administration of naloxone, which is a competitive antagonist of opioids.

7. **What are the drug-drug interactions to be concerned with regarding a particular medication?**

Patients are often prescribed multiple medications, from either the same practitioner or different clinicians. Patients may not be aware of the drug-drug interactions; thus, the clinician must compile, as a component of good clinical practice, a current list of all medications (prescribed, over-the-counter, and herbal) taken by the patient. Thus, the student should be aware of the most common and dangerous interactions; once again, understanding the underlying mechanism allows for lifelong learning rather than short-term rote memorization of facts that are easily forgotten. For example, magnesium sulfate to stop preterm labor should not be used if the patient is taking a calcium-channel-blocking agent such as nifedipine. Magnesium sulfate acts as a competitive inhibitor of calcium, and by decreasing its intracellular availability it slows down smooth muscle contraction such as in the uterus. Calcium-channel blockers potentiate the inhibition of calcium influx and can lead to toxic effects, such as respiratory depression.

COMPREHENSION QUESTIONS

[I.1]   Bioavailability of an agent is maximal when the drug has which of the following qualities?

A. Highly lipid soluble
B. More than 100 Daltons in molecular weight
C. Highly bound to plasma proteins
D. Highly ionized

[I.2] An agent is noted to have a very low calculated volume of distribution (V_d). Which of the following is the best explanation?

A. The agent is eliminated by the kidneys, and the patient has renal insufficiency.
B. The agent is extensively bound to plasma proteins.
C. The agent is extensively sequestered in tissue.
D. The agent is eliminated by zero-order kinetics.

[I.3] Which of the following describes the first-pass effect?

A. Inactivation of a drug as a result of the gastric acids.
B. Absorption of a drug through the duodenum.
C. Drug given orally is metabolized by the liver before entering the circulation.
D. Drug given IV accumulates quickly in the central nervous system (CNS).

[I.4] A laboratory experiment is being conducted in which a mammal is injected with a noncompetitive antagonist to the histamine receptor. Which of the following best describes this agent?

A. The drug binds to the histamine receptor and partially activates it.
B. The drug binds to the histamine receptor but does not activate it.
C. The drug binds to the receptor, but not where histamine binds, and prevents the receptor from being activated.
D. The drug irreversibly binds to the histamine receptor and renders it ineffective.

[I.5] A 25-year-old medical student is given a prescription for asthma, which the physician states has a very high therapeutic index. Which of the statements best characterizes the drug as it relates to the therapeutic index?

A. The drug's serum levels will likely need to be carefully monitored.
B. The drug is likely to cross the blood-brain barrier.
C. The drug is likely to have extensive drug-drug interactions.
D. The drug is unlikely to have any serious adverse effects.

[I.6] A drug M is injected IV into a laboratory subject. It is noted to have high serum protein binding. Which of the following is most likely to be increased as a result?

A. Drug interaction
B. Distribution of the drug to tissue sites
C. Renal excretion
D. Liver metabolism

[I.7] A bolus of drug K is given IV. The drug is noted to follow first-order kinetics. Which of the following describes the elimination of drug K?

   A. The rate of elimination of drug K is constant.
   B. The rate of elimination of drug K is proportional to the patient's renal function.
   C. The rate of elimination of drug K is proportional to its concentration in the patient's plasma.
   D. The rate of elimination of drug K is dependent on a nonlinear relationship to the plasma protein concentration.

Answers

[I.1] **A.** Transport across biologic membranes and thus bioavailability is maximal with high lipid solubility.

[I.2] **B.** The volume of distribution is calculated by administering a known dose of drug (mg) IV and then measuring an initial plasma concentration (mg/L). The ratio of the mass of drug given (mg) divided by the initial plasma concentration (mg/L) gives the V_d. A very low V_d may indicate extensive protein binding (drug is sequestered in the bloodstream), whereas a high V_d may indicate extensive tissue binding (drug is sequestered in the tissue).

[I.3] **C.** The first-pass effect refers to the process in which following oral administration a drug is extensively metabolized as it initially passes through the liver, before it enters the general circulation. Liver enzymes may metabolize the agent to such an extent that the drug cannot be administered orally.

[I.4] **C.** A noncompetitive antagonist binds to the receptor at a site other than the agonist-binding site and renders it less effective by preventing agonist binding or preventing activation.

[I.5] **D.** An agent with a high therapeutic index means the toxic dose is very much higher than the therapeutic dose, and it is less likely to produce toxic effects at therapeutic levels.

[I.6] **A.** High protein binding means less drug to the tissue, the kidney, and the liver. Drug interaction may occur if the agent binds to the same protein site as other drugs, thus displacing drugs and increasing serum levels.

[I.7] **C.** First-order kinetics means the rate of elimination of a drug is proportional to the plasma concentration.

PHARMACOLOGY PEARLS

  Understanding the pharmacologic mechanisms of medications allows for rational choices for therapy, fewer medication errors, and rapid recognition and reversal of toxic effects.

  The therapeutic index, certain safety factor (TD_1/ED_{99}), and median lethal dose are various methods of describing the potential toxicity of medications.

❖ There are seven key questions to stimulate the application of basic science information to the clinical arena.

REFERENCES

Braunwald E, Fauci AS, Kasper KL, et al., eds. Harrison's Principles of Internal Medicine, 16th ed. New York: McGraw-Hill, 2004.

Rosenfeld GC, Loose-Mitchell DS. Pharmacology, 4th ed. Philadelphia, PA: Lippincott, Williams & Wilkins, 2007:1.

Clinical Cases

❖ CASE 1

A 12-year-old girl presents to your office with a sore throat and fever. You diagnose her with pharyngitis caused by group A β-hemolytic *Streptococcus*. She is given an IM injection of penicillin. Approximately 5 minutes later, she is found to be in respiratory distress and audibly wheezing. Her skin is mottled and cool, she is tachycardic (rapid heart rate), and her blood pressure has fallen to 70/20 mm Hg. You immediately diagnose her as having an anaphylactic reaction to the penicillin and give an SC injection of epinephrine.

◆ **What effect will epinephrine have on this patient's vascular system?**

◆ **Which adrenoceptor primarily mediates the vascular response?**

◆ **What effect will epinephrine have on her respiratory system?**

◆ **Which adrenoceptor primarily mediates the respiratory system response?**

ANSWERS TO CASE 1: AUTONOMIC SYMPATHETIC NERVOUS SYSTEM

Summary: A 12-year-old girl with "strep throat" is given an injection of penicillin and develops an acute anaphylactic reaction.

◆ **Effect of epinephrine on vascular system:** Vasoconstriction.

◆ **Adrenoceptor which primarily mediates the vascular response:** Alpha-1 (α_1).

◆ **Effect of epinephrine on the pulmonary system:** Bronchial muscle relaxation.

◆ **Adrenoceptor which primarily mediates the pulmonary response:** Beta-2 (β_2).

CLINICAL CORRELATION

Anaphylaxis is an acute, immune-mediated response to an allergen characterized by bronchospasm, wheezing, tachycardia, and hypotension. Epinephrine is the drug of choice used to treat this condition because it appears, through the activation of alpha (α)- and beta (β)-adrenoceptors, to counteract the pathophysiologic processes underlying anaphylaxis. As with all emergencies, the ABCs (airway, breathing, circulation) should be addressed first. Occasionally, the anaphylaxis causes laryngeal edema to the extent that the airway is compromised, and intubation (placement of a tube in the trachea) is impossible. In these circumstances, an emergency airway, such as a surgical cricothyroidotomy (creating an opening from the skin through the cricoid cartilage), is required.

APPROACH TO THE AUTONOMIC SYMPATHETIC NERVOUS SYSTEM

Objectives

1. List the neurotransmitters of the autonomic sympathetic nervous system and describe their anatomical localization.
2. List the receptors and receptor-subtypes of the autonomic sympathetic nervous system.
3. Predict the responses to activation and inhibition of autonomic sympathetic nervous system receptors.

Definitions

Autonomic nervous system: Subdivision of the efferent peripheral nervous system that is largely under unconscious control (the somatic subdivision of the peripheral nervous system is largely under conscious control), shown in Figure 1-1.

Sympathetic nervous system: A division of the autonomic nervous system (the other is the parasympathetic nervous system) that originates in nuclei of the CNS. Preganglionic fibers exit through the **thoracic and lumbar spinal nerves** to synapse on ganglia close to the spinal cord and also on the adrenal medulla (considered modified ganglia). Postganglionic fibers innervate a wide variety of effector organs and tissues, including arteriole and bronchial smooth muscles.

Agonist: A drug that activates a receptor and results in a pharmacologic response.

Antagonist: A drug that binds to receptors with little or no effect of its own, but that can block the action of an agonist that binds to the same receptors.

DISCUSSION

Class

The neurotransmitter **norepinephrine** is released from the efferent nerves of the **sympathetic autonomic nervous system** at postganglionic sympathetic (also known as "adrenergic") nerve endings, whereas **epinephrine and some norepinephrine** are released from the **adrenal medulla.**

These endogenous catecholamine neurotransmitter agonists interact at postjunctional specialized cell membrane components called **adrenoceptors** (named after the adrenergic nerves that innervate them) that are classified as either alpha (α) or beta (β).

There are two **subtypes of the α-adrenoceptor, α_1 and α_2,** each of which has variants of unclear pharmacologic importance. Activation of the autonomic sympathetic nervous system α_1-adrenoceptors by adrenergic agonists results in, among other effects, **contraction of most vascular smooth muscle (α_1)** causing increased peripheral resistance and blood pressure, **contraction of the pupillary dilator muscle** resulting in **mydriasis,** an indirectly mediated (through inhibition of acetylcholine [Ach] release) **relaxation of gastrointestinal smooth muscle and contraction of gastrointestinal sphincters** (α_1), and activation of the seminal vesicles, prostate gland, and ductus deferens that results in **ejaculation.** Activation of prejunctional adrenoceptor autoreceptors (α_2) by catecholamines results in (feedback) inhibition of the release of norepinephrine and other neurotransmitters from their respective nerve endings.

There are also **three subtypes of the β-adrenoceptor, β_1, β_2, and β_3.** Activation of the autonomic sympathetic nervous system α-adrenoceptors by adrenergic agonists results in, among other effects, increased rate and **force of**

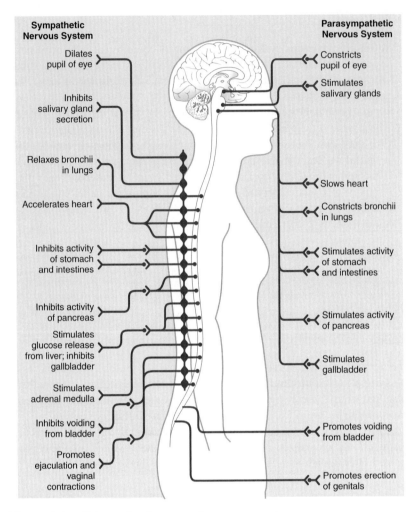

Sympathetic Nervous System

Dilates pupil of eye

Inhibits salivary gland secretion

Relaxes bronchii in lungs

Accelerates heart

Inhibits activity of stomach and intestines

Inhibits activity of pancreas

Stimulates glucose release from liver; inhibits gallbladder

Stimulates adrenal medulla

Inhibits voiding from bladder

Promotes ejaculation and vaginal contractions

Parasympathetic Nervous System

Constricts pupil of eye

Stimulates salivary glands

Slows heart

Constricts bronchii in lungs

Stimulates activity of stomach and intestines

Stimulates activity of pancreas

Stimulates gallbladder

Promotes voiding from bladder

Promotes erection of genitals

Figure 1-1. Schematic of autonomic nervous system.

contraction of the heart (β_1), smooth muscle relaxation of bronchi causing bronchodilation (β_2), and activation of fat cell lipolysis (β_3).

Because the catecholamines epinephrine and norepinephrine have important physiologic roles, drugs that block their actions, that is, adrenoceptor antagonists, can have important pharmacologic effects, many of which are clinically useful. α-Adrenoceptor nonselective antagonists (e.g., phentolamine) are used to treat the hypertension of pheochromocytoma (a tumor that secretes catecholamines) and male erectile dysfunction, whereas the more selective α_1-adrenoceptor antagonists (e.g., prazosin, terazosin, doxazosin) are used to treat hypertension and benign prostatic hyperplasia (Table 1-1).

Table 1-1
SELECTED EFFECTS OF ADRENOCEPTOR ACTIVATION

ORGAN	EFFECTS (ADRENOCEPTOR SUBTYPE)
Bronchial smooth muscle	Dilates (β_2)
Heart rate and contractile force	Increases (β_1)
Eye (pupil size)	Dilates (α_1)[*]
Blood vessels	Constrict (α_1)[†,‡]
Gastrointestinal tract (tone, motility, secretions)	Decrease (α_1, β_2)
Pancreas (insulin release)	Decrease (α_2)

[*]**Dilation (mydriasis)** results from α_1-adrenoceptor stimulation of the radial muscle.
[†]Skeletal muscle blood vessels have β_2-adrenoceptors that, when activated, result in **vessel constriction.**
[‡]Coronary arteries also have β-adrenoceptors that, when activated, result in **vessel dilation,** which is the dominant effect.

Structure

Epinephrine and norepinephrine are catecholamines, **synthesized from tyrosine,** that possess a catechol nucleus with an ethylamine side chain (epinephrine is the methylated side chain derivative of norepinephrine). The **rate-limiting enzyme** in this process is **tyrosine hydroxylase.**

Mechanism of Action

Epinephrine binds to α_1-adrenoceptors and, through a G-protein (Gq-type GTP-binding protein [Gq])-mediated activation of phospholipase C and stimulation of polyphosphoinositide hydrolysis, results in formation of inositol 1,4,5-trisphosphate (IP_3) that promotes the release of stored intracellular Ca^{2+}. Epinephrine interaction with α_2-adrenoceptors results in activation of a Gi-type GTP-binding protein (Gi) to inhibit adenylyl cyclase activity, thereby decreasing cyclic adenosine monophosphate (cAMP) levels. Epinephrine perhaps also increases β_1-adrenoceptor-mediated influx of Ca^{2+} across membrane channels. In addition to the increased formation of the **"second messenger" IP_3,** epinephrine also increases the phospholipase-mediated formation of another second messenger diacylglycerol (DAG) that activates protein kinase C that influences the activity of a number of other signaling pathways. Epinephrine also activates β_1- and β_2-adrenoceptors to increase a G-protein-mediated stimulation of adenylyl cyclase activity, thereby increasing intracellular cAMP levels and the activity of cAMP-dependent protein kinases.

Administration

Epinephrine is generally administered **parenterally** (IM) for treatment of anaphylactic shock. For this and other conditions, it is also available as IV, SC, ophthalmic, nasal, and aerosol preparations. Norepinephrine is only available for parenteral, generally IV, administration.

Pharmacokinetics

Epinephrine released from the adrenal gland is metabolized primarily by catechol-*O*-methyltransferase (COMT) and monoamine oxidase (MAO). The action of norepinephrine released from nerve endings is terminated primarily by reuptake into nerve terminals (uptake 1) and other cells (uptake 2).

COMPREHENSION QUESTIONS

[1.1]   A patient with septic shock is noted to have persistent hypotension despite dopamine infusion. Epinephrine in an IV infusion is used. With which adrenoceptor does epinephrine act to constrict vascular smooth muscle?

   A. α_1-Adrenoceptors
   B. α_2-Adrenoceptors
   C. β_1-Adrenoceptors
   D. β_2-Adrenoceptors

[1.2]   A 16-year-old male is having an acute asthmatic attack. Epinephrine is given SC. With which of the following adrenoceptors does epinephrine act to dilate bronchial smooth muscle?

   A. α_1-Adrenoceptors
   B. α_2-Adrenoceptors
   C. β_1-Adrenoceptors
   D. β_2-Adrenoceptors

[1.3]   Which of the following best describes the cellular action of epinephrine?

   A. Activation of adenylyl cyclase
   B. Decreased activity of cAMP-dependent protein kinases
   C. Increased intracellular stores of Ca^{2+}
   D. Inhibition of the activity of phospholipase

[1.4]   Epinephrine-mediated β_1-adrenoceptor activation results in which of the following?

   A. Constriction of bronchial smooth muscle
   B. Decreased gastrointestinal motility
   C. Dilation of the pupils
   D. Increased heart rate

Answers

[1.1]   **A.** α_1-Adrenoceptors mediate vasoconstriction in many vascular beds. In skeletal muscle, epinephrine can act at β_2-adrenoceptors to cause vasodilation.

[1.2]   **D.** Epinephrine acts on β_2-adrenoceptors to cause smooth muscle relaxation of bronchi resulting in bronchodilation. Because of adverse cardiovascular effects of epinephrine (β_1), more selective β_2-adrenoceptor agonists are now used (e.g., albuterol).

[1.3]   **A.** Epinephrine activates α_1-adrenoceptors to cause a release of intracellular stored Ca^{2+} and β_1- and β_2-adrenoceptors to activate adenylyl cyclase.

[1.4]   **D.** Epinephrine activation of β_1-adrenoceptors results in an increase in heart rate. Activation of α_1-adrenoceptors results in dilation of the pupil. Activation of β_2-adrenoceptors causes dilation of bronchial smooth muscle and decreased gastrointestinal (GI) motility.

PHARMACOLOGY PEARLS

❖ Physiologically epinephrine acts as a hormone on distant cells after its release from the adrenal medulla.

❖ As exceptions, sympathetic postganglionic neurons that innervate sweat glands and renal vascular smooth muscle release, respectively, ACh and dopamine rather than norepinephrine.

❖ Exogenously administered epinephrine increases blood pressure through its action on β_1-adrenoceptors in the heart, resulting in increased heart rate and force of contraction and through its action on α_1-adrenoceptors in many vascular beds that results in vasoconstriction.

❖ In skeletal muscle, epinephrine injection can result in vasodilation (β_2) that in some cases may lead to a decreased total peripheral resistance and a decrease in diastolic pressure.

❖ Norepinephrine has little, if any, effect on β_2-adrenoceptors (norepinephrine and epinephrine have similar effects on α- and β_1-adrenoceptors), thus increasing both systolic and diastolic blood pressure.

REFERENCES

Goldstein DS, Robertson D, Straus SE, et al. Dysautonomias: clinical disorders of the autonomic nervous system. Ann Intern Med 2002;137(9):753–63.

Brown SG. Cardiovascular aspects of anaphylaxis: implications for treatment and diagnosis. Curr Opin Allergy Clin Immunol 2005;5(4):359–64.

Clark AL, Cleland JG. The control of adrenergic function in heart failure: therapeutic intervention. Heart Fail Rev 2000;5(1):101–14.

August P. Initial treatment of hypertension. N Engl J Med 2003;348(7):610–7.

A 61-year-old man is noted to have increased intraocular pressure on a routine eye examination. The visual acuity is normal in both eyes. The dilated eye examination reveals no evidence of optic nerve damage. Visual field testing shows mild loss of peripheral vision. He is diagnosed with primary open-angle glaucoma and is started on pilocarpine ophthalmic drops.

◆ **What is the action of pilocarpine on the muscles of the iris and cilia?**

◆ **What receptor mediates this action?**

◆ **Is pilocarpine the appropriate first-line drug for treatment of primary open-angle glaucoma?**

ANSWERS TO CASE 2: MUSCARINIC CHOLINOMIMETIC AGENTS

Summary: A 61-year-old man with open-angle glaucoma is prescribed pilocarpine ophthalmic drops.

◆ **Action of pilocarpine on muscles of the iris and cilia:** Constriction of the muscles

◆ **Receptor that mediates this action:** Muscarinic cholinoreceptor

◆ **First-line drugs to treat primary open-angle glaucoma:** Prostaglandin analogs

CLINICAL CORRELATION

Open-angle glaucoma is a disease caused by obstruction of the outflow of aqueous humor into the canal of Schlemm, causing an increase in intraocular pressure. The use of a direct-acting muscarinic agonist, such as pilocarpine, causes contraction of the muscles of the cilia and iris. Because these are circular muscles, the pupil is constricted, which helps to relieve the outflow obstruction and lower the intraocular pressure. Although not common with the use of topical ophthalmic drops, bronchospasm and pulmonary edema has been noted with the use of pilocarpine drops. More commonly, blurred vision and myopia (nearsightedness) occur as a result of the impairment of accommodation caused by the contraction of the iris and ciliary muscles.

The use of a direct-acting muscarinic agonist such as pilocarpine to treat open-angle glaucoma is now not common due to its numerous side effects, the need to administer it up to four times per day, and the availability of other agents. Prostaglandin analogs such as latanoprost are now considered first-line therapy for this condition followed by β-adrenoceptor agonists.

APPROACH TO MUSCARINIC CHOLINOMIMETIC AGENTS

Objectives

1. Be able to list the receptors of the parasympathetic nervous system.
2. Contrast the actions and effects of direct and indirect stimulation of muscarinic cholinoreceptors.
3. List the therapeutic uses of parasympathomimetic agents.
4. List the adverse effects of parasympathomimetic agents.

Definitions

Parasympathetic nervous system: An anatomic division of the autonomic nervous system (the other is the sympathetic nervous system) that originates in nuclei of the CNS. Preganglionic fibers exit through **cranial and sacral spinal nerves** to synapse via short postganglionic nerve fibers on ganglia, many of which are in the organs they innervate.

Cholinomimetic agents: Agents that **mimic the action of ACh.** These act directly or indirectly to activate **cholinoreceptors.** Some directly acting agents (pilocarpine, bethanechol, carbachol) are designed to act selectively on either muscarinic or nicotinic cholinoreceptors, whereas indirectly acting agents (such as neostigmine, physostigmine, edrophonium, demecarium), which inhibit the enzyme acetylcholinesterase (AChE) that is responsible for the inactivation of ACh, can activate both. Pilocarpine is a directly acting cholinomimetic agent that acts chiefly at muscarinic cholinoreceptors. Additional selectivity of pilocarpine and other cholinomimetics in the treatment of glaucoma is achieved by the use of an ophthalmic (topical) preparation.

DISCUSSION

Class

The **efferent nerves of the parasympathetic autonomic nervous system** release the **neurotransmitter ACh** at both preganglionic and postganglionic (i.e., "cholinergic") nerve endings, and also at somatic nerve endings. Nitric oxide is a cotransmitter at many of the parasympathetic postganglionic sites.

The **ACh** released from nerve endings of the parasympathetic nervous system interacts at specialized cell membrane components called cholinoreceptors that are classified as either **nicotinic or muscarinic** after the alkaloids initially used to distinguish them.

Nicotinic cholinoreceptors are localized at **all postganglionic neurons** (the autonomic ganglia), including the adrenal medulla, and skeletal muscle endplates innervated by somatic nerves. **Muscarinic cholinoreceptors** are localized at **organs** innervated by parasympathetic postganglionic nerve endings, for example, on **cardiac atrial muscle, sinoatrial node cells, and atrioventricular node cells,** where activation can cause a **negative chronotropic effect** and delayed atrioventricular conduction. Cholinergic stimulation of **muscarinic receptors** in the **smooth muscle, exocrine glands, and vascular endothelium** can cause, respectively, **bronchoconstriction, increased acid secretion, and vasodilation** (Table 2-1).

There are **two subtypes of the nicotinic cholinoreceptors: N_N,** localized to **postganglionic neurons, and N_M,** localized to **the skeletal muscle endplates.** There are three pharmacologically important subtypes of the **muscarinic cholinoreceptors, M_1, M_2, and M_3** (two additional subtypes have been identified by

Table 2-1
EFFECTS OF CHOLINORECEPTOR ACTIVATION

ORGAN	EFFECTS
Bronchial smooth muscle	Contracts
Heart rate	Decreases
Eye smooth muscles Pupil size Accommodation	Contracts Contracts
Blood vessels	Dilate[*]
Gastrointestinal tract (tone, motility, secretions)	Increase

[*]There is no parasympathetic innervation of blood vessels. However, they have cholinoreceptors that when activated result in their dilation.

cloning), that alone or in combination are localized to sympathetic postganglionic neurons (and the CNS), to the atrial muscle, sinoatrial (SA) cells, and atrioventricular (AV) node of the heart, to smooth muscle, to exocrine glands, and to the vascular endothelium that does not receive parasympathetic innervation.

Directly and indirectly acting parasympathetic cholinomimetic agents, primarily pilocarpine and bethanechol, and neostigmine, are used most often therapeutically to treat certain diseases of the eye (acute angle-closure glaucoma), the urinary tract (urinary tract retention), the gastrointestinal tract (postoperative ileus), salivary glands (xerostomia), and the neuromuscular junction (myasthenia gravis). The **ACh** is generally not used clinically because of its numerous actions and **very rapid hydrolysis by AChE and pseudocholinesterase.**

The adverse effects of direct- and indirect-acting cholinomimetics result from cholinergic excess and may include **diarrhea, salivation, sweating, bronchial constriction, vasodilation, and bradycardia.** Nausea and vomiting are also common. Adverse effects of cholinesterase inhibitors (most often as a result of toxicity from pesticide exposure, e.g., **organophosphates**) also may include **muscle weakness, convulsions, and respiratory failure.**

Structure

ACh is a choline ester that is not very lipid soluble because of its **charged quaternary ammonium group.** It **interacts with both muscarinic and nicotinic cholinoreceptors.** Choline esters similar in structure to ACh that are used therapeutically include methacholine, carbachol, and bethanechol. Unlike ACh and carbachol, **methacholine and bethanechol are highly selective for muscarinic cholinoreceptors.** Pilocarpine is a tertiary amine alkaloid.

Mechanism of Action

Muscarinic cholinoreceptors activate **inhibitory G-proteins (G_i)** to stimulate the activity of **phospholipase C,** which, through increased phospholipid metabolism, results in **production of inositol triphosphate (IP_3)** and **DAG** that lead to the mobilization, respectively, of **intracellular calcium** from the endoplasmic and sarcoplasmic reticulum and, through activation of protein kinase C (PK-C), the opening of smooth muscle calcium channels with an influx of extracellular calcium. Activation of muscarinic cholinoreceptors also results in altered potassium flux that results in cell hyperpolarization, and in inhibition of adenylyl cyclase activity and cAMP accumulation induced by other hormones, including the catecholamines.

The **nicotinic receptor** functions as a **cell membrane ligand-gated ion channel pore.** On interaction with ACh, the receptor undergoes a conformational change that results in **influx of sodium** with membrane depolarization of the nerve cell or the skeletal muscle neuromuscular endplate.

Indirectly acting parasympathetic cholinomimetic agents inhibit AChE and thereby increase ACh levels at both muscarinic and nicotinic cholinoreceptors.

Administration

Directly acting muscarinic cholinomimetic agents may be administered topically as ophthalmic preparations (pilocarpine, carbachol), orally (bethanechol, pilocarpine), or parenterally (bethanechol). Depending on the agent, an indirectly acting cholinesterase inhibitor may be administered topically, orally, or parenterally.

Pharmacokinetics

ACh is synthesized from choline and acetyl-coenzyme A (acetyl-CoA) by the enzyme choline acetyltransferase and then transported into nerve ending vesicles. Like ACh, methacholine, carbachol, and bethanechol are poorly absorbed by the oral route and have limited penetration into the CNS. **Pilocarpine is more lipid soluble and can be absorbed and can penetrate the CNS.**

After release from nerve endings, ACh is rapidly metabolized into choline and acetate, and its effects are terminated by the action of the enzymes AChE and pseudocholinesterase. Methacholine and particularly carbachol and bethanechol are resistant to the action of cholinesterases.

COMPREHENSION QUESTIONS

[2.1]   A 62-year-old woman is noted to have open-angle glaucoma. She inadvertently applies excessive pilocarpine to her eyes. This may result in which of the following?

    A. Bronchial smooth muscle dilation
    B. Decreased gastrointestinal motility
    C. Dilation of blood vessels
    D. Mydriasis

[2.2]   Muscarinic cholinergic agonists

    A. Activate inhibitory G-proteins (G_i)
    B. Decrease production of IP_3
    C. Decrease release of intracellular calcium
    D. Inhibit the activity of phospholipase C

[2.3]   Choline esters like carbachol are most likely to cause which of the following adverse effects?

    A. Anhydrosis (dry skin)
    B. Delirium
    C. Salivation
    D. Tachycardia (rapid heart rate)

Answers

[2.1]   **C.** Excessive pilocarpine may initially result in dilation of blood vessels with a drop in blood pressure and a compensatory reflex stimulation of heart rate. Higher levels will directly inhibit the heart rate. In addition, pilocarpine stimulation of muscarinic cholinoreceptors can result in miosis, bronchial smooth muscle dilation, and increased GI motility.

[2.2]   **A.** In addition to activating inhibitory G-proteins (G_i), muscarinic cholinergic agonists stimulate the activity of phospholipase C, increase production of IP_3, and increase release of intracellular calcium.

[2.3]   **C.** Diarrhea, salivation, and lacrimation may be seen. The heart rate is usually slowed. Choline esters do not cross the blood-brain barrier, and therefore delirium is not an adverse effect.

PHARMACOLOGY PEARLS

❖ Cholinoreceptors are classified as either nicotinic or muscarinic.

❖ Muscarinic cholinoreceptors are localized at organs such as the heart, causing a negative chronotropic effect.

❖ Stimulation of muscarinic receptors in the smooth muscle, exocrine glands, and vascular endothelium cause bronchoconstriction, increased acid secretion, and vasodilation.

❖ Methacholine and bethanechol are highly selective for muscarinic cholinoreceptors.

❖ Cholinomimetic agents, including anticholinesterase inhibitors, are precluded for treatment of gastrointestinal or urinary tract disease because of mechanical obstruction, where therapy can result in increased pressure and possible perforation. They are also not indicated for patients with asthma.

REFERENCES

Felder C. Muscarinic acetylcholine receptors: signal transduction through multiple effectors. FASEB J 1995;9(8):619–25.

Marquis RE, Whitson JT. Management of glaucoma: focus on pharmacological therapy. Drugs Aging 2005;22(1):1–21.

Millard CB, Broomfield CA. Anticholinesterases: medical applications of neurochemical principles. J Neurochem 1995;64(5):1909–18.

A 53-year-old woman comes to see you for a consultation. She is scheduled to take a Caribbean cruise in 2 weeks but is concerned about sea sickness. She has been on boats before and is very sensitive to motion sickness. A friend mentioned to her that there is a patch that is effective for this problem. She is in good health and takes no medications regularly. Her examination is normal. You prescribe a scopolamine transdermal patch for her.

◆ **What is the mechanism of action of scopolamine?**

◆ **What are the common side effects of this medication?**

◆ **What are some relative contraindications to its use?**

ANSWERS TO CASE 3: MUSCARINIC CHOLINORECEPTOR ANTAGONISTS

Summary: A 53-year-old woman with motion sickness is prescribed transdermal scopolamine before she takes a sea cruise.

◆ **Mechanism of action of scopolamine:** Competitive antagonist of muscarinic cholinoreceptors in the vestibular system and the CNS

◆ **Common side effects:** Mydriasis, dry mouth, tachycardia, urinary retention, confusion, drowsiness

◆ **Relative contraindications:** Glaucoma, urinary obstruction, heart disease

CLINICAL CORRELATION

Scopolamine, like other antimuscarinic agents, including the prototype atropine, is a selective competitive (surmountable) antagonist of ACh at muscarinic cholinoreceptors. Its actions can be overcome by increased concentrations of ACh or other muscarinic cholinoreceptor agonists. **Scopolamine blocks muscarinic cholinoreceptors in the vestibular system and CNS to prevent motion sickness.** It has a relatively long duration of action and can be given as a transdermal patch, making it well suited for the treatment of motion sickness. Histamine H_1-receptor antagonists, such as cyclizine, are also used to treat motion sickness.

In addition to motion sickness, muscarinic cholinoreceptor antagonists (e.g., benztropine) are used therapeutically to treat **Parkinson disease.** Short-acting topical agents or ointments are used to facilitate ophthalmoscopic examination (e.g., cyclopentolate, tropicamide). Ipratropium bromide, a quaternary ammonium compound that does not cross the blood-brain barrier, is used to treat asthma and has efficacy in chronic obstructive pulmonary disease (COPD). They (e.g., trospium, tolterodine) are also used to treat certain bladder disorders. Because it penetrates the CNS, the tertiary amine atropine is used to counter the muscarinic cholinoreceptor effects of cholinergic excess resulting from organophosphate insecticide poisoning.

The **adverse effects of scopolamine and other muscarinic cholinoreceptor antagonists** are related to inhibition of muscarinic cholinoreceptors in organ systems of the body. **Drowsiness and sedation are caused by actions on the CNS. Mydriasis** is caused by blocking parasympathetic tone in the muscles of the cilia and iris. This could increase intraocular pressure in a person with **glaucoma.** Cholinoreceptor blockade at the sinoatrial node results in **tachycardia.** This could cause **arrhythmias,** especially in someone with underlying heart disease. The **urinary bladder is relaxed** and the **urinary sphincter constricted,** which may promote **urinary retention.** Blockade of muscarinic cholinoreceptors in the salivary glands **reduces salivation,** causing **dry mouth.** Blockade of other muscarinic cholinoreceptors in the CNS can lead to **impairment of memory, confusion, restlessness, drowsiness, or hallucinations.**

Muscarinic cholinoreceptor antagonist drugs are used cautiously in patients with **angle-closure glaucoma (contraindicated), open-angle glaucoma, urinary tract obstruction** (e.g., prostatic hypertrophy), **cardiac disease, and gastrointestinal infections,** among other conditions. Elderly patients are particularly sensitive to CNS effects.

APPROACH TO MUSCARINIC CHOLINORECEPTOR ANTAGONISTS

Objectives

1. Describe the mechanism of action of muscarinic cholinoreceptor antagonists.
2. Describe the physiologic effects of muscarinic cholinoreceptor antagonists.
3. List important therapeutic uses of muscarinic cholinoreceptor antagonists.
4. List the adverse effects and contraindications for muscarinic cholinoreceptor antagonists.

Definitions

Chronic obstructive pulmonary disease [COPD]: Progressive, inflammatory lung conditions, including both chronic bronchitis and emphysema, which result in airway obstruction that is not fully reversible. Most COPD is due to smoking.

Asthma: An inflammatory lung condition characterized by reversible airway obstruction that can be precipitated by irritants such as environmental allergens, cigarette smoke, cold air or exercise.

Muscarinic Cholinoreceptor antagonists: Drugs that block the actions of acetylcholine.

DISCUSSION

Class

Cholinoreceptor antagonists are distinguished by their specificity for muscarinic and nicotinic cholinoreceptors. Muscarinic cholinoreceptor antagonists block the effects of ACh at muscarinic cholinoreceptors in the parasympathetic autonomic nervous system and in the CNS. Nicotinic cholinoreceptor antagonists block the effects of ACh at ganglia of the parasympathetic and sympathetic nervous system (and medulla), and at the neuromuscular junction.

Structure

Like atropine, the prototype muscarinic cholinoreceptor antagonist **scopolamine is a tertiary amine.** As such, it has **ready access to the CNS** when administered parenterally, and it can be absorbed across the skin when combined with a suitable vehicle in a transdermal patch. **Quaternary amine antimuscarinic agents,** including **tiotropium bromide,** have **limited access to the CNS** and thus are used therapeutically for their peripheral effects.

Mechanism of Action

Interaction of scopolamine, atropine, or other antimuscarinic agents with muscarinic cholinoreceptors prevents the typical actions of ACh, such as activation of G-proteins and subsequent production of IP_3, and DAG that results in mobilization of calcium.

Administration

The patch formulation of scopolamine for motion sickness provides for up to 72 hours of pharmacologic activity. Scopolamine can also be administered IV, IM, or PO. Ipratropium bromide and tiotropium are administered topically to the airways as a metered-dose inhaler for COPD.

Pharmacokinetics

The duration of action of antimuscarinic agents ranges from less than a day (tropicamide) to 3–10 days (scopolamine, atropine).

COMPREHENSION QUESTIONS

[3.1]   Prescription of a muscarinic cholinoreceptor antagonist with a quaternary amine group is most appropriate for the patient with which of the following conditions?

A. A 50-year-old woman with angle-closure glaucoma
B. A 34-year-old man with gastrointestinal infectious enteritis
C. A 66-year-old man with mild dementia
D. A 56-year-old diabetic woman with urinary tract obstruction

[3.2]   A 16-year-old teenager is going on his first deep sea fishing trip and is using a scopolamine patch to ward off sea sickness. Which of the following is the most likely adverse effect he will experience?

A. Bradycardia
B. Drowsiness
C. Miosis
D. Urinary urgency

[3.3]   Cholinergic excess resulting from organophosphate insecticide poisoning can be treated with which of the following?

   A. Atropine
   B. Digoxin
   C. Ipratropium bromide
   D. Tropicamide

Answers

[3.1]   **C.** Muscarinic cholinoreceptor antagonists with quaternary amine groups do not penetrate the CNS and are therefore unlikely to impair memory. By blocking gastrointestinal motility, these agents can cause increased retention of infecting organisms.

[3.2]   **B.** Scopolamine penetrates the CNS and can cause drowsiness and sedation. It also can cause mydriasis, tachycardia, and urinary retention.

[3.3]   **A.** Atropine is a tertiary amine that can penetrate the CNS. In addition to its peripheral blocking actions, it can also block the adverse CNS effects as a result of cholinergic excess. Tropicamide is also a tertiary amine. However, it has a very short duration of action and would be an unsuitable antidote. Ipratropium bromide is a charged quaternary ammonium compound that does not penetrate the CNS.

PHARMACOLOGY PEARLS

 Many antihistaminic agents, antipsychotic agents, and antidepressant agents have muscarinic cholinoreceptor antagonist (antimuscarinic) activity.

 Scopolamine is a tertiary amine and has ready access to the CNS when administered parenterally, whereas quaternary amine antimuscarinic agents, such as ipratropium bromide, have limited access to the CNS.

 Scopolamine can cause drowsiness and sedation, as well as mydriasis, tachycardia, and urinary retention.

 Cholinoreceptor agonists cause symptoms of SLUD—**s**alivation, **l**acrimation, **u**rination, **d**iarrhea—whereas cholinoreceptor antagonists have the opposite effects—dry mouth, dry eyes, urinary retention, constipation.

REFERENCES

Alhasso AA, McKinlay J, Patrick K et al. Anticholinergic drugs versus non-drug active therapies for overactive bladder syndrome in adults. Cochrane Database Syst Rev 2006;18(4):CD003193.

Eglen RM, Choppin A, Watson N. Therapeutic opportunities from muscarinic receptor research. Trends Pharmacol Sci 2001;22(8):409–14.

Nachum Z, Shupak A, Gordon C. Transdermal scopolamine for prevention of motion sickness: clinical pharmacokinetics and therapeutic applications. Clin Pharmacokinet 2006;45(6):543–66.

❖ CASE 4

A healthy 25-year-old man is undergoing a brief surgical procedure requiring general anesthesia. He underwent an unremarkable intubation and induction of anesthesia using IV succinylcholine and inhaled halothane. During the surgery the patient develops muscle rigidity and tachycardia, and his temperature rapidly rises.

◆ **What is the mechanism of action of succinylcholine?**

◆ **What reaction is occurring in the patient?**

◆ **What drug should immediately be given to the patient, and what is its mechanism of action?**

ANSWERS TO CASE 4: SKELETAL MUSCLE RELAXANTS

Summary: A 25-year-old man develops muscle rigidity, tachycardia, and high fever during surgery.

◆ **Mechanism of action of succinylcholine:** Nicotinic receptor agonist at the motor endplate of the neuromuscular junction, which causes persistent stimulation and depolarization of muscle cells.

◆ **Reaction that is occurring:** Malignant hyperthermia.

◆ **Drug given for treatment and its mechanism of action:** Dantrolene, which acts by interfering with calcium release from the sarcoplasmic reticulum.

CLINICAL CORRELATION

Succinylcholine is the only depolarizing neuromuscular agent in wide clinical use. It is used for the rapid induction of a brief flaccid paralysis. It works as an agonist of the nicotinic receptor at the motor endplate of the neuromuscular junction. This causes a persistent stimulation and depolarization of the muscle, preventing stimulation of contraction by ACh. It has a rapid onset and short duration of action because it is quickly hydrolyzed by plasma and liver cholinesterase. **Malignant hyperthermia,** a rare but significant cause of anesthetic morbidity and mortality, is an inherited **autosomal dominant disorder** that results in **tachycardia, muscle rigidity, and high body temperatures** in response to the use of certain **inhaled anesthetics** in combination with **muscle relaxants, usually succinylcholine.** It is caused by a **release of calcium ions from the sarcoplasmic reticulum in muscle cells.** **Dantrolene** interferes with this release and is therefore the treatment of choice for this condition.

APPROACH TO PHARMACOLOGY OF SKELETAL MUSCLE RELAXANTS

Objectives

1. Contrast the mechanism of action of depolarizing and nondepolarizing neuromuscular junction-blocking agents.
2. List the therapeutic uses and adverse effects of skeletal muscle relaxants.

Definitions

Hyperkalemia: Elevated levels of the electrolyte potassium in the serum
Myalgia: Pain originating in skeletal muscle
Depolarizing neuromuscular agent: A drug that acts at the neuromuscular junction to prevent the initiation of an action potential by ACh.

DISCUSSION

Class

Neuromuscular blocking agents are classified as either **depolarizing** or **non-depolarizing** (Table 4-1) and are used mostly as adjuncts with general anesthetics to block motor endplate activity of ACh at the neuromuscular junction. **Succinylcholine** is the prototype for **depolarizing agents** and used for **brief paralysis** for surgery and for intubation. **Tubocurarine,** the prototype, and other **nondepolarizing agents** (e.g., cisatracurium, vecuronium, rocuronium) are used for **longer term paralysis** for surgery.

In addition to malignant hyperthermia, succinylcholine administration may result in **hyperkalemia,** particularly in patients with **burn and trauma,** which could result in **cardiac arrest.** Myalgia is also commonly reported.

Certain **nondepolarizing agents** may produce **hypotension,** as a result of histamine release and some ganglionic blocking activity, and tachycardia as a result of vagolytic activity.

Numerous drug interactions between neuromuscular blocking agents and other drugs have been reported that lead to increased neuromuscular blockade, particularly with certain antibiotics and inhaled anesthetics.

Table 4-1
SELECTED SKELETAL MUSCLE RELAXANTS

TYPE OF AGENT	MECHANISM OF ACTION	SELECTED ADVERSE EFFECTS
Depolarizing agents (succinylcholine)	Persistent endplate depolarization and desensitization	Malignant hyperthermia, hyperkalemia, myalgia
Nondepolarizing agents (tubocurarine, cisatracurium vecuronium, rocuronium)	Reversible competitive antagonists that block the action of ACh at nicotinic cholinoreceptor	Hypotension, tachycardia

Structure

The **neuromuscular blocking agents resemble ACh** (succinylcholine contains two linked ACh molecules) and contain **one or two quaternary nitrogens** that **limit entry into the CNS.**

Mechanism of Action

After a single dose, **succinylcholine occupies the nicotinic receptor** to produce a **persistent endplate depolarization** (phase I block) that results in flaccid paralysis because the muscles become unresponsive to endogenously released ACh. The initial depolarization is accompanied by muscle fasciculations. **Continued exposure of endplates to succinylcholine results in their repolarization.** However, through an unclear mechanism, they become relatively insensitive to subsequent depolarization (so-called desensitization, or phase II block).

Nondepolarizing blocking agents act as reversible competitive antagonists that block the action of ACh at nicotinic cholinoreceptors in muscle endplates and autonomic ganglia.

Cholinesterase inhibitors (e.g., neostigmine, pyridostigmine) can effectively **antagonize and reverse the neuromuscular blocking action of nondepolarizing agents and succinylcholine during phase II.** However, they will augment the action of succinylcholine during phase I.

Administration

The neuromuscular blocking agents are **highly polar** and therefore must be administered parenterally. Most nondepolarizing agents are eliminated through the kidney. Succinylcholine is eliminated by the hydrolytic action of plasma butyrylcholinesterase (pseudocholinesterase).

Pharmacokinetics

Neuromuscular blocking agents are **highly ionized** and therefore have limited volume of distribution and **limited access to the CNS.**

COMPREHENSION QUESTIONS

[4.1]   The use of succinylcholine as an adjunct to general anesthetics during
        surgery is based on its ability to:

        A. Block the action of ACh at the motor endplate
        B. Increase release of ACh from autonomic ganglia
        C. Increase release of histamine from mast cells
        D. Inhibit cholinesterase

[4.2]   Continued exposure of muscle endplates to succinylcholine results in their:

A. Conversion to ion channels
B. Enhanced sensitivity to ACh
C. Regeneration of ACh receptors
D. Repolarization

[4.3]   Cholinesterase inhibitors can reverse the action of which of the following?

A. Cisatracurium
B. Succinylcholine
C. Both A and B
D. Neither A or B

[4.4]   A 35-year-old man undergoes surgery for a hernia repair. After the surgery, he complains of diffuse muscle aches, which the anesthesiologist states is likely caused by the skeletal muscle relaxant. He has a temperature of 37.8°C (100°F). Which of the following is the most accurate statement?

A. The agent also commonly causes hypokalemia.
B. The agent blocks ACh at the nicotinic receptor.
C. The agent causes persistent endplate depolarization and desensitization.
D. The patient likely has malignant hyperthermia.

Answers

[4.1]   **A.** Succinylcholine acts like ACh to cause depolarization of the muscle endplate. However, unlike ACh, succinylcholine is not metabolized at the synapse. Therefore, the endplate remains depolarized and unresponsive to endogenous ACh, resulting in muscle paralysis.

[4.2]   **D.** Continued exposure of the muscle endplate to succinylcholine results in desensitization (phase II block) where the endplate repolarizes but cannot readily be depolarized.

[4.3]   **C.** Cholinesterase inhibitors like neostigmine can effectively antagonize and reverse the neuromuscular blocking action of nondepolarizing agents and succinylcholine during phase II. However, they will augment the action of succinylcholine during phase I.

[4.4]   **C.** Myalgia (muscle aches) is a common adverse reaction of depolarizing agents such as succinylcholine; these agents also may induce hyperkalemia and malignant hyperthermia.

PHARMACOLOGY PEARLS

 Malignant hyperthermia is a rare autosomal dominant disorder characterized by tachycardia, muscle rigidity, and high body temperatures, which occurs when the patient is exposed to inhaled
anesthetics in combination with muscle relaxants, usually succinylcholine.

 Dantrolene interferes with the release of intracellular calcium and is
therefore used to treat the muscle rigidity and hyperthermia associated with malignant hyperthermia.

 The neuromuscular blocking agents are highly polar and highly ionized and therefore, must be administered parenterally and have
limited volume of distribution and limited access to the CNS.

 A small number of patients (1:10,000) with atypical cholinesterase
experience long-lasting apnea of 1–4 hours following succinylcholine (or the nondepolarizing neuromuscular blocking drug
mivacurium that is also eliminated by the action of butyrylcholinesterase). Mechanical ventilation is used to manage the
apnea even though prescreening could detect this rare condition.

REFERENCES

Bowman WC. Neuromuscular block. Br J Pharmacol 2006;147(Suppl 1):S277–86.
Lee C. Structure, conformation, and action of neuromuscular blocking drugs. Br J
Anaesth 2001;87(5):755–69.
Sparr HJ, Beaufort TM, Fuchs-Buder T. Newer neuromuscular blocking agents.
How do they compare with established drugs? Drugs 2001;61(7):919–42.

❖ CASE 5

A 65-year-old woman is admitted to the intensive care unit (ICU) of the hospital with sepsis caused by a urinary tract infection. She is hypotensive, with a blood pressure of 80/40 mm Hg and has an elevated heart rate (tachycardia) and decreased urine output (oliguria). Along with the institution of appropriate antibiotic therapy and IV fluids, a decision is made to start her on an IV infusion of dopamine to attempt to raise her blood pressure.

◆ **What effects can be expected with low-dose dopamine?**

◆ **Which receptors mediate these effects?**

◆ **What effects occur with higher dose dopamine and which receptors mediate these?**

ANSWERS TO CASE 5: SYMPATHOMIMETIC AGENTS

Summary: A 65-year-old woman in septic shock has persistent hypotension and oliguria requiring IV dopamine.

◆ **Effects of low-dose dopamine:** Reduces arterial resistance and increases blood flow in renal, coronary, and splanchnic systems; positive inotropic effect.

◆ **Receptors involved:** β_1-receptors and specific dopamine receptors.

◆ **Effects of higher dose dopamine and receptors involved:** Vasoconstriction mediated by α-receptors.

CLINICAL CORRELATION

Dopamine is frequently used to treat cardiogenic or septic shock. The β_1-adrenoceptor-mediated effects in the heart result in an increase in cardiac output with minimal peripheral vasoconstriction. This contributes to dopamine's ability to raise systolic blood pressure with no effect or only a slight effect on diastolic pressure. Specific dopamine receptors in the vasculature of the renal, coronary, and splanchnic systems allow for reduced arterial resistance and increased blood flow. At higher doses there is a peripheral α-adrenoceptor effect that overrides dopamine receptor-mediated vasodilation and results in vasoconstriction. The combination of renal blood-flow preservation, while supporting the blood pressure, is desirable in conditions of shock. This also contributes to increasing blood pressure. Prolonged high doses of dopamine can result in peripheral tissue necrosis because of the α-adrenoceptor-mediated vasoconstriction that reduces blood flow to the extremities, particularly in the digits.

APPROACH TO PHARMACOLOGY OF AUTONOMIC SYMPATHETIC AGENTS

Objectives

1. Outline the effects of sympathomimetic agents on peripheral organ systems.
2. List the major sympathomimetic agonists and their routes of administration.
3. Describe the therapeutic and adverse effects of the major sympathomimetic drugs.

Definitions

Sympathomimetic agents: Drugs that either directly or indirectly mimic all or some of the effects of epinephrine or norepinephrine.

Receptor selectivity: Preferential binding (greater affinity) of a drug to a specific receptor group or receptor subtype at concentrations below which there is little, if any, interaction with another receptor group or subtype.

DISCUSSION

Class

Sympathomimetic agents act **directly** (e.g., epinephrine, norepinephrine, dopamine, dobutamine, phenylephrine, metaraminol, methoxamine, albuterol, terbutaline) or indirectly (amphetamine, ephedrine) to activate **α- and β-adrenoceptors** (Table 5-1). Sympathomimetic agent adrenoceptor

Table 5-1
AUTONOMIC NERVOUS SYSTEM EFFECTS*

ORGAN	ADRENERGIC RECEPTOR/ACTION	MUSCARINIC CHOLINERGIC RECEPTOR/ACTION
Heart	β_1—increased heart rate and contractility	Decreased heart rate and contractility
Blood vessels[†]	α_1—constriction β_2—dilation	Dilation
Bronchi	β_2—bronchial smooth muscle relaxation	Bronchial smooth muscle contraction
GI tract	α_1—sphincter contraction β_2—relaxation	Overall contraction relaxation of sphincter
Kidney	β_1—renin release	No effect
Urinary bladder	α_1—sphincter contraction β_2—wall relaxation	Wall contraction sphincter relaxation
Adipose tissue	β_1—increased lipolysis	No effect
Eye	α_1—radial muscle contraction with pupil dilation	Sphincter muscle contraction with pupil constriction ciliary muscle contraction

*See also Figure 1-1.
[†]No direct parasympathetic innervation.

selectivity varies. Some are **nonselective** (e.g., ephedrine), whereas some have greater affinity for α-adrenoceptors (e.g., phenylephrine, metaraminol, methoxamine) or $β_1$-adrenoceptor (e.g., dobutamine) or $β_2$-adrenoceptor (e.g., terbutaline, albuterol) subgroups. However, selectivity is often lost as the dose of a sympathomimetic agent is increased. Compared to nonselective β-receptor agonists (isoproterenol), **$β_1$-selective sympathomimetic agents may increase cardiac output with minimal reflex tachycardia. $α_2$-Selective agents,** which **decrease blood pressure** by a prejunctional action in the CNS (clonidine, methyldopa), are used to treat hypertension. Fenoldopam is a potent D_1 agonist with a short half-life, useful in severe hypertension; its effects include decreasing systemic vascular resistance.

Dopamine interacts with specific subtypes of **dopamine receptors** in the **periphery (D_1 and D_2).** Stimulation of the D_1 receptor on the vasculature is principally vasodilation, and on the renal proximal tubules leads to natriuresis and diuresis; stimulation of the D_2 receptor on the presynaptic sympathetic nerve endings inhibits norepinephrine release. It also has direct and indirect sympathomimetic activity where, at lower doses, it has greater affinity for β-adrenoceptors than it does for α-adrenoceptors.

The clinical utility of a particular sympathomimetic agent depends on, among other factors, the specific organ system and receptor subtypes that are involved. In the **cardiovascular** system, a reduction in blood flow by relatively selective α-adrenoceptor sympathomimetic agents is used to achieve surgical hemostasis, reduced diffusion of local anesthetics, and a reduction of mucous membrane congestion in hay fever and for the common cold. An increase in blood flow or blood pressure by α-adrenoceptor sympathomimetic agents is beneficial for the management of hypotensive emergencies (e.g., phenylephrine, methoxamine, norepinephrine) and chronic orthostatic hypotension (oral ephedrine). Sympathomimetic agents such as isoproterenol (and epinephrine) are also used for emergency short-term treatment of complete heart block and cardiac arrest.

Treatment of **bronchial asthma** represents a major use of **$β_2$-selective sympathomimetic agents** (e.g., terbutaline, albuterol). Its effect is bronchodilation and relaxation of the smooth muscles of the bronchioles.

Ophthalmic examination is facilitated with the use of the **directly acting α-adrenoceptor sympathomimetic agonist,** phenylephrine. Phenylephrine (and the indirectly acting sympathomimetic agent, cocaine) is also used to localize the lesion in Horner syndrome. In addition to β-adrenoceptor-blocking agents, $α_2$-selective agents (e.g., apraclonidine) are used to lower intraocular pressure in glaucoma.

The peripheral adverse effects of the sympathomimetic agents are generally an extension of their pharmacologic effects. These are most often cardiovascular in nature, particularly when they are administered parenterally, and may include increased blood pressure, arrhythmias, and cardiac failure.

Structure

Sympathomimetic agents, as well as norepinephrine and epinephrine, are **derived from phenylethylamine.** Substitutions on the amino group, the benzene ring or the α- or β-carbon, markedly alter the selectivity, activity, and metabolism of the sympathomimetic agents. For example, alkyl substitutions on the amino group tend to markedly increase β-adrenoceptor selectivity.

Mechanism of Action

Directly acting sympathomimetic agents bind to and activate adrenoceptors to mimic the actions of epinephrine or norepinephrine. Indirectly acting sympathomimetic agents mimic the actions of norepinephrine by either displacing it or inhibiting its reuptake from adrenergic nerve endings.

Administration

Sympathomimetic agents are available for administration by **topical, nasal, oral, ophthalmic, and parenteral routes** depending on the drug and condition being treated.

Pharmacokinetics

Like the catecholamines norepinephrine and epinephrine, direct and indirect sympathomimetic agent may be subject to **metabolism and inactivation** by **COMT and MAO.** Phenylephrine is not metabolized by COMT, whereas metaraminol and methoxamine are not substrates for either COMT or MAO. Their durations of action, therefore, are relatively long (20–60 minutes).

COMPREHENSION QUESTIONS

[5.1]   A 25-year-old man is noted to be in septic shock. A low-dose dopamine infusion is administered, and will likely result in which of the following?

A. Decrease cardiac output
B. Decrease systolic blood pressure
C. Increase renal blood flow
D. Produce significant peripheral vasoconstriction

[5.2]   In contrast to norepinephrine, metaraminol, and methoxamine are metabolized by which of the following?

A. COMT
B. MAO
C. Both
D. Neither

[5.3]   Which of the following is the most accurate statement?

A. α-Adrenoceptor sympathomimetic agonists are used to reduce mucous membrane congestion.

B. α-Adrenoceptor agonists are used to treat bronchospasm.

C. β-Adrenoceptor agonists are used to reduce surgical bleeding.

D. β_2-Adrenoceptor agonist agents are used to prolong local anesthesia.

Answers

[5.1]   **C.** Dopamine binding to specific dopamine receptors in the vasculature in the kidney increases renal blood flow. Cardiac output is increased by dopamine action on β_1-adrenoceptors. Dopamine causes minimal peripheral vasoconstriction.

[5.2]   **D.** Metaraminol and methoxamine are not substrates for either COMT or MAO and have a longer duration of action than norepinephrine, which is a substrate for both.

[5.3]   **A.** α-Adrenoceptor sympathomimetic agents will cause vasoconstriction and thereby reduce mucous membrane congestion.

PHARMACOLOGY PEARLS

 β_1-Selective sympathomimetic agents may increase cardiac output with minimal reflex tachycardia.

 α_2-Selective agents decrease blood pressure by a prejunctional action in the CNS.

 Terbutaline and albuterol are preferred over ephedrine for relieving the bronchoconstriction of asthma, and other bronchial conditions, because of their greater bronchiolar selectivity.

 Dopamine binding to specific dopamine receptors in the vasculature in the kidney increases renal blood flow. Cardiac output is increased by dopamine action on β_1-adrenoceptors. Low-dose dopamine causes minimal peripheral vasoconstriction.

REFERENCES

Cleland JG. Beta-blockers for heart failure: why, which, when, and where. Med Clin North Am 2003;87(2):339–71.

Graham RM, Perez DM, Hwa J, et al. Alpha₁-adrenergic receptor subtypes. Molecular structure, function and signaling. Circ Res 1996;78(5):737–49.

Mann HJ, Nolan PE. Update on the management of cardiogenic shock. Curr Opin Crit Care 2006;12(5):431–6.

❖ CASE 6

A 70-year-old man is seen in follow-up at your office after he has been hospitalized for a myocardial infarction (MI). He underwent successful angioplasty and is currently asymptomatic. Prior to his MI, he was not on medications. He is not a smoker and is not diabetic. During his hospitalization, he was noted to have persistently elevated blood pressure readings. He had asthma as a child, but has not had any recent wheezing episodes. While in the hospital, he was started on oral metoprolol.

◆ **Metoprolol is selective for which adrenoceptor?**

◆ **What effects do agents such as metoprolol have on the cardiovascular system?**

◆ **In which organ is metoprolol primarily metabolized?**

◆ **Why must β-adrenergic antagonists be used with caution in asthmatics?**

ANSWERS TO CASE 6: ADRENOCEPTOR ANTAGONISTS

Summary: A 70-year-old hypertensive man with a childhood history of asthma had a recent myocardial infarction and is prescribed metoprolol.

◆ **Adrenoceptor selectively antagonized by metoprolol:** β_1.

◆ **Effect of β-adrenoceptor antagonists on the cardiovascular system:** Reduction of sympathetic-stimulated increases in heart rate, contractility, and cardiac output; lower blood pressure as a result of effects on the heart, renin-angiotensin system, and CNS; increased atrioventricular (AV) conduction time and refractoriness.

◆ **Organ in which metoprolol is metabolized:** Liver.

◆ **Reason for caution in use in asthmatics:** Blockade of β_2-adrenoceptor in bronchial smooth muscle may cause increased airway resistance and bronchospasm.

CLINICAL CORRELATION

β-Adrenergic receptor antagonists are widely used in medicine, primarily for their beneficial effects on the cardiovascular system and for lowering intraocular pressure in patients with glaucoma. Both the nonselective β-adrenoreceptor antagonists and the relatively β_1-adrenoceptor selective antagonists are used to treat hypertension. The mechanism of their action is multifactorial, probably including reduction in cardiac output, reduction in renin release, and some CNS effect. They are also beneficial for treating coronary artery disease and postmyocardial infarction patients as they reduce sympathetic-stimulated increases in heart rate and contractility. This helps to reduce myocardial oxygen demand, providing prophylaxis for angina. **β-Adrenoceptor antagonists have a proven benefit in prolonging survival after heart attacks.** They lengthen AV conduction time and refractoriness and suppress automaticity. This helps to prevent both supraventricular and ventricular arrhythmias. Caution must be used when giving β-blockers to patients with asthma, COPD, and diabetes. All β-adrenoceptor blockers, including those that are β_1-adrenoceptor selective, have some β_2-adrenoceptor antagonist activity and **may cause bronchospasm** by their effects on bronchial smooth muscle. They **can also mask the symptoms of hypoglycemia** in a diabetic by blocking the adrenergic stimulated symptoms of tremor, tachycardia, and nervousness that would normally occur.

APPROACH TO PHARMACOLOGY
OF ADRENOCEPTOR AGONISTS

Objectives

1. Describe the therapeutic uses and adverse effects of α-adrenoceptor antagonists.
2. Describe the therapeutic uses and adverse effects of β-adrenoceptor antagonists.
3. Contrast the differences between the nonselective and relatively β_1-selective adrenoceptor antagonists.

Definitions

Pheochromocytoma: A tumor of the adrenal medulla that releases excess levels of epinephrine and norepinephrine that can result in hypertension, cardiac anomalies, and severe headache.

Myocardial infarction: Death of cardiac muscle as a result of ischemia.

DISCUSSION

Class

There are two classes of clinically important α-adrenoceptor antagonists: nonselective antagonists and selective α_1-antagonists. **Phentolamine, a nonselective, competitive α-adrenoceptor antagonist,** and **phenoxybenzamine,** a **nonselective, noncompetitive α-adrenoceptor antagonist** are used for the preoperative management of the marked catecholamine-induced **vasoconstriction** associated with **pheochromocytoma. Prazosin** and other α_1-**adrenoceptor selective antagonists** (doxazosin, terazosin) are used to manage **chronic mild-to-moderate hypertension** and **benign prostatic hypertrophy.**

In addition to the nonselective β-adrenoceptor antagonists, there are two classes of clinically important selective β-adrenoceptor antagonists, β_1 and β_2 (Table 6-1). The major clinical uses for β-adrenoceptor antagonists include ischemic heart disease, cardiac arrhythmias, hypertension, hyperthyroidism, and glaucoma. Ischemic heart disease is managed with nonselective β-adrenoceptor antagonists, propranolol, timolol, and nadolol, as well as β_1-adrenoceptor selective antagonists, metoprolol, atenolol, and esmolol. **Cardiac arrhythmias** are managed, depending on the arrhythmia, with **propranolol and esmolol. Hypertension** is managed with a wide variety of **nonselective and β_1-adrenoceptor selective antagonists,** except esmolol. **Timolol** and other β-adrenoceptor antagonists are used to manage **glaucoma** by decreasing aqueous humor production and thereby reducing intraocular pressure.

Table 6-1

β-ADRENOCEPTOR ANTAGONIST SELECTIVITY

Nonselective β-Adrenoceptor Antagonists
Propranol
Nadolol
Timolol

Selective β$_1$-Adrenoceptor Antagonists
Atenolol
Metoprolol
Esmolol

Nonselective β- and α$_1$-Adrenoceptor Antagonists
Labetalol
Carvedilol

Labetalol (and several other agents, including carvedilol), in formulations used clinically, **blocks both β- and α$_1$-adrenoceptors in a 3:1 ratio.** It also has some β$_2$-adrenoceptor agonist activity. Labetalol **lowers blood pressure** by **decreasing systemic vascular resistance** without any major effect on heart rate or cardiac output. It is used to treat hypertensive emergencies and hypertension from **pheochromocytoma.** Table 6-2 has a listing of selected sympathomimetic agents.

The **major adverse effects of nonselective α-adrenoceptor antagonists** are **cardiac stimulation,** primarily **tachycardia** because of baroreflex-mediated sympathetic discharge, and **postural hypotension.** Additional cardiac stimulation by phentolamine may be caused by antagonist activity at prejunctional α$_2$-adrenoceptors that result in increased norepinephrine release. (Prazosin and other selective α$_1$-adrenoceptor selective antagonists are less likely to cause reflex tachycardia.) A β-adrenoceptor antagonist may be required to counter the cardiac effects. α-Antagonists are rarely used as first-line agents for hypertension, as they are associated with a higher rate of congestive heart failure than other agents.

The **major adverse effects of nonselective β-adrenoceptor antagonists** are related to their effects on **bronchial smooth muscle and on carbohydrate metabolism. Blockade of β$_2$-receptors in smooth muscle may increase airway resistance in patients with asthma or other airway obstruction diseases.** Although the clinical use of a selective β$_1$-adrenoceptor antagonist may offer some protection in patients with asthma, the selectivity of these agents is not great, and therefore they should be used judiciously, if at all. In patients with **insulin-dependent diabetes, nonselective β-adrenoceptor antagonists** increase the incidence and severity of **hypoglycemic episodes.** The use of selective β$_1$-adrenoceptor antagonists in patients with this condition offers some potential benefit.

Table 6-2
SELECTED DRUGS AND THEIR EFFECTS ON THE AUTONOMIC NERVOUS SYSTEM

DRUG	ADRENOCEPTOR ACTIVITY	MECHANISM OF ACTION	CLINICAL USE
Epinephrine	Nonselective α- and β-adrenoceptor agonist	Bronchial smooth muscle dilation	Asthma and other allergic diseases to relax airways and reduce swelling
Phenylephrine	α_1-Adrenoreceptor stimulation	Vasoconstriction	Rhinitis and colds as decongestant
Propranolol	Nonselective β-adrenoceptor agonist	Decreases heart rate, cardiac contractility	Hypertension, coronary heart disease
Albuterol	β_2-Adrenoceptor agonist	Bronchial smooth muscle dilation	Asthma
Phentolamine	Nonselective competitive α-adrenoceptor antagonist	Vasodilation	Preoperative management of the marked catecholamine-induced vasoconstriction associated with pheochromocytoma
Prazosin	α_1-Adrenoreceptor selective antagonists	Vasodilation	Chronic mild to moderate hypertension and benign prostatic hypertrophy

Mechanism of Action

α-Adrenoceptor antagonists and β-adrenoceptor antagonists interact directly, and either competitively or irreversibly with, respectively, α-adrenoceptors and β-adrenoceptors to block actions of the endogenous catecholamines (norepinephrine and epinephrine), and exogenously administered sympathomimetic agents.

Administration

α- and β-adrenoceptor antagonists are administered orally or parenterally. β-Adrenoceptor antagonists are also available for ophthalmic application.

Pharmacokinetics

Metoprolol and propranolol undergo extensive and variable interindividual first-pass hepatic metabolism resulting in relatively low bioavailability. Oral sustained-release preparations of these agents are available. Drugs that inhibit cytochrome P_{450} 2D6 may decrease the metabolism of carvedilol. Esmolol is ultra-short-acting as a result of its ester linkage that is rapidly metabolized by plasma esterases.

COMPREHENSION QUESTIONS

[6.1]   Which of the following actions of epinephrine are blocked by prazosin?

A. Bronchial dilation
B. Increased cardiac stroke volume
C. Increased heart rate
D. Mydriasis

[6.2]   A 34-year-old man is prescribed labetalol for hypertension. The effect on the cardiovascular system is a result of its action as an antagonist at which of the following?

A. α-Adrenoceptors
B. β-Adrenoceptors
C. Both α- and β-adrenoceptors
D. Muscarinic cholinoreceptors

[6.3]   Which of the following is the least likely clinical use for β-adrenoceptor antagonists?

A. Benign prostatic hypertrophy
B. Cardiac arrhythmias
C. Hypertension
D. Ischemic heart disease

Answers

[6.1]   **D.** Prazosin is an α-adrenoceptor antagonist that will block epinephrine-mediated contraction of the radial smooth muscle of the eye that results in mydriasis. All the other actions listed are mediated by β-adrenoceptors, which would be blocked by β-adrenoceptor antagonists like propranolol.

[6.2]   **C.** Labetalol blocks both β- and α-adrenoceptors. It lowers blood pressure by decreasing systemic vascular resistance (α-adrenoceptor antagonist activity), without any major effect on heart rate or cardiac output (β-adrenoceptor antagonist activity).

[6.3]   **A.** β-Adrenoceptor antagonists are used therapeutically to manage ischemic heart disease, cardiac arrhythmias, and hypertension. α_1-Adrenoceptor selective antagonists are used to manage benign prostatic hypertrophy.

PHARMACOLOGY PEARLS

 α_1-Adrenoceptor selective antagonists, such as doxazosin and terazosin, are used for mild chronic hypertension and benign prostatic hypertrophy.

 The major clinical uses for β-adrenoceptor antagonists include ischemic heart disease, cardiac arrhythmias, hypertension, hyperthyroidism, and glaucoma.

 The **major adverse effects of nonselective β-adrenoceptor antagonists** are related to their effects on **bronchial smooth muscle** (increased airway resistance in asthmatics) and on **carbohydrate metabolism** (hypoglycemia in **insulin-dependent diabetics**).

REFERENCES

Shin J, Johnson JA. Pharmacogenetics of beta-blockers. Pharmacotherapy 2007;27(6):874–87.

Piascik MT, Perez DM. Alpha 1-adrenergic receptors: new insights and directions. J Pharmacol Exp Ther 2001;293(2):403–10.

A 64-year-old woman with a history of two previous myocardial infarctions (MIs) comes to the emergency room with shortness of breath. In the previous 2 weeks, she has developed dyspnea with exertion and swelling of her legs. She sleeps on three pillows because she coughs and gets short of breath if she tries to lie flat. In the emergency department, she is sitting upright, appears to be in moderate respiratory distress, and is tachycardic and hypertensive. She has jugular venous distension to the angle of her jaw. On auscultation of her lungs, wet rales are heard bilaterally. She has pitting edema of both lower legs up to her knees. A chest x-ray confirms the diagnosis of pulmonary edema. She is placed on oxygen and immediately given an IV injection of furosemide.

◆ **What is the mechanism of action of furosemide?**

◆ **What electrolyte abnormalities can be caused by furosemide?**

ANSWERS TO CASE 7: DIURETICS

Summary: A 64-year-old woman with pulmonary edema is prescribed furosemide.

◆ **Mechanism of action of furosemide:** Inhibit active NaCl reabsorption in the ascending limb of the loop of Henle, increasing water and electrolyte excretion.

◆ **Potential electrolyte abnormalities:** Hypokalemia, hypomagnesemia, and metabolic alkalosis because of enhanced H^+ excretion.

CLINICAL CORRELATION

Loop diuretics given intravenously promote diuresis within minutes, making them ideal for the treatment of acute pulmonary edema. Furosemide is the prototype and most widely used drug in this class. Loop diuretics inhibit NaCl reabsorption in the ascending limb of the loop of Henle. This causes a marked *increase* in the excretion of both water and electrolytes. **The excretion of potassium, magnesium, and calcium ions are all increased,** which may cause clinically significant adverse effects. A metabolic alkalosis may also occur as a result of the excretion of hydrogen ions. However, the ability to cause excretion of these electrolytes may also provide a clinical benefit in certain situations. **Forced diuresis by giving IV saline and furosemide is a primary method of treatment of hypercalcemia.**

APPROACH TO PHARMACOLOGY OF THE LOOP DIURETICS

Objectives

1. Know the site and mechanism of action of diuretic agents.
2. Know the electrolyte effects of the various diuretic agents.
3. Know the therapeutic uses, adverse effects, and contraindications to diuretic use.

Definitions

Diuretic: An agent that increases the production of urine. The most common are natriuretic diuretics, agents that increase urine production by interfering with sodium reabsorption in the kidney.

Edema: Accumulation of water in interstitial spaces. Causes include elevated blood pressure, a decrease in plasma oncotic pressure caused by a reduction in hepatic protein synthesis, or an increase in the oncotic pressure within the interstitial space.

DISCUSSION

Class

Natriuretic diuretics all act within the kidney to reduce the reabsorption of Na^+ and Cl^-. There are **four sites within the kidney** where various diuretics act; these correspond to four anatomic regions of the nephron. The **proximal tubule (site 1)** is the site of approximately 60 percent Na^+ reabsorption, but diuretics acting here are relatively ineffective because of the sodium-reabsorbing capacity in more distal regions of the nephron. The **ascending loop of Henle (site 2)** has active reabsorption of approximately 35 percent of the filtered Na^+. This is mediated by a cotransporter termed NKCC2 that transports 1 Na^+, 1 K^+, and 2 Cl^-, and this is the molecular target of **furosemide** and other loop or "high-ceiling" diuretics. The **distal convoluted tubule (site 3)** is responsible for transport of approximately 15 percent of filtered sodium. **Thiazide** diuretics act in this segment of the nephron by interfering with another cotransporter, NCC, which cotransports Na^+ and Cl^-. **Site 4 diuretics** act in the **collecting tubule** by interfering with Na^+ reabsorption through a specific channel, the epithelial sodium channel (ENaC), also called the amiloride-sensitive sodium channel (Figure 7-1).

   Loop diuretics—furosemide, ethacrynic acid, bumetanide, and torsemide—are highly acidic drugs that act on the **luminal side of the tubule.** They reach this site by being secreted into the tubule by anion secretion in the proximal tubule. Compared with other diuretics, loop diuretics cause the greatest diuresis because the Na^+ K^- $2Cl^-$ transporter is responsible for a large fraction of Na^+ reabsorption, and regions distal to the ascending limb have more limited capacity for sodium transport. Loop diuretics are useful for the treatment of peripheral and pulmonary edema, which may occur secondarily as a consequence of cardiac failure, liver failure, or renal failure. Loop diuretics increase the excretion of Na^+, Cl^-, K^+, Mg^{2+}, Ca^{2+} and decrease the excretion of Li^+. The increased excretion of Ca^{2+} is clinically relevant, and loop diuretics can be used to treat hypercalcemia. Some of the diuretic actions of furosemide are mediated via prostaglandins because inhibitors of prostaglandin biosynthesis diminish the increase in diuresis produced by the drug. In addition, furosemide has actions on the vascular system that occur prior to diuresis and this action may be mediated by prostaglandins. Other effects include changes in renal blood flow and a reduction in left-ventricular-filling pressure. Loop diuretics increase urine production and decrease plasma K^+ in patients with acute renal failure.

   Major adverse effects of loop diuretics are electrolyte imbalances. Increased delivery of Na^+ to the collecting duct increases K^+ and H^+ excretion. Loop diuretics therefore cause **hypokalemia, hypochloridemia, and metabolic alkalosis. Hyperuricemia** may be caused by the volume contraction and enhanced uric acid reabsorption by the proximal tubule. Loop diuretics can produce dose-dependent **ototoxicity.**

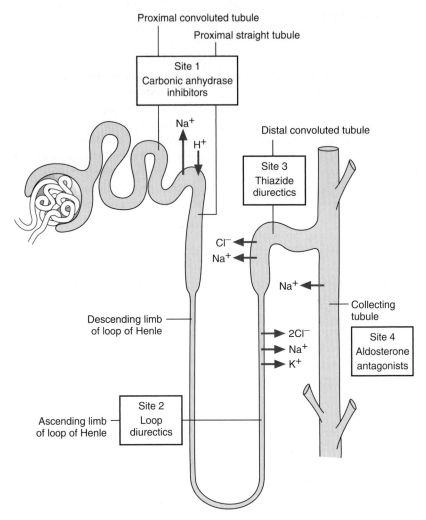

Figure 7-1. Sites of action of the nephron and diuretic agents.

Structure

Most loop diuretics are **sulfonamide derivatives;** the exceptions are ethacrynic acid, which is a phenoxyacetic acid derivative, and torsemide, which is a sulfonylurea.

Mechanism of Action

The molecular target of furosemide and other loop or high-ceiling diuretics is the sodium-potassium-2 chloride cotransporter (NKCC2), which transports 1 Na^+, 1 K^+, and 2 Cl^-. The activity of this transporter is blocked by loop diuretics.

Administration

All loop diuretics can be administered orally, and their onset of action is approximately 1 hour (torsemide) to 2 hours (furosemide). Loop diuretics can also be administered IV, and for furosemide, this produces vasodilation in as little as 5 minutes and diuresis in 20 minutes.

Pharmacokinetics

All loop diuretics are extensively bound to plasma proteins. Half-lives vary from 45 minutes (bumetanide) to 3.5 hours (torsemide). Approximately 65 percent of a dose of furosemide is eliminated by the kidney, and the remainder is metabolized. Only 20 percent of torsemide is eliminated by the kidney, and 80 percent is metabolized.

COMPREHENSION QUESTIONS

[7.1] Furosemide acts to inhibit Na^+ reabsorption in which of the following locations?

    A. Ascending limb of the loop of Henle
    B. Collecting duct
    C. Descending limb of the loop of Henle
    D. Distal convoluted tubule

[7.2] A patient arrives in the emergency room in a coma and has a serum Ca^{2+} of 4.5 mM. You start a saline infusion of which of the following drugs?

    A. Calcitonin
    B. Ethacrynic acid
    C. Hydrochlorothiazide
    D. Spironolactone

[7.3] A 55-year-old man with congestive heart failure is noted to be taking furosemide each day. Which of the following is most likely to be found in the serum?

    A. Decreased potassium level
    B. Decreased uric acid level
    C. Elevated magnesium level
    D. Low bicarbonate level

Answers

[7.1] **A.** Furosemide acts specifically on a Na^+ K^+ $2Cl^-$ transporter in the ascending limb of the loop of Henle.

[7.2] **B.** Loop diuretics such as ethacrynic acid increase the excretion of Ca^{2+}.

[7.3] **A.** Furosemide leads to hypokalemia, hypomagnesemia, and metabolic alkylosis (elevated bicarbonate level).

PHARMACOLOGY PEARLS

 Furosemide, which acts on the loop of Henle, is the most efficacious diuretic.

 Hypokalemia is a frequent adverse effect encountered with loop diuretics, and this can be managed with the concomitant use of potassium-sparing diuretics such as triamterene or spironolactone.

 Loop diuretics can produce dose-dependent ototoxicity.

REFERENCES

Paul RV. Rational diuretic management in congestive heart failure: a case-based review. Crit Care Nurs Clin North Am 2003;15(4):453–60.

Padilla MC, Armas-Hernandez MJ, Hernandez RJ, et al. Update of diuretics in the treatment of hypertension. Am J Ther 2007;14(4): 331–5.

Following his third episode of gouty arthritis, a 50-year-old man sees you in the clinic. Each case was successfully treated acutely; however, your patient is interested in trying to prevent future episodes. He is not on regular medications and has a normal physical examination today. Blood work reveals an elevated serum uric acid level and otherwise normal renal function and electrolytes. A 24-hour urine collection for uric acid reveals that he is under-excreting uric acid. Suspecting that this is the cause of his recurrent gout, you place him on probenecid.

◆ **What is the mechanism of action of probenecid?**

◆ **Which drugs could have their excretion inhibited by probenecid?**

ANSWERS TO CASE 8: NONDIURETIC INHIBITORS OF TUBULAR TRANSPORT

Summary: A 50-year-old man with recurrent gout is prescribed probenecid.

◆ **Mechanism of action of probenecid:** Inhibits secretion of organic acids and decreases reabsorption of uric acid, causing a net increase in secretion.

◆ **Other drugs whose secretion could be inhibited:** Penicillin, indomethacin, and methotrexate.

CLINICAL CORRELATION

Gout is a disease in which uric acid crystals deposit in joints, causing an extremely painful acute inflammatory arthritis. Persons with recurrent gout often have chronically elevated levels of uric acid in their blood. This hyperuricemia is frequently caused by either overproduction of uric acid or underexcretion of uric acid by the kidneys. Probenecid (and other uricosuric drugs) promotes the excretion of uric acid. It works by inhibiting the secretion of organic acids from the plasma into the tubular lumen and blocking the reuptake of uric acid. The net result of this is an **increase in the secretion of uric acid.** The benefit of this is the prevention of recurrent gout attacks in chronic underexcreters of uric acid. In those individuals who overproduce uric acid, allopurinol is used. This inhibits xanthine oxidase, a key enzyme in the production of uric acid.

APPROACH TO PHARMACOLOGY OF URICOSURIC AGENTS

Objectives

1. Understand the mechanism of action of uricosuric agents.
2. Know the therapeutic uses, adverse effects, and contraindications to uricosurics.
3. Know the mechanism of action and use of allopurinol.

Definitions

Uricosuric agents: Increase the mass of uric acid that is excreted in the urine.
Renal secretion: Moves solutes such as urate from the plasma into the urine.
Renal reabsorption: Moves solutes from the urine back into the plasma.

DISCUSSION

Class

Urate is both secreted and reabsorbed by at least three independent molecular transporters located in the proximal tubule. Urate is nearly completely secreted into the lumen of the nephron against an electrochemical gradient by the action of **organic acid transporter-1 (OAT-1) and organic acid transporter-3 (OAT-3).** These cotransporters exchange α-ketoglutarate and urate (or other organic anions) and move urate from the plasma into the tubular cell. The protein UAT is an electrically neutral channel that permits uric acid to leave tubular cells and enter either the tubular lumen or the plasma. URAT1, located on the apical membrane of tubular cells, is thought to be responsible for most of the reabsorption of urate from the filtrate. URAT1 is a transporter that is capable of exchanging a variety of anions with urate in an electrically neutral manner. Interaction of uricosuric agents such as probenecid with URAT1 diminishes the reabsorption of urate and increases urate excretion. All of these transporters or channels are relatively nonselective with respect to the organic acid transported. OAT-1 and OAT-3 are capable of secreting most organic acids including probenecid, penicillin, aspirin, furosemide, and hydrochlorothiazide.

In patients with **gout, probenecid can be used prophylactically; uricosuric drugs will not diminish the severity of an acute attack. An acute gouty attack** may be **precipitated** by the **initiation of probenecid treatment** as uric acid is mobilized out of joints. **Adequate hydration** should be ensured, because probenecid predisposes patients to the formation of **uric acid kidney stones.**

The alternate therapeutic approach to the treatment of gout is to reduce the **production of uric acid with allopurinol.** The enzyme **xanthine oxidase** produces uric acid in a two-step reaction from the purine hypoxanthine. Allopurinol is metabolized to alloxanthine by xanthine oxidase, and this metabolite is a long-lasting inhibitor of the enzyme.

Probenecid is also useful for decreasing the excretion of penicillin, because **penicillin is eliminated** primarily by renal secretion mediated by **OAT-1 and OAT-3.** Probenecid competes for this secretion and thereby reduces the rate of elimination and **increases both the biological half-life of penicillin and the plasma concentration** of the antibiotic more than twofold. This adjunct use of probenecid is particularly useful in single-dose regimens for the treatment of gonococcal infections with long-acting penicillins such as penicillin G.

Secretion of organic acids is quite nonspecific, and most acidic drugs are secreted by the same transporters OAT-1 and OAT-3. This implies that nearly any combination of acidic drugs will compete for elimination at the level of the transporters, and the effects on elimination of each individual drug must be considered. For example, the half-life of diuretics such as furosemide will be increased by probenecid, and this may require dosage adjustment. **Aspirin,** another acidic drug, **will compete with probenecid for secretion.** This reduces the action of probenecid to increase uric acid excretion and thus increases plasma urate. Therefore **aspirin is contraindicated in patients with gout who are taking probenecid.**

The most common adverse effect of probenecid is gastrointestinal (GI) upset, and approximately 2 percent of patients experience a hypersensitivity reaction usually manifest as a skin rash. The incidence of hypersensitivity is lower with sulfinpyrazone, but the incidence of GI upset is higher.

Structure

Probenecid is a lipid-soluble benzoic acid derivative with a pKa of 3.4. Another agent in this class is sulfinpyrazone, a pyrazolone derivative similar to the anti-inflammatory agent phenylbutazone. It has a pKa of 2.8 but is no longer marketed in the United States.

Mechanism of Action

Both probenecid and sulfinpyrazone are secreted into the lumen of the nephron via OAT-1 and OAT-3 where the drugs can diminish the ability of URAT1 to reabsorb urate.

Administration

Both drugs are active orally, and both are nearly completely absorbed.

Pharmacokinetics

The half-life of probenecid is 5–8 hours; sulfinpyrazone is approximately 3 hours, but its uricosuric actions can last as long as 10 hours. Increased excretion of uric acid occurs promptly after oral administration. Both agents are eliminated in the urine.

COMPREHENSION QUESTIONS

[8.1] Probenecid is effective in treating gout because it decreases which of the following?

A. Inflammation in affected joints
B. Production of uric acid
C. Reabsorption of uric acid
D. Secretion of uric acid

[8.2]   Which of the following describes the action of allopurinol?

   A. Inhibits metabolism of purines to uric acid
   B. Inhibits prostaglandin biosynthesis
   C. Inhibits uric acid reabsorption
   D. Interferes with cytokine production

[8.3]   An 18-year-old man who is known to have non-penicillinase-producing gonococcal urethritis is given an injection of penicillin and probenecid. What is the mechanism used by probenecid that makes penicillin more efficacious?

   A. Decreases the bacterial resistance by inhibiting penicillinase production
   B   Increases the half-life and serum level by decreasing the renal excretion of penicillin
   C. Prolongs the duration of action by affecting the liver metabolism of penicillin
   D. Promotes entry of the penicillin into the bacteria

Answers

[8.1]   **C.** Probenecid does inhibit renal tubular secretion of urate, but at therapeutic doses it inhibits reabsorption to a greater degree, thereby increasing net excretion urate.

[8.2]   **A.** Allopurinol interferes with the metabolism of purines by inhibiting the enzyme xanthine oxidase.

[8.3]   **B.** Probenecid decreases the renal excretion of penicillin, thereby increasing both the half-life and the serum level.

PHARMACOLOGY PEARLS

❖   At low doses, probenecid inhibition of urate secretion predominates, and this paradoxically increases plasma urate.
❖   At higher doses, inhibition of reabsorption predominates, leading to the therapeutically useful **increased** excretion of urate.
❖   An acute gouty attack may be precipitated by the initiation of probenecid treatment as uric acid is mobilized out of joints.
❖   Probenecid is also useful for decreasing the excretion of penicillin and cephalosporins.
❖   Patients are typically begun on a high loading dose to ensure the action on reabsorption is achieved.

REFERENCES

Dantzler WH. Regulation of renal proximal and distal tubule transport: sodium, chloride and organic ions. Comp Biochem Physiol Part A 2003;136:453–78.
Stamp LK, O'Donnell JL, Chapman PT. Emerging therapies in the long-term management of hyperuricemia and gout. Intern Med J 2007;37:258–66.

A 72-year-old man presents to the office for routine follow-up. He is under treatment for hypertension and congestive heart failure with enalapril and a diuretic. His blood pressure is under acceptable control and he has no symptoms of heart failure at present. He does complain that he has been coughing frequently in the past few months. History and examination reveal no other cause of a chronic cough, so you decide to discontinue his enalapril and start him on losartan.

◆ **What is the mechanism of action of enalapril?**

◆ **By what mechanism does enalapril convert to its active form enalaprilat?**

◆ **What is the likely cause of the cough?**

◆ **What is the mechanism of action of losartan?**

ANSWERS TO CASE 9: DRUGS ACTIVE ON THE RENIN-ANGIOTENSIN SYSTEM

Summary: A 72-year-old man with hypertension and congestive heart failure presents with an ACE inhibitor-induced cough, and is switched to losartan.

◆ **Mechanism of action of enalapril:** Inhibits the conversion of angiotensin I to angiotensin II, this also inhibits the angiotensin II-stimulated release of aldosterone. Angiotensin-converting enzyme (ACE) inhibitors also impair the inactivation of bradykinin.

◆ **Mechanism of converting enalapril to enalaprilat:** Deesterification in the liver.

◆ **Mechanism of ACE inhibitor-induced cough:** Secondary to the increased bradykinin levels, which is caused by reduction in the inactivation of bradykinin.

◆ **Mechanism of action of angiotensin receptor blockers (ARBs):** Antagonists of angiotensin-1 (AT-1) receptors which mediate the pressor effects of angiotensin II.

CLINICAL CORRELATION

ACE inhibitors have gained wide-scale use in medicine for their effectiveness in hypertension, congestive heart failure, coronary artery disease, and renal protection in diabetics. They inhibit the conversion of angiotensin I to angiotensin II. Angiotensin II is a *potent* vasoconstrictor and stimulates the release of aldosterone, which promotes sodium retention. Angiotensin II also increases catecholamine release by the adrenal medulla and at sympathetic nerves. *Inhibition of the production of angiotensin II* reduces vascular resistance and sodium and water retention. Another effect of ACE inhibitors is to reduce the inactivation of bradykinin. Active bradykinin is a vasodilator, providing an additive effect in lowering blood pressure. However, raising bradykinin levels contributes to one of the ACE inhibitors' most bothersome side effects, chronic dry cough. ACE inhibitors in general are well tolerated, but along with cough, can cause hyperkalemia and should be used with caution with potassium-sparing diuretics or in persons with impaired renal function. ARBs are antagonists of the angiotensin I receptor, which mediates the direct vasoconstrictor effect of angiotensin II. This also blocks the release of aldosterone. ARBs do not affect the bradykinin system and therefore do not cause a cough. They are also well tolerated but, like ACE inhibitors, can cause hyperkalemia. Aliskiren (Tekturna), a renin inhibitor has recently been introduced in the United States. It appears to be as efficacious as ACE inhibitors or ARBs, but clinical experience is limited.

APPROACH TO PHARMACOLOGY OF THE RENIN-ANGIOTENSIN SYSTEM

Objectives

1. Know the mechanism of action of ACE inhibitors.
2. Know the therapeutic uses, side effects, and contraindications to ACE inhibitor use.
3. Know the mechanism of action of ARBs.
4. Know the therapeutic uses, side effects, and contraindications to ARB use.

Definitions

Hypertension: From the Seventh Report, Joint National Committee on Detection, Evaluation, and Treatment of High Blood Pressure, normal blood pressure is 120/80 mm Hg. Progressive disease may be staged as prehypertensive (120–139/80–89), Stage 1 (140–159/90–99), and Stage 2 (> 160/> 100).

Bradykinin: A member of a class of peptides, the kinins, that have a variety of effects on the cardiovascular system, including vasodilatation and inflammation.

ARB: Angiotensin receptor blocker, more precisely angiotensin AT-1 receptor blockers.

DISCUSSION

Class

The **renin-angiotensin-aldosterone system provides a humoral system for controlling blood pressure and electrolyte levels.** The "sensors" in this **system monitor Na$^+$, K$^+$, vascular volume, and blood pressure.** A reduction in blood pressure, detected by intrarenal stretch receptors, or a fall in the delivery of Na$^+$ to the distal portions of the nephron results in release of renin from the juxtaglomerular apparatus (JGA). Renin secretion can also be increased through the baroreceptor reflex mediated by increased central nervous system (CNS) outflow and β_1-adrenergic receptors on the JGA. Renin is an aspartyl protease that cleaves angiotensinogen, a 56-kD polypeptide produced in the liver, to the decapeptide angiotensin I (Figure 9-1, "classic" pathway).

Angiotensin I is biologically inactive and is **rapidly converted to the octapeptide angiotensin II** by the action of **ACE,** a dipeptidyl peptidase. Angiotensin II is further metabolized within the brain and in the plasma by aminopeptidase A, which removes the *N*-terminal aspartic acid to produce **angiotensin III**, which may itself be further metabolized by aminopeptidase N, which removes the *N*-terminal arginine yielding angiotensin IV. The latter

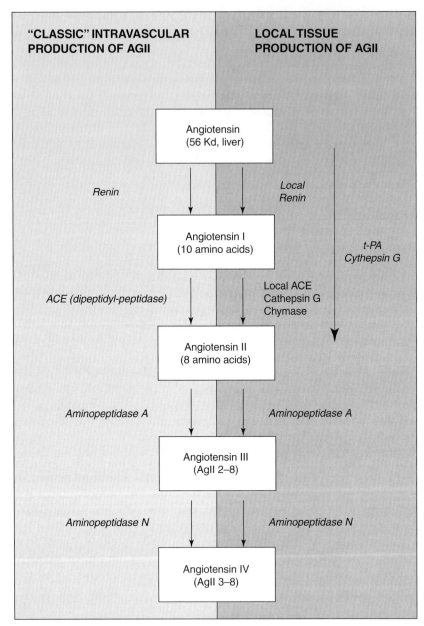

Figure 9-1. Schematic of angiotensin pathway.

two metabolites may play a critical role in regulating blood pressure in the brain. Distinct from this classic intravascular pathway for the formation of angiotensins, evidence has accumulated indicating that angiotensins can also be produced within various tissues by a local conversion to angiotensins II, III, and IV (see Figure 9-1).

Angiotensin II has multiple actions that act in concert to increase blood pressure and alter electrolyte levels. **Angiotensin II is a potent vasoconstrictor,** 10–40 times more potent than epinephrine, an effect **mediated by receptor-coupled Ca^{2+} channels** in **vascular smooth muscle cells,** as described below. **Angiotensin II enhances the release of catecholamines** from both the adrenal medulla and at peripheral nerve endings. Within the adrenal cortex, angiotensin II increases the biosynthesis of aldosterone, which leads to an increase in Na^+ and water reabsorption in the kidneys and volume expansion. Angiotensin II has several actions within the CNS including altering vagal tone to increase blood pressure, increasing thirst, and increasing the release of antidiuretic hormone.

Angiotensin II also has effects on the heart and the vasculature that do not directly affect blood pressure. **Angiotensin II induces cardiac hypertrophy,** is proproliferative, and enhances matrix remodeling and the deposition of matrix proteins, which leads to **increased myocardial stiffness.** Within vessel walls, angiotensin II is proinflammatory and can stimulate the release of several chemokines.

Three angiotensin receptors mediate these actions. The AT-1 and angiotensin-2 (AT-2) receptors have been described in various tissues. Both are seven-transmembrane receptors that appear to couple to various signaling pathways. AT-1 receptors bind angiotensin II, angiotensin III, and angiotensin IV. This receptor mediates most of the cardiovascular and central responses to angiotensin II, including vasoconstriction of vascular smooth muscle and aldosterone biosynthesis in the adrenal medulla. AT-1 receptors also mediate the cardiac hypertrophic and proproliferative responses to angiotensin II. AT-2 receptors also bind angiotensin II and play a role in the development of the cardiovascular system. In general, activation of AT-2 receptors is physiologically antagonistic to the action of AT-1 receptors. Activation of AT-2 receptors is hypotensive and antiproliferative and is coupled to distinctly different signaling pathways compared to AT-1 receptors. Angiotensin-4 (AT-4) receptors appear to be identical to transmembrane aminopeptidase insulin-regulated aminopeptidase (IRAP) and have a single transmembrane domain. AT-4 receptors are expressed in the numerous tissues and bind angiotensin IV. Activation of these receptors has been reported to regulate cerebral blood flow, and to stimulate endothelial cell expression of plasminogen activator inhibitor, and has effects on both memory and learning.

Inhibition of the renin-angiotension system (RAS) is accomplished pharmacologically in three ways: inhibition of the production of angiotensin II, blockade of AT-1 receptors, or inhibition of renin activity. **ACE inhibitors**, or peptidyl dipeptidase (PDP) inhibitors, include **enalapril, lisinopril, fosinopril,**

captopril, and seven others. These drugs differ in their chemistry and pharmacokinetic properties, but all are orally active, have the same range of activities, and are equally effective clinically. **ACE is the enzyme responsible for both *activation* of angiotensin I (metabolism to angiotensin II) and *inactivation* of bradykinin.** The decreased metabolism of bradykinin is partly responsible for the hypotensive action of ACE inhibitors, and is also responsible for enhancing the irritability of airways that leads to the **dry cough** associated with ACE inhibitors.

ARBs block the action of angiotensin II by acting as antagonists at AT-1 receptors. These nonpeptide antagonists include **losartan, valsartan, candesartan,** and others. ARBs bind with high affinity to AT-1 receptors without interfering with AT-2 or AT-4 receptors.

The **ACE inhibitors and ARBs are equally effective in reducing blood pressure.** More clinical experience exists with the ACE inhibitors and it has been well established that this class of drugs reduces the risk of second events in patients who have had an MI and in reducing renal damage in patients with diabetic nephropathy. **Hypotension and hyperkalemia are adverse effects seen with both classes of RAS inhibitors. Cough and angioedema, caused by increased bradykinin** levels, are more frequently seen with the **ACE inhibitors.**

A newly approved agent, aliskiren, has been approved for use in the treatment of hypertension. Aliskiren is a small molecule inhibitor of renin. In clinical trials of more than 2000 patients, aliskiren was effective in 24-hour blood pressure control. The effect was maintained for at least a year. Aliskiren was about as effective as ACE inhibitors or ARBs but may cause a greater rebound in renin production when discontinued than the other agents.

Structure

Although the various ACE inhibitors have different chemical structures, they are mostly based on extensive modifications of L-proline. The ARBs are also quite distinct chemically: Valsartan is an L-valine derivative, and losartan is an imidazole derivative. Aliskiren was designed based on the crystal structure of renin and is a nonpeptide, small molecule, transition-state mimetic that binds to the active site of the enzyme.

Mechanism of Action

ACE inhibitors are all competitive inhibitors of angiotensin-converting enzyme. ARBs are competitive antagonists of the angiotensin II type 1 receptor (AT-1)

Administration

All ACE inhibitors are available for oral administration. Enalaprilat, the active metabolite of enalapril, is available for intravenous infusion. Aliskiren is an oral agent.

Pharmacokinetics

Most of the current ACE inhibitors are prodrugs and require conversion to the active metabolite in the liver. For example, enalapril is converted to enalaprilat, fosinopril is converted into fosinoprilat. Captopril and lisinopril are active drugs that do not require metabolism. The onset of action of ACE inhibitors is 0.5–2 hours, and the duration of action is typically 24 hours (captopril is 6 hours). Most are eliminated in the urine.

COMPREHENSION QUESTIONS

[9.1] Losartan acts to decrease which of the following?

A. AT-1 receptor activity
B. Bradykinin production
C. Production of angiotensin II
D. Renin production

[9.2] Which of the following is a limiting adverse effect of ACE inhibitors?

A. Acidosis
B. Hyperkalemia
C. Hypernatremia
D. Hypokalemia
E. Hyponatremia

[9.3] Which of the following is an advantage of losartan over enalapril?

A. Better efficacy in lower blood pressure
B. Better prevention of secondary myocardial events
C. Less cost
D. Less incidence of angioedema

Answers

[9.1] **A.** Losartan is a prototypical angiotensin AT-1 receptor antagonist.

[9.2] **B.** By reducing aldosterone levels, ACE inhibitors decrease K^+ excretion in the distal nephron.

[9.3] **D.** Losartan does not lead to elevated bradykinin levels; thus, there is less of an incidence of angioedema and dry cough. The effects on blood pressure are equal. The track record for prevention of secondary cardiovascular events is well established for ACE inhibitors, although the same is speculated for ARBs.

PHARMACOLOGY PEARLS

❖ Elevation of the bradykinin levels is thought to be the etiology of the dry cough and angioedema of ACE inhibitors.

❖ ACE inhibitors improve outcome in patients with cardiovascular disease and have been recommended as therapy in several guidelines.

❖ Clinical experience suggests that inhibitors of the renin-angiotensin system are somewhat less effective in African Americans.

❖ ARBs block the action of angiotensin II by acting as antagonists at AT-1 receptors.

REFERENCES

Yusuf S, Sleight P, Pogue J, et al. Effects of an angiotensin-converting-enzyme inhibitor, ramipril, on cardiovascular events in high-risk patients: the heart outcomes prevention evaluation study investigators. N Engl J Med 2000;342: 145–53.

Stojiljkovic L, Behnia R. Role of angiotensin system inhibitors in cardiovascular and renal protection: a lesson from clinical trials. Curr Pharm Des 2007;13: 1335–45.

A 69-year-old man sees you in the office for follow-up of his chronic conges-tive heart failure. He has a marked reduction in his ejection fraction following a series of MIs. He also has hypertension and type II diabetes mellitus. His symptoms include dyspnea on exertion, orthopnea, paroxysmal nocturnal dys-pnea, and peripheral edema. He has normal renal function. He is on appropriate treatment of his diabetes, along with an ACE inhibitor and a loop diuretic. You decide to add digoxin to his regimen.

◆ **What is the effect of digoxin on the normal heart?**

◆ **What is the effect of digoxin on the failing heart?**

◆ **What neural effects does digoxin have?**

◆ **What are the side effects and toxicities of digoxin?**

ANSWERS TO CASE 10: AGENTS USED TO TREAT CONGESTIVE HEART FAILURE

Summary: A 69-year-old man with congestive heart failure, hypertension, and diabetes mellitus has a markedly low ejection fraction and is prescribed digoxin.

◆ **Effect on a normal heart:** Increased systemic vascular resistance and constriction of smooth muscle in veins, which may decrease cardiac output.

◆ **Effect on a failing heart:** Increased stroke volume and increased cardiac output.

◆ **Neural effects:** Decreased sympathetic tone and increased vagal activity, resulting in inhibition of sinoatrial (SA) node and delayed conduction through atrioventricular (AV) node.

◆ **Side effects and toxicities:** Induction of arrhythmias, anorexia, nausea, vomiting, diarrhea, disorientation, and visual disturbance.

CLINICAL CORRELATION

Digoxin can be useful in improving some of the symptoms of congestive heart failure, but its use must be closely monitored. Digoxin works by inhibiting the sodium-potassium adenosine triphosphatase (ATPase), primarily in cardiac muscle cells. This causes increased intracellular sodium and decreased intracellular potassium. The increased sodium reduces the exchange of intracellular calcium for extracellular sodium, causing an increased intracellular calcium level. The overall effect of this is to allow for a greater release of calcium with each action potential. This has a positive inotropic effect. In a failing heart, stroke volume and cardiac output are increased. End-diastolic volume, venous pressure, and blood volume are decreased. These circulatory improvements also result in a reduction of sympathetic tone. This further improves circulation by lowering systemic vascular resistance. **Digoxin also has the effect of increasing vagal activity,** which inhibits the SA node and slows conduction through the AV node. This is beneficial in patients with atrial tachyarrhythmias such as atrial fibrillation, atrial flutter, and atrial tachycardias. **Digoxin has a narrow therapeutic index,** and its **level in the blood must be closely monitored.** The **dose must be adjusted for renal impairment,** because it is cleared by the kidney. Toxic digoxin levels may produce many types of **arrhythmias,** with **AV blocks and bradycardia** being common. Mental status changes and gastrointestinal symptoms are common as well. Asymptomatic elevations in digoxin levels are usually treated by discontinuing or reducing the drug's dosage. Symptomatic toxicity, particularly arrhythmias, is **most often treated by the IV infusion of digoxin-binding antibodies.**

APPROACH TO PHARMACOLOGY
OF THE CARDIAC GLYCOSIDES

Objectives

1. Know the mechanism of action of the cardiac glycosides.
2. Know the therapeutic uses, adverse effects, and toxicities of cardiac glycosides.
3. Know the other agents used frequently in the treatment of congestive heart failure.

Definitions

Cardiac glycosides: The cardenolides include digitalis, digoxin, digitoxin, and ouabain.

Inotropic: Affecting myocardial contractility.

Chronotropic: Affecting heart rate.

Congestive heart failure: A syndrome with multiple causes that may affect either systole or diastole. Left heart failure leads to pulmonary congestion and reduced cardiac output and appears in patients with MI, aortic and mitral valve disease, and hypertension. Right heart failure leads to peripheral edema and ascites and appears in patients with tricuspid valve disease, cor pulmonale, and prolonged left heart failure. The New York Heart Association classification of congestive heart failure includes class I (mild disease) to class IV (severe disease).

DISCUSSION

Class

The medicinal actions of the cardiac glycosides, digitalis, have been used successfully for over 200 years, and they have both positive inotropic and antiarrhythmic properties. **Digoxin is the most commonly used cardiac glycoside. Cardiac glycosides act to indirectly increase intracellular calcium** (Figure 10-1). **Digitalis binds to a specific site on the outside of the Na^+-K^+-ATPase** and this reduces the activity of the enzyme. All cells express Na^+/K^+-ATPase but there are several different isoforms of the enzyme; the isoforms expressed by **cardiac myocytes and vagal neurons are the most susceptible to digitalis.** Inhibition of the enzyme by digitalis causes an increase in intracellular Na^+ and decreases the Na^+ concentration gradient across the plasma membrane. It is this Na^+ concentration that provides the driving force for the Na^+-Ca^{2+} antiporter. The rate of transport of Ca^{2+} out of the cell is reduced, and this leads to an increase in intracellular Ca^{2+}, greater activation of contractile elements, and an increase in the force of contraction of the heart. The **electrical characteristics of myocardial cells** are also **altered by**

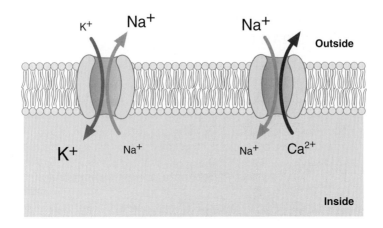

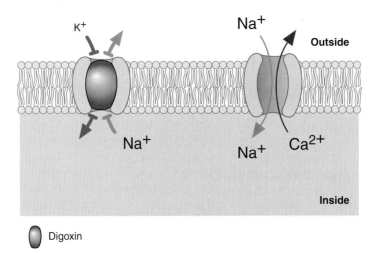

○ Digoxin

Figure 10-1. Digoxin acts to indirectly increase intracellular calcium levels by binding to the Na$^+$-K$^+$-ATPase.

the **cardiac glycosides.** The most important effect is a **shortening of the action potential** that produces a **shortening of both atrial and ventricular refractoriness.** There is also an **increase in the automaticity of the heart,** both within the AV node and in the cardiac myocytes.

Within the nervous system cardiac glycosides affect both the sympathetic and parasympathetic systems, and parasympatheticomimetic effects predominate at therapeutic doses. **Increased vagal activity inhibits the SA node and delays conduction through the AV node.**

In **acute heart failure, digitalis clearly improves contractility.** Ejection fraction and cardiac output is increased and symptoms are decreased. **In congestive** heart failure, digitalis is used primarily in patients who are symptomatic after optimal therapy with diuretics, ACE inhibitors, and beta blockers. In this setting, digitalis decreases symptoms and increases exercise tolerance. However, in patients with **normal sinus rhythm,** there is **no decline in overall mortality** because of deaths associated with digitalis toxicity.

Because of its action in **increasing vagal tone, cardiac glycosides** are useful in the treatment of **several supraventricular arrhythmias** including **atrial flutter** and **atrial fibrillation. Digitalis can control paroxysmal atrial and AV nodal tachycardia.** Its use is **contraindicated in Wolff-Parkinson-White syndrome,** where it can induce arrhythmias in the alternate pathway.

Cardiac glycosides have a **narrow therapeutic index. Toxic levels of cardiac glycosides lead to depletion of intracellular K^+ and accumulation of Na^+** (because of inhibition of Na^+/K^+-ATPase). This leads to partial depolarization of the cell and increased excitability, both of which can lead to arrhythmias including supraventricular and ventricular tachyarrhythmias. Bradycardia and heart block are also manifestations of digitalis toxicity in the heart. **Adverse effects of digitalis on the gastrointestinal (GI) tract** are common including **anorexia, vomiting, pain, and diarrhea.** Central nervous system effects include **yellowed and blurred vision, dizziness, fatigue, and delirium.** At very high toxic ranges digitalis inhibits Na^+/K^+-ATPase in skeletal muscle, resulting in hyperkalemia.

K^+ competes with digitalis for binding to the Na^+/K^+-ATPase; **hypokalemia increases the effectiveness of digitalis and increases toxicity.** Hypercalcemia can also increase the action of digitalis and increase toxicity.

Dopamine and dobutamine are positive inotropic agents that can be used on a **short-term basis in congestive heart failure. Dobutamine stimulates D_1- and D_2-adrenergic receptors.** The action on β_1-**adrenoreceptors** is responsible for **most of the beneficial actions of dobutamine.** It is useful in patients with acute left ventricular failure or to prevent pulmonary edema in heart failure. At sufficient doses, **dopamine** interacts with β_1 **receptors** and **increases myocardial contractility.** It is useful in the treatment of **cardiogenic and septic shock.**

Structure

These compounds share two structural features: an aglycone steroid nucleus with a lactone at carbon 17 in the D ring, which confers the cardiotonic properties, and polymeric sugar moieties attached to carbon 3 of the A ring. Both features are necessary for pharmacologic activity; the sugar groups are largely responsible for the pharmacokinetic properties of these drugs.

Mechanism of Action

Inhibition of the activity of the Na^+-K^+-ATPase; this indirectly increases intracellular Ca^{2+}.

Administration

Digoxin can be administered IV or orally. Oral bioavailability is approximately 75 percent. Digitoxin is available only as an oral agent and its bioavailability is greater than 90 percent. Ouabain has limited bioavailability and is not used clinically.

Pharmacokinetics

Digoxin is excreted by the **kidney** and is not metabolized. Patients with compromised renal function must be monitored carefully for digoxin toxicity. Digitoxin is metabolized in the **liver** and renal impairment does not affect the half-life of the drug.

COMPREHENSION QUESTIONS

[10.1] Digoxin increases cardiac contractility by directly engaging in which of the following?

    A. Activating L-type Ca^{2+} channels
    B. Inhibiting cardiac phosphodiesterase
    C. Inhibiting myocardial Na^+/Ca^{2+}-ATPase
    D. Inhibiting myocardial Na^+/K^+-ATPase

[10.2] Which of the following drugs may be used to increase cardiac output in a patient with pulmonary edema secondary to MI?

    A. Captopril
    B. Dobutamine
    C. Metoprolol
    D. Verapamil

[10.3] Which of the following is the most accurate statement regarding digoxin?

    A. Decreased mortality in patients with congestive heart failure with normal sinus rhythm
    B. Increases vagal tone and decreases AV node conduction
    C. Lengthens the action potential and increases the refractoriness of the heart
    D. Useful in the treatment of Wolff-Parkinson-White syndrome

Answers

[10.1]   **D.** While digoxin reduces the amount of Na^+-Ca^{2+} exchange, this effect is indirect and mediated by the inhibition of the Na^+/K^+-ATPase.

[10.2]   **B.** Dobutamine is useful in this setting; the other choices would not increase cardiac output.

[10.3]   **B.** Cardiac glycosides increase vagal tone and decrease AV node conduction. The action potential is decreased and the refractoriness of the heart is decreased. Mortality is not decreased in patients with normal sinus rhythm because of digoxin toxicity. Digoxin is contraindicated in Wolff-Parkinson-White syndrome.

PHARMACOLOGY PEARLS

❖ Cardiac glycosides inhibit the activity the Na^+-K^+-ATPase; this indirectly increases intracellular Ca^{2+}.

❖ While several studies have found that digitalis does not improve mortality, it is still useful in reducing symptoms in congestive heart failure.

❖ The increased effectiveness of digitalis as serum K^+ falls is significant because most patients with congestive heart failure are also frequently treated with diuretics that cause potassium loss.

❖ Hypokalemia exacerbates digoxin toxicity.

REFERENCE

Hood W, Jr, Dans A, Guyatt G, et al. Digitalis for treatment of congestive heart failure in patients in sinus rhythm. Cochrane Database Syst Rev 2004;2:CD002901.

A 62-year-old man is being managed in the intensive care unit following a large anterior wall MI. He has been appropriately managed with oxygen, aspirin, nitrates, and β-adrenergic receptor blockers but has developed recurrent episodes of ventricular tachycardia. During these episodes he remains conscious but feels dizzy, and he becomes diaphoretic and hypotensive. He is given an IV bolus of lidocaine and started on an IV lidocaine infusion.

◆ **To what class of antiarrhythmic does lidocaine belong?**

◆ **What is lidocaine's mechanism of action?**

ANSWERS TO CASE 11: ANTIARRHYTHMIC DRUGS

Summary: A 62-year-old man develops symptomatic ventricular tachycardia after an MI. He is begun on IV lidocaine.

◆   **Class of antiarrhythmic to which lidocaine belongs:** Ib.

◆   **Mechanism of action:** Specific Na$^+$ channel blocker, reduces the rate of phase 0 depolarization, primarily in damaged tissue.

CLINICAL CORRELATION

Lidocaine is a common treatment for ventricular tachycardia in a patient who is symptomatic and remains conscious. It works by blocking Na$^+$ channels and is highly selective for damaged tissue. This makes it useful for the treatment of ventricular ectopy associated with an MI. It is administered as an IV bolus followed by a continuous drip infusion. It is metabolized in the liver and undergoes a large first-pass effect. It has many neurological side effects, including agitation, confusion, and tremors, and can precipitate seizures.

APPROACH TO PHARMACOLOGY OF THE ANTIARRHYTHMICS

Objectives

1. Know the classes of antiarrhythmic agents and their mechanisms of action.
2. Know the indications for the use of antiarrhythmic agents.
3. Know the adverse effects and toxicities of the antiarrhythmic agents.

Definitions

Paroxysmal atrial tachycardias (PAT): Arrhythmia caused by reentry through the AV node.
Heart block: Failure of normal conduction from atria to ventricles.
WPW: Wolff-Parkinson-White syndrome.

DISCUSSION

Class

Arrhythmias arise as a result of improper impulse generation or improper impulse conduction. The abnormal action potentials cause disturbances in the rate of contraction or in the coordination of myocardial contraction. The molecular targets of antiarrhythmics are ion channels in the myocardium or conduction pathways; these may be direct or indirect effects.

There are four ion channels of pharmacologic importance in the heart:

Voltage-activated Na^+ channel—SCN5A
Voltage-activated Ca^{2+} channel—L-type
Voltage-activated K^+ channel—IKr
Voltage-activated K^+ channel—IKs

Most antiarrhythmic drugs either bind directly to sites within the pore of a channel or indirectly alter channel activity. There are approximately 20 antiarrhythmics approved for use today. They are classified according to which of the ion channels they affect and their mechanism of action (Table 11-1).

Table 11-1
SELECTED ANTIARRHYTHMIC AGENTS

CLASS	PROTOTYPE DRUG	Na^+	K^+	Ca^{2+}	EFFECT
Ia	Quinidine	X	X		Increases refractory period, slows conduction
Ib	Lidocaine	X			Shortens duration of refractory period
Ic	Flecainide	X	X		Slows conduction
II	Propranolol			X*	Blocks β_1-adrenergic receptors
III	Amiodarone	X		X	Increases refractory period
IV	Verapamil			X	Increases refractory period AV node
Other					
	Adenosine		X	X*	Decreases AV node conduction
	Moricizine	X†			
	Atropine				Decreases vagal tone
	Digoxin				Increases vagal tone
	Sotalol		X‡		Also nonselective beta blocker

*Indirect effect mediated by decreasing cAMP.

†Moricizine blocks Na^+ channels and is usually considered a class 1 antiarrhythmic, but it has properties of Ia, Ib, and Ic drugs.

‡Solotol has α- and β-adrenergic antagonist properties and also inhibits K^+ channels.

The major arrhythmias of clinical concern are ventricular arrhythmias, atrial arrhythmias, bradycardias, and heart blocks. There is also the pharmacologic need to convert an abnormal rhythm to normal sinus rhythm (cardioconversion). The class of antiarrhythmics used for any particular arrhythmia depends on the clinical circumstances. The treatment of acute, life-threatening disease, in contrast with the long-term management of chronic disease, requires a different selection of antiarrhythmics.

Class I Antiarrhythmics

Class I antiarrhythmics bind to Na^+ channels and prevent their activation. This increases their effective refractory period and decreases conduction velocity. Class I antiarrhythmics have a greater effect on damaged tissue compared to normal tissue. This may be because of several factors:

Depolarization. Damaged tissues tend to be depolarized because of K^+ leakage—many class I antiarrhythmics preferentially bind to depolarized tissues.

pH. Ischemic tissues are more acidic, and many class I antiarrhythmics preferentially bind to membranes at low pH.

Inactivation frequency. During arrhythmias, Na^+ channels undergo more rapid cycles of activation/inactivation. At any given time there will be an increase in the number of inactive channels compared to normal tissues in a normal rhythm. Class I antiarrhythmics generally bind preferentially to Na^+ channels in the inactive state.

The subclasses a, b, and c of class I antiarrhythmics are distinguished based on their ability to inhibit K^+ channels.

Class Ia. Procainamide is a prototype class Ia antiarrhythmic that suppresses the activity of Na^+ and also suppresses K^+-channel activity. **Administered IV**, it is used for the acute suppression of supraventricular and ventricular arrhythmias and for suppressing episodes of atrial flutter and atrial fibrillation. **It may be administered orally for the long-term suppression of both supraventricular and ventricular arrhythmia, but toxicity limits this application. Procainamide can suppress sinoatrial (SA) and AV nodal activity, especially in patients with nodal disease, and cause heart block. Prolonged use of procainamide is associated with increased risk of ventricular tachycardias. Procainamide has some ganglionic blocking activity and can cause hypotension and decreased myocardial contractility.** A limiting adverse effect of procainamide is the development of lupus-like syndrome characterized by skin rash, arthritis, and serositis. **All patients on procainamide will develop antinuclear antibodies within 2 years.** Procainamide is metabolized to *N*-acetyl procainamide (NAPA), **which has K^+-channel-blocking effects. NAPA is excreted by the kidney, and plasma levels of procainamide and** NAPA should both be monitored especially in patients with renal disease.

Class Ib. Lidocaine is very specific for the Na^+ channel and it blocks both activated and inactivated states of the channel. **It must be administered parenterally. Lidocaine has been used extensively to suppress ventricular arrhythmias associated with acute MI** or cardiac damage (surgery). **It has been used prophylactically to prevent arrhythmias in patients with MI, but there is controversy as to the overall benefit in decreasing mortality. Lidocaine is metabolized in the liver and has relatively short half-life (60 minutes). This limits its adverse effects which generally are mild and rapidly reversible.** Overdose can produce sedation, hallucinations, and convulsions.

Class Ic. Flecainide inhibits both Na^+ and K^+ channels but shows no preference for inactivated Na^+ channels. It delays conduction and increases refractoriness. **It is effective for the control of atrial arrhythmias and it is very effective in suppressing supraventricular arrhythmias.** A recent large clinical trial with patients with **ischemic heart disease** demonstrated that flecainide is **associated with increased mortality. Currently its use is restricted to patients with atrial arrhythmias without underlying ischemic heart disease.**

Class II Agents

Endogenous catecholamines increase myocardial excitability and can trigger ventricular arrhythmias. β-Adrenergic receptor blockade indirectly suppresses L-type Ca^{2+}-channel activity. This slows phase 3 repolarization and lengthens the refractory period. Reduction in sympathetic tone depresses automaticity, decreases AV conduction, and decreases heart rate and contractility. **Beta blockers are useful for the long-term suppression of ventricular arrhythmias particularly in patients at risk for sudden cardiac arrest.** Beta blockers are most effective in patients with increased adrenergic activity:

- Surgical or anesthetic stress.
- Anginal pain and MI.
- Congestive heart failure and ischemic heart disease.
- Hyperthyroidism.
- Beta blockers have been shown to reduce mortality and second cardiovascular events by 25–40% in patients with post-MI.

There are a large number of beta blockers approved for use as antiarrhythmics. Two of particular interest are

1. **d,l-sotalol,** which is particularly effective as an antiarrhythmic agent because it combines inhibition of K^+ channels with beta-blocker activity
2. Metoprolol, a specific β_1 antagonist, which reduces the risk of pulmonary complications

d,l-sotalol is a racemic mixture; l-sotalol is an effective, **nonselective β-adrenergic antagonist;** and d-sotalol is a class III antiarrhythmic that inhibits K^+ channels. It is an oral agent with a long half-life (20 hours) that can maintain therapeutic blood levels with once a day dosing. d,l-sotalol is useful for the long-term suppression of ventricular arrhythmias, especially in patients at risk of sudden death. It is also used to suppress atrial flutter and fibrillation and paroxysmal atrial tachycardia. It is a valuable adjunct in the use of implantable cardiac defibrillators, decreasing the number of events that require defibrillation. At low doses, the β-adrenergic-blocking activity, and associated adverse effects, predominates. At higher doses, the K$^+$-channel inhibitory effects predominate with the risk of developing ventricular tachycardia.

Class III Antiarrhythmics

Drugs in this class **include bretylium, dofetilide, and amiodarone.** These agents act predominantly to **inhibit cardiac K$^+$ channels (IKr).** This lengthens the time to repolarize and prolongs the refractory period. Amiodarone is also a potent inhibitor of Na$^+$ channels and has α- and β-adrenergic antagonist activity.

Amiodarone has an unusual structure related to thyroxine. It can be administered IV or orally, but its actions differ depending on route of administration. IV-administered amiodarone has acute effects to inhibit K$^+$-channel activity, slowing repolarization, and increasing the refractory period of all myocardial cell types. Administered orally in a more chronic setting, it leads to long-term alterations in membrane properties with a reduction in both Na$^+$- and K$^+$-channel activity and decrease in adrenergic receptor activity. **Amiodarone is used extensively for ventricular and atrial arrhythmias and has little myocardial depressant activity,** allowing it to be used in patients with diminished cardiac function. Administered IV, amiodarone is effective in treating ventricular tachycardia and to prevent recurrent ventricular tachycardia, and to suppress atrial fibrillation. Oral amiodarone is useful for arrhythmias that have not responded to other drugs (such as adenosine) and for long-term suppression of arrhythmias in patients at risk of sudden cardiac death.

Amiodarone has little myocardial toxicity, does not impair contractility, and rarely induces arrhythmias. Most of the adverse effects of amiodarone result from its **long half-life** (13–103 days) and **poor solubility. Amiodarone deposits in the lung** and can cause **irreversible pulmonary damage.** Similarly, **amiodarone can be deposited in the cornea causing visual disturbances or in the skin where it can cause a bluish tinge.**

Class IV Antiarrhythmics

The class IV antiarrhythmics act by directly blocking the activity of L-type Ca^{2+} channels. Verapamil and **diltiazem** are the major members of this class, and they have a similar pharmacology. **Verapamil blocks both active and inactive Ca^{2+} channels** and has effects that are equipotent in cardiac and peripheral tissues. The **dihydropyridines** such as **nifedipine** have **little effect on Ca^{2+} channels in the myocardium, but are effective in blocking Ca^{2+}**

channels in the vasculature. **Verapamil** has marked effects on both **SA and AV nodes** because these tissues are highly dependent on Ca^{2+} currents. AV node conduction and refractory period are prolonged and the SA node is slowed. **Verapamil and diltiazem are useful for reentrant supraventricular tachycardias** and can also be used to reduce the ventricular rate in atrial flutter or fibrillation. The **major adverse effect of verapamil** is related to its **inhibition of myocardial contractility.** It can cause heart block at high doses.

Other Antiarrhythmics

Adenosine is a **very short-acting drug (approximately 10 seconds)** used specifically to **block PAT. Adenosine binds to purinergic A1 receptors.** Activation of these receptors leads to increased potassium conductance and decreased in calcium influx. This results in hyperpolarization and a decrease in Ca^{2+}-dependent action potentials. The effect in the AV node is marked with a decrease in conduction and an increase in nodal refractory period. Effects on the SA node are smaller. Adenosine is nearly 100 percent effective in converting PAT to sinus rhythm. Adenosine must be given IV, and because of its short half-life, it has few adverse effects. Flushing and chest pain are frequent but typically resolve quickly.

Digoxin (see Case 10) blocks Na^+-K^+-ATPase and indirectly increases intracellular Ca^{2+}. In the myocardium this causes an increase in contractility; in nerve tissue the predominant effect is to increase neurotransmitter release; and the parasympathetic system (vagus) is affected more than the sympathetic system. The increased vagal tone results in increased stimulation of muscarinic acetylcholine receptors that slow conduction in the AV node. **Digoxin is very effective controlling the ventricular response rate in patients with atrial fibrillation or flutter.** Digoxin can be administered IV to acutely treat atrial arrhythmias or orally for long-term suppression of abnormal atrial rhythms. Digitalis is less effective than adenosine in PAT and **should not be used in** Wolff-Parkinson-White syndrome.

Atropine is **a muscarinic antagonist that can be used in some bradycardias and heart blocks. It can be administered to reverse heart block caused by increased vagal tone such as an MI or digitalis toxicity. Atropine is administered IV, and it exerts its effect within minutes.**

COMPREHENSION QUESTIONS

[11.1] Which of the following is the most effective agent for converting paroxysmal atrial tachycardia to normal sinus rhythm?

    A. Adenosine
    B. Atropine
    C. Digoxin
    D. Lidocaine

[11.2] Which of the following best describes a pharmacologic property of amiodarone?

A. α-Adrenergic agonist
B. β-Adrenergic agonist
C. Activation of Ca^{2+} channels
D. Inhibition of K^+ channels

[11.3] A 45-year-old man is noted to have dilated cardiomyopathy with atrial fibrillation and a rapid ventricular rate. An agent is used to control the ventricular rate, but the cardiac contractility is also affected, placing him in pulmonary edema. Which of the following agents was most likely used?

A. Amiodarone
B. Digoxin
C. Nifedipine
D. Verapamil

Answers

[11.1]   **A.** Adenosine is nearly 100 percent effective in converting PAT. Digoxin could be used but is less effective.

[11.2]   **D.** Amiodarone blocks both Na^+ and K^+ channels and has α- and β-adrenoreceptor **antagonist** activities. The latter would indirectly decrease Ca^{2+}-channel activity.

[11.3]   **D.** Verapamil is a calcium-channel-blocking agent that slows conduction in the AV node, but it also has a negative inotropic effect on the heart.

PHARMACOLOGY PEARLS

 Amiodarone is typically the first choice in acute ventricular arrhythmias.

 Adenosine is the best choice to convert PAT to sinus rhythm.

 Long-term benefit of using class I antiarrhythmics is uncertain, but mortality is not decreased.

 Beta blockers have been shown to reduce mortality and second cardiovascular events by 25–40% in patients post-MI.

REFERENCES

Cooper HA, Bloomfield DA, Bush DE, et al. Relation between achieved heart rate and outcomes in patients with atrial fibrillation (from the atrial fibrillation follow-up investigation of rhythm management [AFFIRM] study): AFFIRM investigators. Am J Cardiol 2004;93(10):1247–53.

Boriani G, Diemberger I, Biffi M et al. Pharmacological cardioversion of atrial fibrillation: current management and treatment options. Drugs 2007;64:2641–62.

A 50-year-old man presents for follow-up of his hypertension. He is maintaining a low-sodium diet, exercising regularly, and taking metoprolol at maximum dosage. He is on no other medications. His blood pressure remains elevated at 150/100 mm Hg. His examination is otherwise unremarkable. You decide to add a thiazide diuretic to his regimen.

◆ **What is the mechanism of action of metoprolol?**

◆ **What is the mechanism of action of thiazide diuretics?**

◆ **What electrolyte abnormalities commonly occur with thiazide diuretics?**

ANSWERS TO CASE 12: ANTIHYPERTENSIVE AGENTS

Summary: A 50-year-old man with inadequately controlled hypertension is prescribed a thiazide diuretic.

◆ **Mechanism of action of metoprolol:** β_1-Selective adrenoreceptor antagonist.

◆ **Mechanism of action of thiazide diuretics:** Inhibit active reabsorption of NaCl in the distal convoluted tubule by interfering with a specific Na^+/Cl^- cotransporter.

◆ **Electrolyte abnormalities seen with thiazide diuretics:** Hypokalemia, hyponatremia, hypochloremia.

CLINICAL CORRELATION

Thiazide diuretics are the recommended first-line agents for most people with hypertension. They are frequently used in combination with other classes of antihypertensives. Thiazides inhibit the active reabsorption of Na^+. This causes an increase in the excretion of Na^+, Cl^-, and K^+. They also reduce the excretion of Ca^{2+} by increasing its absorption. The excretion of sodium and water reduces intravascular volume and contributes to their antihypertensive effect. Thiazides are used as single agents primarily in mild to moderate hypertension. They are often added as second agents when other drugs alone cannot control a patient's hypertension. The electrolyte abnormalities caused by thiazides can be clinically important. Hypokalemia occurs frequently, especially when higher doses of thiazides are used. Patients need to be instructed to follow a high potassium diet and frequently require potassium supplementation. Thiazides can also elevate serum uric acid levels, which can precipitate gout in susceptible individuals.

APPROACH TO PHARMACOLOGY OF ANTIHYPERTENSIVE AGENTS

Objectives

1. Know the classes of antihypertensive medications and their mechanisms of action.
2. Know the common side effects of the antihypertensive agents.

Definitions

Hypertension: Blood pressure continuously elevated to levels greater than 120/80 mm Hg. Pressures of 130/90 mm Hg are considered prehypertensive.

Essential hypertension: Hypertension of unknown etiology makes up approximately 90 percent of hypertensive patients.

DISCUSSION

Class

There are 12 major classes of drugs that are used as oral antihypertensive drugs, and these include drugs that act centrally and those that work in the periphery. Antihypertensive drugs may cause vascular smooth-muscle relaxation, vascular volume reduction, or a decrease in cardiac output. This is accomplished by decreasing Ca^{2+} in vascular smooth muscle cells or by reducing Na^+ reabsorption on the kidney. Table 12-1 lists these major classes. **Lifestyle modifications include smoking cessation, weight management, and commencement of an exercise program.**

The Joint National Commission (JNC) also emphasized the need to recognize and treat **systolic hypertension,** which is associated with a **higher degree of risk of MI** in patients **older than 45 years.** Systolic hypertension is more difficult to treat than diastolic hypertension and frequently requires multiple drugs acting via different mechanisms.

The JNC-7 report and other recent studies recommend thiazide diuretics as the first-line agent for the treatment of hypertension in most cases **(Table 12-2).** This conservative approach is based on data supporting the fact that these **agents decrease morbidity and mortality** in clinical trials. The other agents that should be considered for initial **monotherapy** include the beta blockers, the renin-angiotensin system inhibitors (either ACE inhibitors or ARBs), α-adrenoreceptor antagonists, calcium-channel antagonists, and arterial vasodilators. All have been shown to reduce blood pressure by 10–15 mm Hg.

Diuretics

Diuretics cause an initial reduction in blood pressure by **facilitating loss of Na^+ and water.** This leads to a decrease in cardiac output and blood pressure. However, after 8 weeks, cardiac output returns to normal while blood pressure remains reduced. This is thought to be caused by a **reduction in the vasoconstrictive activities of Na^+ on vascular smooth muscles** that include **elevation of intracellular Ca^{2+} via the Ca^{2+}/Na^+ antiporter. Thiazide** diuretics, which reduce the activity of a specific Na^+Cl^- cotransporter (NCC2) in the **distal convoluted tubule,** are the class of diuretics most often used for hypertension. In refractory cases or in patients with concomitant edema, loop diuretics can be used with caution. Loop diuretics reduce Na^+ reabsorption in the ascending limb of the loop of Henle by reducing the activity of another Na^+-K^+-$2Cl^-$ cotransporter (NKCC) and can produce a profound loss of Na^+ and K^+. **Both thiazides and loop diuretics can cause hypokalemia and hyponatremia.** A common complaint associated with diuretic use is the increased **frequency of**

Table 12-1
SELECTIVE CLASSES OF ANTIHYPERTENSIVE AGENTS

CLASS	PROTOTYPE DRUG	MOA	COMMON ADVERSE EFFECT
Beta blocker	Propranolol	Adrenergic β-receptor antagonist	Fatigue, reduction on libido
α_1-Antagonist	Prazosin	Adrenergic receptor antagonist	Orthostatic hypotension
ACE inhibitor	Enalapril	Reduces production of angiotensin II	Hyperkalemia
ARB (angiotenson receptor blocker)	Losartan	AT-1 receptor antagonist	Hyperkalemia
Renin inhibitor	Aliskiren	Inhibits renin activity	Angioedema, headache, dizziness, gastrointestinal events
Specific aldosterone-receptor antagonist	Eplerenone	Aldosterone-receptor antagonists	Hyperkalemia
Diuretic—loop	Furosemide	Reduces Na^+ reabsorption in loop of Henle	Hypokalemia
Diuretic—distal tubule	Hydrochlorothiazide	Reduces Na^+ reabsorption at site 3	Hypokalemia
Ca^{2+} channel blocker	Nifedipine	Blocks Ca^{2+} entry in vascular smooth muscle cells	Hypotension arrhythmias
Arterial vasodilators	Minoxidil	Hyperpolarizes VSMC	Orthostatic hypotension
Central acting vasodilator	Clonidine	α_2-Adrenergic agonist, I_2-receptor agonist	Sedation, depression
Adrenergic neuron blockers	Guanethidine	Inhibits release of norepinephrine	Postural hypotension
Neuronal uptake inhibitor	Reserpine	Depletes neurons of neurotransmitters	Sedation

Table 12-2
THE JOINT NATIONAL COMMITTEE ON HYPERTENSION HAS DEFINED FOUR CATEGORIES OF HYPERTENSION

STAGE	BLOOD PRESSURE SYSTOLIC (mm Hg)	BLOOD PRESSURE DIASTOLIC (mm Hg)	RECOMMENDED TREATMENT
Normal	<120	and <80	—
Prehypertensive	120–139	or 80–89	Lifestyle modification
Hypertensive stage 1	140–159	or 90–99	Lifestyle modification, R_x
Hypertensive stage 2	≥160	or ≥100	Lifestyle modification, R_x

urination. Spironolactone and eplerenone are antagonists of the aldosterone receptor and are weakly diuretic. Eplerenone is much more specific for the alososterone receptor compared to spironolactone.

Beta (β) Blockers

Use of β-adrenoreceptor blockers for hypertension relies on **decreasing cardiac output and decreasing peripheral vascular resistance.** The various drugs in this class vary in their potency on β_1 receptors; **metoprolol is more than 1000 times more potent in blocking β_1 compared to β_2 receptors,** giving this drug a relative **cardioselectivity.** Blockade of β_1-adrenoreceptors in the JGA of the kidney reduces renin secretion, and this reduces the production of angiotensin II. Nonselective beta blockers such as propranolol cause a number of predictable adverse effects including bronchoconstriction (contraindicating use in asthmatics); a decrease in the production of insulin (contraindicating use in diabetics); and central nervous system (CNS) effects including depression, insomnia, and a decline in male potency. In addition, the nonselective agents increase both triglycerides and low-density lipoprotein (LDL). These effects are reduced but not eliminated with the more β_1-selective agents.

Alpha₁ (α₁) Blockers

Prazosin, doxazosin, and terazosin reduce blood pressure by **antagonizing α_1-adrenoreceptors in vascular smooth muscle.** Blockade of this receptor reduces intracellular **cyclic adenosine monophosphate** (cAMP) and leads to a reduction in intracellular Ca^{2+}. **Orthostatic hypotension** is common on initiation of therapy but diminishes. Dizziness and headache are also adverse effects. α_1-Blockers appear to reduce LDL cholesterol. **Alpha blockers** are used primarily for hypertension in patients who also have symptomatic **prostatic hyperplasia**. Because of excess cases of **congestive heart failure** in users of alpha blockers, these agents should not be used as first-line therapy in hypertension.

Calcium Channel Blockers

Calcium channel (Ca^{2+}-channel) blockers are useful antihypertensives and can reduce blood pressure by 10–15 mm Hg. These agents exert their antihypertensive effect by **blocking L-type (voltage-sensitive) Ca^{2+} channels.** By blocking the entry of Ca^{2+} into the cell, less is available to activate the contractile apparatus, and within vascular smooth muscle, this produces a reduction in vascular tone. Three distinct chemical classes comprise the Ca^{2+}-channel antagonists, **dihydropyridines** include nifedipine, diphenylalkylamines include verapamil, and **benzothiazepines** include diltiazem. All are approved for treating hypertension. Nifedipine and the other dihydropyridines have less of an effect on the heart than verapamil and diltiazem. **Verapamil has the greatest effect on the heart and can significantly reduce contractility.** Because of its effect on the heart, verapamil can be used to treat supraventricular arrhythmias as well as variant angina. Depression of cardiac function is the greatest adverse effect of the Ca^{2+}-channel blockers, and this is markedly diminished with the dihydropyridines. Dihydropyridines can induce a reflex tachycardia in response to their blood pressure–lowering effect. However, clinical trials with short-acting nifedipine suggested that there was an increase in the risk of MI in patients treated for hypertension, and these agents should not be used to treat the disease.

Renin-Angiotensin System Inhibitors

Inhibitors of the renin-angiotensin system, both **ACE inhibitors and ARBs** are effective for hypertension monotherapy. ACE inhibitors block the conversion of the inactive angiotensin I to the potent angiotensin II. Angiotensin II acts to increase blood pressure in several ways. In vascular smooth muscle it increases intracellular Ca^{2+} and produces pronounced vasoconstriction. At peripheral nerve endings and in the adrenal medulla it increases the amount of catecholamines released on stimulation. In the zona glomerulosa of the adrenal cortex it acts to stimulate the biosynthesis of aldosterone, which increases renal Na^+ and water retention. Adverse effects include hypotension, dizziness, and fatigue; rarely, hyperkalemia may occur. A dry cough and angioedema may occur as a result of the reduction in degradation of bradykinin that is brought about by these drugs.

Aliskiren (Tekturna) reduces the activity of renin; this in turn causes a reduction in the production of angiotensin II. Clinical experience is lacking for aliskiren, but it appears about as effective as ACE inhibitors and has fewer side effects. During clinical trials, headache, dizziness, and some gastrointestinal events were the most common side effects, and angioedema was observed in a few patients.

Angiotensin II acts through AT-1 and AT-2 receptors, which in turn couple to numerous signal transduction pathways. The hypertensive actions of angiotensin II are mediated by AT-1 receptors. Losartan, valsartan, and other AT-1 receptor blockers are also effective in reducing blood pressure by 10–15 mm Hg. The adverse-effect profile is similar to the ACE inhibitors but without the cough or angioedema.

Direct Arterial Vasodilators

Arterial vasodilators act by increasing the efflux of potassium from the cell. This causes **hyperpolarization** across the plasma membrane that diminishes the activity of the voltage-regulated L-type calcium channel. In vascular smooth muscle cells this produces a reduction in vascular tone. **Minoxidil and hydralazine** are the two most commonly used oral vasodilators used to treat hypertension. Both have pronounced effects on the resistance vessels and little effect on veins. Because of their predominant effect on arterioles, these agents provoke the **baroreceptor reflex that includes tachycardia, vasoconstriction, and the release of renin.** For this reason, these agents are usually combined with a beta blocker and a diuretic.

Centrally Acting Agents

Centrally acting vasodilators such as clonidine and methyldopa act as **α_2-adrenergic receptor agonists in the vasomotor center within the medulla.** These agents decrease sympathetic outflow and thereby decrease vascular tone and cardiac output. The use of these agents as antihypertensives has been overshadowed by the introduction of ACE inhibitors and ARBs and Ca^{2+}-channel blockers. This is largely a result of the adverse effects, which are mostly in the CNS and include sedation, depression, and dry mouth. However, they are still used in cases of refractory hypertension.

Peripheral Sympathetic Inhibitors

Peripheral sympatholytic agents used for hypertension include guanethidine and reserpine. Guanethidine enters sympathetic nerve terminals by transport and replaces norepinephrine in transmitter vesicles. Release of norepinephrine is thereby diminished. Reserpine blocks the uptake and storage of biogenic amines, and this diminishes the amount of transmitter released on stimulation. Because of much higher rates of adverse effects, these agents are rarely used to treat simple hypertension but may be combined in the treatment of refractory hypertension.

COMPREHENSION QUESTIONS

[12.1] The inclusion of spironolactone with a thiazide diuretic in a regimen to treat hypertension is done to achieve which of the following?

A. Reduce hyperuricemia
B. Reduce Mg^+ loss
C. Decrease the loss of Na^+
D. Reduce K^+ loss

[12.2] Which of the following drugs would be the best to treat moderate hypertension in a diabetic patient with mild proteinuria?

A. Enalapril
B. Propranolol
C. Hydrochlorothiazide
D Nifedipine

[12.3] A 33-year-old man is diagnosed with essential hypertension. He is started on a blood pressure medication, and after 6 weeks, he notes fatigue, rash over his face, joint aches, and effusions. A serum antinuclear antibody (ANA) test is positive. Which of the following is the most likely agent?

A. Hydralazine
B. Propranolol
C. Thiazide diuretic
D. Nifedipine
E. Enalapril

Answers

[12.1]   **D.** Spironolactone is a "potassium-sparing" diuretic that reduces K^+ excretion in the collecting duct. It diminishes the K^+-wasting effects of thiazide diuretics.

[12.2]   **A.** ACE inhibitors, such as enalapril, have been shown to reduce the progressive loss of renal function that is often seen in diabetic patients. The nonselective beta blocker, propranolol, would worsen the diabetes.

[12.3]   **A.** Hydralazine is associated with a lupus-like presentation, with photosensitivity, malar rash, joint pain, and sometimes pericardial effusion or pleural effusion.

PHARMACOLOGY PEARLS

 The ALLHAT clinical trial (Antihypertensive and lipid-lowering treatment to prevent heart attack) compared amlodipine, a dihydropyridine Ca^{2+}-channel blocker, lisinopril, an ACE inhibitor, doxazosin, an α_1-adrenergic antagonist with chlorthalidone, a thiazide diuretic.

 Thiazide diuretics are the preferred initial therapy for hypertension in most cases.

 Beta-blocking agents can cause depression, insomnia, male impotency, bronchoconstriction, and decreased production of insulin.

REFERENCES

Kostis JB. The importance of managing hypertension and dyslipemia to decrease cardiovascular disease. Cardiovasc Drugs Ther Epub; 21(4):297–309:2007.

ALLHAT Officers and Coordinators for the ALLHAT Collaborative Research Group. Major outcomes in moderately hypercholesterolemic, hypertensive patients randomized to pravastatin vs usual care: the antihypertensive and lipid-lowering treatment to prevent heart attack trial (ALLHAT-LLT). The antihypertensive and lipid-lowering treatment to prevent heart attack trial. JAMA 2002;288(23):2998–3007.

A 60-year-old man with hypertension and type II diabetes comes in for a follow-up visit. Along with making appropriate diet and lifestyle changes, he is taking an ACE inhibitor-thiazide diuretic combination for his hypertension and metformin for his diabetes. His blood pressure and diabetes are under acceptable control. Routine blood work revealed normal electrolytes, renal function, and liver enzymes. He is noted to have elevated total cholesterol and low-density lipoprotein (LDL) levels, which have remained high in spite of his lifestyle changes. In an effort to reduce his risk of developing coronary artery disease, you start him on a 3-hydroxy-3-methylglutaryl-coenzyme A (HMG-CoA) reductase inhibitor.

◆ **What is the mechanism of action of HMG-CoA reductase inhibitors?**

◆ **What effect do they have on total and LDL cholesterol levels?**

◆ **What are the common adverse effects of HMG-CoA reductase inhibitors?**

ANSWERS TO CASE 13: LIPID-LOWERING AGENTS

Summary: A 60-year-old man has hypertension, diabetes, and hyperlipidemia and is started on an HMG-CoA reductase inhibitor.

◆ **Mechanism of action of HMG-CoA reductase inhibitors:** Competitive inhibition of the rate-limiting enzyme in cholesterol biosynthesis results in compensatory increase in plasma cholesterol uptake in the liver mediated by an increase in the number of LDL receptors.

◆ **Effect on total cholesterol:** Up to 30 percent reduction.

◆ **Effect on LDL cholesterol:** Up to 50 percent reduction.

◆ **Common adverse events:** Elevated liver enzymes and hepatotoxicity, myalgia and myositis, irritability, sleep disturbance, anxiety.

CLINICAL CORRELATION

HMG-CoA reductase inhibitors are in wide clinical use with proven benefit in lowering cholesterol levels and reducing the risk of coronary artery disease in susceptible individuals. **They competitively antagonize the rate-limiting enzyme in cholesterol biosynthesis.** Reduced cholesterol synthesis spurs a compensatory increase in hepatic uptake of plasma cholesterol mediated by an increase in the number of LDL receptors. The net effect of this is to lower the plasma levels of lipoproteins, especially LDL cholesterol. The effect on high-density lipoprotein (HDL) cholesterol is less pronounced. Although generally very well tolerated, **severe hepatotoxicity** has occurred, and monitoring of liver enzymes is mandatory while taking these medications. **Myalgia** is a common side effect, but rarely severe, myositis and rhabdomyolysis have occurred. **Hepatotoxicity and myositis** can occur while using an HMG-CoA reductase inhibitor alone, but they become more likely when combinations of medications are used.

APPROACH TO PHARMACOLOGY
OF LIPID-LOWERING DRUGS

Objectives

1. Know the drugs used to treat hyperlipoproteinemias.
2. Know the adverse effects and toxicities of the drugs.
3. Know the therapeutic uses of each of the lipid-lowering agents.

Definitions

Hyperlipidemia: An elevation in either plasma cholesterol or plasma triglycerides or both.

Myopathy: General term for any disease of muscle.

Myositis: Muscle pain with increased creatinine kinase levels.

Rhabdomyolysis: Muscle pain accompanied by a greater than tenfold increase in creatinine kinase above upper limits of normal, indicating serious muscle damage.

LDL cholesterol: Low-density lipoprotein. Atherogenic lipoprotein particle. Several subfractions have been identified, and the smallest are the most atherogenic. It contains apolipoproteins B_{100} (apo B_{100}; interacts with LDL receptor), Apo E (interacts with LDL receptor and Apo E receptor), and Apo C (activates lipoprotein lipase).

HDL cholesterol: High-density lipoprotein particle involved in transporting cholesterol from the periphery back to the liver. Has antiatherosclerotic activity. Contains Apo A, C, and D.

VLDL: Very-low-density lipoprotein, a triglyceride-rich lipoprotein particle synthesized in the liver.

DISCUSSSION

Class

Drugs that decrease plasma lipids are among the most commonly prescribed today. Some of these affect primarily cholesterol (e.g., the statins) and are useful in the treatment of hypercholesterolemia while other agents affect primarily triglycerides (e.g., gemfibrozil).

The National Cholesterol Education Program (NCEP) has classified levels of plasma cholesterol (Table 13-1). The LDL cholesterol treatment goal is determined by assessing the risk of cardiovascular disease of individual patients. The major risk factors that modify LDL goals are listed in Table 13-2.

Known CHD include patients who have had an infarction or angina or a surgical procedure for cardiovascular disease. In addition, patients with peripheral arterial disease, abdominal aortic aneurism, or symptomatic carotid artery disease or diabetes are considered to have known CHD or a high risk for CHD. The NCEP classification and the risk assessment are combined and used to modify the LDL cholesterol goals as illustrated in Table 13-3.

Table 13-1
NATIONAL CHOLESTEROL EDUCATION PROGRAM (NCEP) LEVELS OF PLASMA CHOLESTEROL

LDL CHOLESTEROL (mg/dL)	CATEGORIZATION
< 100	Optimal
100–129	Near/above optimal
130–139	Borderline high
160–189	High
> 190	Very high

TOTAL CHOLESTEROL (mg/dL)	
< 200	Desirable
200–239	Borderline high
> 240	High

HDL CHOLESTEROL (mg/dL)	
< 40	Low
> 60	High

Table 13-2
RISK FACTORS FOR CARDIOVASCULAR DISEASE

Clinical CVD
Cigarette Smoking
Hypertension (BP > 140/90 mm Hg) or on an antihypertensive drug
Low HDL cholesterol (< 40 mg/dL)
Family history of premature coronary heart disease
Age (men > 45 years, women > 55 years)
Poor nutrition

Table 13-3
CARDIOVASCULAR RISK AND LDL GOAL

RISK LEVEL	LDL GOAL (mg/dL)
Known CHD	< 100
≥ 2 risk factors	< 130
0–1 risk factors	< 160

Agents Used for Hypercholesterolemia

Statins

Of the drugs that decrease plasma cholesterol, the statins have gained the widest use. The **statins are structural analogs of the substrate HMG-CoA that inhibit the activity of the enzyme HMG-CoA reductase** at nanomolar concentrations. This enzyme is required for the synthesis of isoprenoids and cholesterol. By inhibiting de novo biosynthesis of cholesterol, cellular uptake of cholesterol from plasma via the LDL receptor is increased, reducing plasma cholesterol levels. Because **statins have additional actions to inhibit the production of the triglyceride-rich VLDL,** this makes them useful in the management of patients with hypertriglyceridemia; atorvastatin and rosuvastatin are particularly effective in this regard. There is evidence that statins also have anti-inflammatory activity, and this may contribute to their reduction in cardiovascular events. **Statins may also reduce the rate of bone resorption and thereby lessen osteoporosis.** This effect is thought to be caused by the inhibition of isoprenoid biosynthesis in osteoclast precursors, which inhibits their differentiation into mature osteoclasts. Six statins are approved in the United States: **lovastatin, rosuvastatin, fluvastatin, atorvastatin, pravastatin, and simvastatin.** They differ in efficacy: Rosuvastatin has been reported to reduce LDL cholesterol by more than 60 percent; atorvastatin, approximately 50 percent; and pravastatin and fluvastatin, approximately 35 percent. All of the statins are active orally. Lovastatin and simvastatin are prodrugs that are converted to their active metabolite by the liver.

The two major adverse effects associated with statin use are hepatotoxicity and myopathy. Hepatotoxicity was initially thought to be as high as 1 percent with elevations in hepatic transaminases as high as three times the upper limits. Subsequent clinical trials indicate that the actual incidence of hepatotoxicity is much lower. Hepatic transaminase levels should be monitored on initiation of therapy and at least yearly thereafter. The myopathy associated with statin use occurs in less than 0.1 percent of patients. However, severe rhabdomyolysis has occurred rarely, and one statin, cerivastatin, was removed from the market after several rhabdomyolysis-associated deaths.

Bile-Acid-Binding Resins

The bile acid sequestrants are also useful in reducing plasma cholesterol. **Cholestyramine,** colestipol, and colesevelam are ion-exchange resins that nonspecifically bind bile acids within the intestine and thereby reduce their enterohepatic circulation. This increases de novo hepatic bile acid synthesis and the cholesterol for this synthesis comes, in part, from the plasma via the LDL receptor. **Bile acid sequestrants typically reduce plasma cholesterol by 15–20 percent with no effect on triglycerides.** Because they are not absorbed, the bile acid sequestrants are quite safe, and adverse effects are typically gastrointestinal and include bloating and constipation. In the intestine, these agents bind many molecules other than bile acids and they **impair the absorption of lipid-soluble vitamins and many drugs including digoxin, furosemide, thiazides, coumarin, and some statins.** Patient adherence with these drugs is poor.

Inhibitors of Cholesterol Absorption

Ezetimibe is a **new class of cholesterol-lowering drug** that acts **within the intestine to reduce cholesterol absorption.** Cholesterol is absorbed from the small intestine by a process that includes specific transporters that have not been completely characterized. Ezetimibe **appears to block one or more of these cholesterol transporters, thereby reducing cholesterol absorption.** Ezetimibe used alone produces a reduction in plasma cholesterol of approximately 19 percent and an approximate 10 percent decline in triglyceride levels. When combined with a statin, reductions in plasma cholesterol as high as 72 percent have been reported in clinical trials. The complementary mechanisms—inhibition of cholesterol biosynthesis by statins and inhibition of cholesterol absorption by ezetimibe—may be useful in treating patients with refractory hypercholesterolemia. Few adverse effects have been reported with ezetimibe, but clinical experience is limited. The most frequently reported adverse effects are back and joint pain.

Nicotinic Acid

Niacin, at doses well beyond those used as a vitamin, has effects on all plasma lipids. It reduces LDL cholesterol by 20–30 percent and reduces **triglycerides** by 35–45 percent. It is the best agent available for **increasing HDL.** Niacin inhibits VLDL production in the liver by inhibiting both the synthesis and esterification of fatty acids. LDL levels are reduced as a consequence of the decline in VLDL synthesis. Niacin inhibits lipolysis in adipose tissue which reduces the supply of fatty acids to the liver, further decreasing VLDL synthesis. HDL levels are increased because niacin decreases the catabolism of Apo A_1. Niacin is useful in treating hypertriglyceridemia as well as hypercholesterolemia especially in the presence of low HDL. The limiting adverse effect of niacin is **cutaneous flushing and itching, and dyspepsia** is common at the doses (1 g/day) necessary to affect lipids. More medically serious adverse effects include hepatotoxicity and hyperglycemia. Niacin induces an **insulin-resistant state** causing **hyperglycemia**. For this reason niacin should not be used in diabetic patients.

Agents Used for Hypertriglyceridemia—Fibrates

The fibrates include clofibrate, fenofibrate, ciprofibrate, bezafibrate, and gemfibrozil. These agents predominantly cause a decline plasma **triglycerides** and a small decrease in LDL cholesterol. HDL levels are increased. The fibrates bind to a nuclear receptor peroxisomal proliferator-activator receptor γ (PPAR-γ) mostly in liver and skeletal muscle. Agonist-bound PPAR-γ induces lipoprotein lipase (LPL), which increases the lipolysis of triglyceride-rich VLDL and chylomicrons. Fibrates reduce triglycerides by 35–50 percent and LDL cholesterol by 10–20 percent. HDL levels are increased by 10–15 percent. All of the fibrates are orally active, but their absorption is decreased by food. The major adverse effect is gastrointestinal upset, cutaneous rash, and itching. Fibrates should not be used in patients with compromised renal function.

COMPREHENSION QUESTIONS

[13.1] Lovastatin reduces plasma cholesterol by which of the following processes?

    A. Inhibiting Apo B_{100} biosynthesis
    B. Inhibiting cholesterol absorption
    C. Inhibiting cholesterol biosynthesis
    D. Interfering with bile acid reabsorption

[13.2] Which of the following is a usual effect of niacin?

    A. Increases HDL
    B. Increases LDL
    C. Increases total cholesterol
    D. Increases triglycerides

[13.3] A 33-year-old man has been prescribed medication for hyperlipidemia. He has been noted to have bleeding from his gums and easy bruisability. His prothrombin time is elevated. Which of the following agents is most likely to be involved?

    A. Atorvastatin
    B. Cholestyramine
    C. Gemfibrozil
    D. Niacin

Answers

[13.1] **C.** The statins are competitive inhibitors of HMG-CoA reductase and thereby inhibit de novo cholesterol biosynthesis.

[13.2] **A.** Niacin increases HDL, decreases total and LDL cholesterol, and decreases triglycerides.

[13.3] **B.** Cholestyramine interferes with the absorption of lipid-soluble vitamins such as vitamin K, leading to decreased levels of vitamin K–dependent coagulation factors.

PHARMACOLOGY PEARLS

❖ The HMG-CoA reductase inhibitors, the statins, are the initial choice of drug for the treatment of hypercholesterolemia.

❖ The statins are structural analogs of the substrate HMG-CoA (3-hydroxy-3-methylglutaryl-coenzyme A) that inhibit the activity of the enzyme HMG-CoA reductase.

❖ The two major adverse effects associated with statin use are hepatotoxicity and myopathy.

❖ Bile acid sequestrants impair the absorption of lipid-soluble vitamins and many drugs including digoxin, furosemide, thiazides, coumarin, and some statins.

❖ The fibrates including clofibrate, fenofibrate, ciprofibrate, bezafibrate, and gemfibrozil predominantly cause a decline in plasma triglycerides.

❖ **Niacin** has effects on all plasma lipids and has side effects of flushing and itching.

REFERENCES

NCEP Report. Implications of recent clinical trials for the National Cholesterol Education Program Adult Treatment Panel III guidelines. Circulation 2004;110:227–39.

Wierzbicki AS, Mikhailidis DP, Wray R. Drug treatment of combined hyperlipidemia. Am J Cardiovasc Drugs 2001;1(5):327–36.

❖ CASE 14

A 19-year-old man is brought to the physician's office by his very concerned mother. He has been kicked out of the dormitory at college for his "bizarre" behavior. He has accused several fellow students and professors of spying on him for the CIA. He stopped attending his classes and spends all of his time watching TV because the announcers are sending him secret messages on how to save the world. He has stopped bathing and will only change his clothes once a week. In your office you find him to be disheveled, quiet, and unemotional. The only spontaneous statement he makes is when he asks why his mother brought him to the office of "another government spy." His physical examination and blood tests are normal. A drug screen is negative. You diagnose him with acute psychosis secondary to schizophrenia, admit him to the psychiatric unit of the hospital, and start him on haloperidol.

◆ **What is the mechanism of therapeutic action of haloperidol?**

◆ **What mediates the extrapyramidal side effects (EPSs) of the antipsychotic agents?**

◆ **Which autonomic nervous system receptors are antagonized by antipsychotic agents?**

ANSWERS TO CASE 14: ANTIPSYCHOTIC DRUGS

Summary: A 19-year-old man with acute psychosis from schizophrenia is pre-scribed haloperidol.

◆ **Mechanism of therapeutic action of haloperidol:** Antagonist activity at postjunctional dopamine D_2-receptors in the mesolimbic and mesocortical areas of the brain.

◆ **Mechanism of EPSs:** Antagonist activity at dopamine receptors in the basal ganglia and other dopamine receptor sites in the central nervous system (CNS).

◆ **Autonomic nervous system receptors blocked by antipsychotic agents:** α-Adrenoceptors and muscarinic cholinoreceptors.

CLINICAL CORRELATION

Schizophrenia is a chronic thought disorder that often presents in adolescence or early adulthood. It is characterized by the presence of "positive symptoms," which include delusions, hallucinations, and paranoia, and "negative symp-toms," which include blunt affect, withdrawal, and apathy. The therapeutic effects of the antipsychotic agents result from their antagonist actions on postjunctional dopamine D_2 receptors in the mesolimbic and mesocortical areas of the brain, although their benefits may also be related to their antago-nist activity at dopamine receptors in other areas of the CNS; additionally, atypical antipsychotic agents have efficacy at serotonin receptors. The dopamine receptor antagonist activity of antipsychotic agents at multiple sites in the CNS, and their antagonist activity at various other receptors in the CNS and throughout the body, contributes to the presence of numerous adverse effects. The presence of so many, and frequently severe, side effects makes patient compliance with long-term antipsychotic therapy an important clinical issue. However, newer, "atypical" agents are now available with greater speci-ficity for the receptors that mediate antipsychotic actions than for the receptors that mediate adverse effects.

APPROACH TO PHARMACOLOGY
OF ANTIPSYCHOTIC DRUGS

Objectives

1. List the classes and specific drugs that have antipsychotic activity.
2. Describe the mechanism of therapeutic action of antipsychotic agents.
3. Describe the common side effects of antipsychotic agents and indicate the receptors that mediate them.

Definitions

Acute dystonia: Sustained painful muscle spasms producing twisting abnormal posture usually occurring shortly after taking an antipsychotic medication.

Akathisia: Characterized by feelings of intense muscle restlessness or strong desire to move about, usually during the first 2 weeks of treatment with an antipsychotic medication.

Parkinson syndrome: Characterized by flat affect, shuffling gait, joint rigidity, and tremor that occurs weeks to months after treatment.

Neuroleptic malignant syndrome: Characterized by the acute onset of hyperthermia, muscle rigidity, tremor, tachycardia, mental status changes, diaphoresis, labile blood pressure, and exposure to a neuroleptic. This syndrome is associated with a significant mortality rate and usually occurs within the first few weeks of therapy.

DISCUSSION

Class

Antipsychotic drugs can be classified according to chemical structure as **phenothiazines, butyrophenones,** and an important group with diverse **atypical structures**. The phenothiazines are further subdivided according to side-chain constituents: **aliphatic, piperidine, and piperazine** (Table 14-1).

Although very similar in their therapeutic efficacy, the "low- (oral-) potency" aliphatic and piperidine phenothiazines have a somewhat different

Table 14-1
REPRESENTATIVE ANTIPSYCHOTIC DRUGS (SIDE CHAINS)

Phenothiazines
Chlorpromazine, triflupromazine (aliphatic)
Thioridazine, mesoridazine (piperidine)
Fluphenazine, trifluoperazine (piperazine)
Butyrophenone
Haloperidol
Atypical
Clozapine
Risperidone
Olanzapine
Quetiapine
Aripiprazole
Ziprasidone

adverse effect profile than the "high-potency" agents that include the piperazine phenothiazines, and also thiothixene, and haloperidol.

The newer, atypical agents have generally unique structures; some studies have suggested that they may have greater therapeutic efficacy with regard to the negative symptoms of schizophrenia. They also have been documented to have superior adverse effect profiles. Recent clinical trials have called into question the safety of several of the newer agents. In summary, individual patient response to antipsychotic agents varies widely and often dictates drug selection.

Administration of the low-potency antipsychotic agents is more likely to result in **autonomic adverse effects** that include **orthostatic hypotension** caused by **α-adrenoceptor blockade, and dry mouth, urinary retention, and tachycardia resulting from blockade of muscarinic cholinoreceptors.** Their blockade of **histamine H_1 receptors in the CNS** results in **sedation.** The still widely used high-potency agents, for example, **haloperidol,** are more likely to result in adverse neurologic effects. Among these are the EPSs, **acute dystonia, akathisia, and Parkinson syndrome,** which occur relatively early in therapy and are thought to be primarily mediated by blockade of **dopamine D_2 receptors** in the nigrostriatal dopamine pathway of the basal ganglia. A **late-occurring tardive dyskinesia** that is often irreversible and that may be a result of the slow development of dopamine receptor supersensitivity also in the basal ganglia is more or less likely to occur with all antipsychotic agents except clozapine. A **potentially fatal neuroleptic malignant syndrome is another serious adverse effect of antipsychotic agents in sensitive patients (1%).** Also, **hyperprolactinemia** in women may occur as a result of enhanced prolactin release from the posterior pituitary, because of antipsychotic drug blockade (phenothiazines, butyrophenones, risperidone) of dopamine D_2 receptors of the tuberoinfundibular dopaminergic pathway, which may lead to amenorrhea, galactorrhea, gynecomastia, decreased libido, and impotence. Weight gain is also a likely effect of many of these antipsychotic agents.

The **atypical agents** are **less likely** than the conventional agents to result in adverse **EPSs.** However, **weight gain** (clozapine, olanzapine, quetiapine), hypotension, and **sedation** are not uncommon events. **Seizures** (2–5%) and **agranulocytosis** (2% risk, 10% fatality) limit the use of **clozapine** to patients unresponsive to other agents.

Mechanism of Action

All clinically useful antipsychotic drugs block postjunctional dopamine **D_2 receptors,** although the degree of blockade among the drugs varies greatly in relation to their action on other neuroreceptors, particularly serotonin 5-hydroxytryptamine 2A (5-HT_{2A}) receptors and certain other dopamine receptor subtypes. Antipsychotic drugs appear to exert their therapeutic effect, at least in part, by **inhibition of dopamine's action in the mesocortical and mesolimbic dopaminergic pathways of the CNS.**

Administration

All antipsychotic agents can be administered by either the oral or parenteral route or both. Fluphenazine decanoate and haloperidol decanoate are available as parenteral depot preparations.

Pharmacokinetics

Most antipsychotic agents are readily but incompletely absorbed. They are highly lipid soluble and have longer clinical duration of action than would be expected from their plasma half-life, probably as a consequence of their deposition in fat tissue.

Thioridazine, which is metabolized to mesoridazine, is the exception to the rule that hepatic metabolism of the antipsychotic agents results in less active metabolites.

Concurrent use of certain antipsychotic agents with other drugs that also block cholinoreceptors may result in additive peripheral and CNS dysfunction.

COMPREHENSION QUESTIONS

[14.1] Haloperidol-induced Parkinson syndrome is a result of haloperidol's action in which of the following tracts?

A. Mesocortical tract
B. Mesolimbic tract
C. Nigrostriatal tract
D. Tuberoinfundibular tract

[14.2] The therapeutic effect of haloperidol is mediated, at least in part, by its blockade of which of the following receptors?

A. α-Adrenoceptors
B. Dopamine D_2 receptors
C. Histamine H_1 receptors
D. Muscarinic receptors

[14.3] Compared to the low-potency phenothiazine antipsychotic agents, haloperidol is more like to cause which of the following adverse effects?

A. Akathisia
B. Orthostatic hypotension
C. Sedation
D. Urinary retention

Answers

[14.1]   **C.** Haloperidol-induced Parkinson syndrome is a result of inhibition of dopamine D_2 receptors in the nigrostriatal tract of the CNS.

[14.2]   **B.** Antipsychotic drugs like haloperidol exert their therapeutic effect, at least in part, by inhibition of dopamine's action at dopamine D_2

receptors in the mesocortical and mesolimbic dopaminergic pathways of the CNS. A number of adverse effects of these drugs are caused by inhibition of dopamine action in the nigrostriatal and tuberoinfundibular dopaminergic pathways of the CNS; blockade of histamine, muscarinic, cholinergic, and α-adrenergic receptors in the CNS and the peripheral nervous system are also contributory.

[14.3]   **A.** Haloperidol is most likely to cause dystonia, akathisia, and Parkinson syndrome, whereas the low-potency phenothiazines are more likely to cause autonomic adverse effects that include orthostatic hypotension, sedation, and urinary retention.

PHARMACOLOGY PEARLS

 The low-potency antipsychotic agents are more likely to result in autonomic adverse effects that include orthostatic hypotension as a consequence of α-adrenoceptor blockade, dry mouth, urinary retention, and tachycardia resulting from blockade of muscarinic cholinoreceptors, and sedation (histamine H_1-receptor blockade).

 High-potency agents, for example, haloperidol, are more likely to result in EPSs, acute dystonia, akathisia, and Parkinson syndrome, mediated by blockade of dopamine D_2 receptors in the nigrostriatal pathway of the basal ganglia.

 A late-occurring tardive dyskinesia is often irreversible and is a serious effect of many antipsychotic agents.

 A potentially fatal neuroleptic malignant syndrome is another serious adverse effect of antipsychotic agents in sensitive patients.

 Hyperprolactinemia may occur as a result of enhanced prolactin release from the posterior pituitary, as a result of antipsychotic drug blockade of dopamine D_2 receptors in the tuberoinfundibular tract.

 Agranulocytosis may occur in patients treated with clozapine.

REFERENCES

Ananth J, Burgoyne KS, Gadasalli R, et al. How do atypical antipsychotics work? J Psychiatry Neurosci 2001;26(5):385–94.

Freedman R. Schizophrenia. N Engl J Med 2003;349(13):1738–49.

Lieberman JA, Stroup TS, McEvoy JP, et al. Effectiveness of antipsychotic drugs in patients with chronic schizophrenia. N Engl J Med 2005;353:1209–23.

Thacker GK, Carpenter WT. Advances in schizophrenia. Nature Med 2001;7(6): 667–71.

A 30-year-old woman presents to your office for the evaluation of fatigue. For the past 2 months she has felt run down. She says that she doesn't feel like participating in activities that she previously enjoyed, such as her weekly softball games. She has not been sleeping well and has not had much of an appetite. On questioning, she admits to feeling "down in the dumps" most of the time and has found herself crying frequently. She has never gone through anything like this before. She denies any thoughts of wanting to hurt herself or anyone else. Other than becoming tearful during her interview, her physical examination is normal. Her blood tests, including a complete blood count and thyroid function, are normal. A serum pregnancy test is negative. You diagnose her as having a major depression and, along with referring her for counseling, start her on fluoxetine.

◆ **What is the mechanism of action of fluoxetine?**

◆ **What are the common side effects of fluoxetine?**

ANSWERS TO CASE 15: ANTIDEPRESSANT AGENTS

Summary: A 30-year-old woman with major depression is prescribed fluoxetine.

◆ **Mechanism of action of fluoxetine:** Inhibition of the reuptake of serotonin (5-hydroxytryptamine, or 5-HT) at the prejunctional nerve terminal.

◆ **Common side effects:** Headache, nausea, agitation, insomnia, and sexual disturbances (loss of libido and erectile dysfunction).

CLINICAL CORRELATION

Selective serotonin reuptake inhibitors (SSRIs) are the most frequently pre-scribed antidepressant medications. **They act by inhibiting the reuptake of serotonin by the prejunctional nerve terminal, allowing more serotonin to interact with postjunctional neurons in the central nervous system (CNS).** This is thought to mediate their therapeutic effect. They have been highly effec-tive in the treatment of major depressive disorders and have an excellent safety profile. Unlike tricyclic antidepressants (TCAs), which have multiple severe and potentially fatal effects in an overdose, SSRIs have relatively few severe toxicities and a very low potential for fatality in an overdose. SSRIs do have several side effects of clinical significance. They often cause headache and gas-trointestinal (GI) side effects such as nausea. In some cases, agitation, anxiety, and insomnia can be exacerbated. Many of these SSRI side effects tend to be temporary and can often be improved with dose reduction. Another common side effect of SSRIs is **sexual disturbance.** Decreased libido and erectile dys-function occur frequently and do not generally spontaneously resolve while continuing SSRI therapy, often leading to reduced patient compliance.

APPROACH TO PHARMACOLOGY OF ANTIDEPRESSANT DRUGS

Objectives

1. List the classes of antidepressant agents.
2. Contrast the mechanisms of action of the antidepressant agents.
3. Contrast the adverse effects and toxicities of the antidepressant agents.
4. Describe the indications and contraindications to antidepressant drug use.

Definitions

Major depressive disorder: Unexplained, long-term difficulty coping with life events characterized by an inability to experience pleasure, abnormal sleep, decreased libido and appetite, feelings of guilt, and sui-cidal ideation.

DISCUSSION

Class

Drugs used to treat depression are classified as **TCAs, atypical heterocyclic (second- and third-generation) agents, SSRIs,** and **monoamine oxidase inhibitors (MAOIs).** Other conditions for which certain antidepressant agents are used include panic disorder, obsessive-compulsive disease (OCD), bipolar affective disorder, chronic pain, and enuresis.

SSRIs are the most extensively prescribed antidepressant agents because, unlike tricyclic and heterocyclic agents, they produce **less sedation, have fewer antimuscarinic cholinoreceptor effects,** and are **safer** in overdose. Nevertheless, they **may cause sexual disturbances, GI dysfunction, headache, and stimulation (insomnia, tremor, and anxiety).** TCAs may cause sedation, tremor, insomnia, blurred vision, constipation, urinary hesitancy, weight gain, and sexual disturbances. The MAOI phenelzine may cause weight gain, sexual disturbances, and sleep disturbances. The adverse effects of heterocyclic agents vary depending on the agent. **Bupropion is contraindicated in patients with seizure disorders (Table 15-1).**

Drug interactions of TCAs include additive sedative effects with other sedatives, particularly alcohol. **Phenelzine,** by increasing catecholamine stores, sensitizes patients to indirectly acting sympathomimetic agents, including **tyramine** that is contained in many **fermented foodstuffs (red wine or aged cheese),** and which together can result in a severe and sometimes **fatal hypertensive episode. MAOIs and SSRIs can interact to cause a potentially lethal "serotonin syndrome"** that includes **tremor, hyperthermia, muscle rigidity, and cardiovascular collapse.**

All antidepressant agents now carry a "black-box warning" of an increased risk of suicidality when used in children and adolescents.

Structure

TCAs have a three-ring nucleus similar to that of the antipsychotic phenothiazine agents. The MAOIs are subclassified as hydrazides (phenelzine) or nonhydrazides (tranylcypromine).

Mechanism of Action

The therapeutic activity of most of the available therapeutic antidepressant agents is due, at least in part, to their actions on norepinephrine and serotonin.

The TCAs block, to one degree or another, the prejunctional neuronal uptake transporters in the CNS that terminate norepinephrine and serotonin neurotransmission, thus allowing increased activity at their respective receptors. Amoxapine also blocks dopamine receptors.

Table 15-1
ANTIDEPRESSANT AGENTS

ANTIDEPRESSANT AGENTS	SELECTED ADVERSE EFFECTS
Tricyclic Agents Amitriptyline Amoxapine Clomipramine Desipramine Doxepin Imipramine Nortriptyline Protriptyline Trimipramine	Sedation, tremor, insomnia, blurred vision, constipation, urinary hesitancy, weight gain, and sexual disturbances
Atypical Agents Bupropion Duloxetine Maprotiline Mirtazapine Nefazodone Trazodone Venlafaxine	*Bupropion:* CNS stimulation, seizures at high doses (up to 0.4%) *Maprotiline:* Like TCAs *Mirtazapine:* Sedation, weight gain *Nefazodone:* Mild sedation, drug-drug interactions *Trazodone:* Sedation, dizziness, orthostatic hypotension, priapism *Venlafaxine:* Like SSRIs
Selective Serotonin Reuptake Inhibitors Citalopram Escitalopram Fluoxetine Fluvoxamine Paroxetine Sertraline	Sexual dysfunction, GI dysfunction, insomnia, tremor, anxiety
Monoamine Oxidase Inhibitors Phenelzine Tranylcypromine	Weight gain, sexual disturbances, sleep disturbances

The atypical agents have a variety of pharmacodynamic effects. Some act similar to the TCAs, whereas others act as inhibitors at certain subtypes of the serotonin receptor (trazodone, mirtazapine, nefazodone). Mirtazapine also blocks the prejunctional α_2-adrenoceptor to enhance serotonin and norepinephrine neurotransmission. Duloxetine inhibits norepinephrine and serotonin uptake.

As the name implies, SSRIs selectively block the prejunctional neuronal uptake transporters in the CNS that terminate serotonin neurotransmission thus allowing increased activity at serotonin receptors.

The MAOI hydrazide, phenelzine, and nonhydrazide, tranylcypromine, essentially irreversibly bind to and inhibit the activity of monoamine oxidase (A and B forms). New enzyme must be synthesized to restore activity. As a result of their actions, both drugs prevent prejunctional metabolism of norepinephrine and serotonin, thus allowing more to accumulate and to be released on nerve stimulation.

The neurochemical and biochemical actions described for the antidepressant agents occur soon after their administration. However, the therapeutic effect of these drugs may not be apparent for up to several weeks with continued administration. Thus, considerable attention has been devoted to discovering the long-term neurochemical and biochemical actions of the antidepressant agents that may correlate better with their clinical effectiveness. Decreased numbers of α-adrenoceptors and decreased cyclic adenosine monophosphate (cAMP) accumulation are two such long-term effects. With chronic administration, enhanced serotonin transmission is also implicated in the therapeutic action of antidepressant agents.

The antidepressant agents also produce a myriad of adverse effects that, depending on the agent, may be caused by blockade of histamine receptors, adrenoceptors, and cholinoreceptors in the peripheral and central nervous systems (see Discussion, Class, and Table 15-1).

Administration

Dosing, which may be by the oral or parenteral routes, is determined empirically in relation to the therapeutic response and the patient's tolerance of adverse effects.

Pharmacokinetics

Monodemethylation by the liver of the tertiary amines TCAs amitriptyline and imipramine results in, respectively, the active metabolites nortriptyline and desipramine. Venlafaxine has an active metabolite, *O*-desmethylvenlafaxine.

Metabolism of the SSRI fluoxetine results in an active metabolite, norfluoxetine, which has a long half-life. Fluoxetine and paroxetine inhibit a number of liver microsomal enzymes, particularly P450 2D6, that can cause clinically significant drug-drug interactions. Nefazodone inhibits cytochrome P450 3A4, which can result in increased levels of other drugs that are dependent on this metabolic pathway for their inactivation.

COMPREHENSION QUESTIONS

[15.1] Which of the following agents is contraindicated in a patient with epilepsy?

   A. Bupropion
   B. Fluoxetine
   C. Mirtazapine
   D. Venlafaxine

[15.2] The antidepressant action of imipramine is thought to be caused by which of the following?

   A. Blockade of prejunctional α_2-adrenoceptors
   B. Blockade of prejunctional neuronal norepinephrine and serotonin uptake transporters in the CNS
   C. Increased numbers of β-adrenoceptors
   D. Inhibition of monoamine oxidase

[15.3] Which of the following antidepressant agents inhibits hepatic microsomal enzymes to cause clinically significant drug-drug interactions?

   A. Fluoxetine
   B. Imipramine
   C. Phenelzine
   D. Trazodone

Answers

[15.1]   **A.** Bupropion causes seizures in a small but significant number of patients. This number is reduced with use of the slow-release form.

[15.2]   **B.** Imipramine and other TCAs block prejunctional neuronal norepinephrine and or serotonin uptake transporters in the CNS. Phenelzine and tranylcypromine inhibit monoamine oxidase. The heterocyclic agent mirtazapine blocks prejunctional α_2-adrenoceptors to enhance serotonin and norepinephrine neurotransmission.

[15.3]   **A.** The SSRI fluoxetine inhibits cytochrome P450 and therefore can significantly elevate the level of other drugs metabolized by these hepatic enzymes.

PHARMACOLOGY PEARLS

 SSRIs are the most commonly prescribed antidepressants because of their favorable side effect profile. Sexual disturbances and GI effects are common, however.

 TCAs may lead to toxicity as a result of cardiac arrhythmias.

 The antidepressant agents are roughly equivalent in their therapeutic action. However, individual patients may respond to, or tolerate, one better than another.

 Small beginning doses of many antidepressant agents are usually preferred because with time tolerance may occur to some of their adverse effects.

❖ Bupropion is contraindicated in patients with seizure disorders.

REFERENCES

Ables AZ, Baughman OL. Antidepressants: update on new agents and indications. Am Fam Physician 2003;67(3):547–54.

American Psychiatric Association. Practice guidelines for the treatment of patients with major depressive disorder (revision). Am J Psychiatry 2000;157(suppl 4):1–45.

Feighner JP. Mechanism of action of antidepressant medications. J Clin Psychiatr 1999;60(5):4–11.

Mann JJ. The medical management of depression. N Engl J Med 2005;353:1819–34.

A 29-year-old man is brought to the emergency center in a drunken stupor. He is accompanied by his wife, who states that he hasn't been himself at all for the past few months. According to his wife, he was evaluated for depression by his personal physician about 3 months ago and started on an SSRI. He responded quite well to this therapy over the subsequent 2 months. He started feeling so good and so energetic that he stopped taking his medication. He found that he needed less and less sleep, to the point where he is now only sleeping 2–3 hours a day. He has been showering his wife with very expensive gifts and has hit the maximum limit on all of their credit cards. He has been extremely romantic and more interested in sexual relations than at any time before. He has also started drinking heavily and has passed out drunk more than once. His work has suffered, and his boss said that he is in danger of being fired if things don't straighten out. Other than being drunk, his physical examination and blood tests are normal. He is admitted to the psychiatric unit with a diagnosis of bipolar disorder and started on lithium.

◆ **What is the mechanism of action of lithium?**

◆ **What are the common side effects of lithium?**

◆ **What is the mechanism of lithium-induced polyuria?**

ANSWERS TO CASE 16: LITHIUM

Summary: A 29-year-old man is diagnosed with bipolar disorder and is started on lithium.

◆ **Mechanism of action of lithium:** Not entirely known but may be related to inhibition of membrane phospholipid turnover with a reduction in key second messengers, important in the overactivity of catecholamines thought to be related to mood swings characteristic of bipolar disorder.

◆ **Common side effects of lithium:** Nausea, vomiting, diarrhea, tremor, edema, weight gain, polydipsia, and polyuria.

◆ **Mechanism of lithium-induced polyuria:** Renal collecting tubule becomes resistant to antidiuretic hormone.

CLINICAL CORRELATION

Lithium (Li^+) is an effective treatment for bipolar disorder. It is administered orally as lithium carbonate and eliminated almost entirely through the kidney. **Lithium has a narrow therapeutic window.** Even at therapeutic levels (0.5–1.4 mM/L), there are frequent side effects. These include **GI side effects, tremor, edema, polydipsia, and polyuria,** as well as diabetes insipidus and weight gain. It can cause a **benign thyroid enlargement** and even overt **hypothyroidism** (5%). It has been associated with congenital malformations when used during pregnancy. Frequent monitoring of blood levels is critical. There are potentially serious adverse effects at somewhat higher levels (above 2 mM/L). These include **confusion, dizziness, ataxia, and vomiting at even higher blood levels (above 2.5 mM/L)** progress to **seizures, circulatory collapse, and coma.** Lithium also has significant drug interactions that may increase its blood levels. Increased sodium clearance or depletion, such as caused by thiazide diuretics, some nonsteroidal anti-inflammatory drugs (NSAIDs; but not aspirin or acetaminophen), or severe vomiting and diarrhea, can lead to the increased renal reabsorption of lithium, thus causing toxicity.

APPROACH TO PHARMACOLOGY OF LITHIUM

Objectives

1. Describe the mechanism of action of lithium.
2. List other pharmacologic agents used to treat bipolar disease.

Definitions

Bipolar affective (manic-depressive) disorder: Bipolar disorder is characterized by paranoid thoughts, hyperactivity, and grandiosity, alternating in a cyclic fashion with symptoms of depression that often requires concomitant use of antidepressant agents.

DISCUSSION

Class

In addition to Li$^+$, the antiepileptic drugs valproic acid and carbamazepine, and the antipsychotic agent quetiapine are also first-line drugs that are effective for the treatment of the manic component of bipolar disease, often in patients unresponsive to lithium. These agents are referred to as mood stabilizers. Their adverse effect profiles when used to treat manic-depression are generally milder than for lithium (see Case 18).

Structure

Lithium is a small, monovalent cation that is similar in its properties to sodium and that enters cells through Na$^+$ channels.

Mechanism of Action

Lithium has a number of actions that may have some relationship to its therapeutic activity, including its effects on the synthesis and release of the neurotransmitters norepinephrine, serotonin, and dopamine. Lithium's most common and best-studied effect is on the membrane recycling of phosphoinositides. It inhibits the key inositol phosphatase enzyme, inositol monophosphatase, with depletion of free inositol that is necessary for the activity of the second messengers inositol trisphosphate (IP$_3$) and diacylglycerol (DAG), which mediate the cellular actions of G-protein-coupled muscarinic cholinoreceptors, α-adrenoceptors, and serotonin 5-HT$_2$ receptors.

Administration

Lithium, as lithium carbonate, carbamazepine, and valproic acid are administered orally.

Pharmacokinetics

Lithium has a relatively slow onset of therapeutic action (valproic acid's effects can be achieved in a few days).

More than 90 percent of Li$^+$ is excreted into the urine, but only 20 percent is cleared. Lithium is actively reabsorbed in the proximal tubule in competition with and at the same sites as Na$^+$. Sodium depletion as a result of a low-Na$^+$ diet, as well as diarrhea, concomitant use of diuretics, or even sweating, can lead to increased Li$^+$ retention and toxicity.

Because the renal clearance of lithium increases during pregnancy and then decreases following delivery, careful monitoring of lithium concentrations is necessary to avoid toxicity.

COMPREHENSION QUESTIONS

[16.1] The therapeutic action of Li$^+$ is thought to be caused by direct inhibition of which of the following?

A. Inositol monophosphatase
B. Inositol trisphosphate (IP$_3$)
C. Diacylglycerol (DAG)
D. Muscarinic cholinoreceptors

[16.2] The renal clearance of Li$^+$ may increase with which of the following?

A. Diarrhea
B. Diuretics
C. NSAIDs
D. Pregnancy

[16.3] Which of the following is the most likely adverse effect of Li$^+$ at therapeutic doses?

A. GI dysfunction
B. Hyperthyroidism
C. Oliguria
D. Thrombocytopenia

Answers

[16.1] **A.** The therapeutic action of Li$^+$ is thought to be caused by direct inhibition of inositol monophosphatase. Its effects on IP$_3$, DAG, and muscarinic cholinoceptor activities are an indirect consequence of this inhibition.

[16.2] **D.** The renal clearance of Li$^+$ may increase with pregnancy, which may lead to a reduction in its therapeutic effect. Diarrhea, certain NSAIDs, and diuretics that result in hyponatremia decrease the renal clearance of Li$^+$, which may result in more severe adverse effects.

[16.3] **A.** GI dysfunction, polydipsia (and polyuria), and hypothyroidism are adverse effects of Li$^+$ that may occur at therapeutic doses.

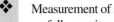

PHARMACOLOGY PEARLS

❖ Measurement of serum lithium concentrations are used routinely to carefully monitor treatment and to evaluate the likelihood of toxicity.

❖ Lithium is associated with thyroid enlargement; hypothyroidism; diabetes insipidus; diarrhea, nausea, and vomiting; and weight gain. It has been associated with congenital malformations when used in pregnancy.

❖ Lithium has a relatively slow onset of therapeutic action, and therefore antipsychotic drugs, such as olanzepine, or benzodiazepines are used acutely to calm seriously agitated patients with bipolar affective disorder.

❖ Antidepressant agents may precipitate mania and induce more rapid cycling in some patients.

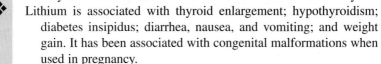

REFERENCES

Manji HK, Potter WZ, Lenox RH. Signal transduction pathways. Molecular targets for lithium's action. Arch Gen Psychiatry 1995;52(7):531–43.

Price LH, Heninger GR. Lithium in the treatment of mood disorders. N Engl J Med 1994;331(9):591–8.

Scherk H, Pajonk FG, Leucht S. Second-generation antipsychotic agents in the treatment of acute mania: a systematic review and meta-analysis of randomized controlled trials. Arch Gen Psychiatry 2007;64(4):442–55.

A 66-year-old man comes in to your office for evaluation of a tremor. He has noticed a progressively worsening tremor in his hands for the past 6 months. The tremor is worse when he is resting and improves a little when he reaches for an object or is using his hands. He has also noticed that it is harder to "get started" when he stands up to walk. He takes several small, "shuffling" steps before he can reach his full stride. He has no significant medical history and takes only an aspirin a day. On examination you note that his face is fairly expressionless, he has a pill-rolling-type tremor of his hands at rest and has cogwheel rigidity of his arms. You diagnose him with Parkinson disease and prescribe a combination of levodopa (L-dopa) and carbidopa.

◆ **What is the most common cause of the symptoms of idiopathic Parkinson disease?**

◆ **What is the mechanism of action of L-dopa?**

◆ **Why is L-dopa usually given in combination with carbidopa?**

ANSWERS TO CASE 17: DRUGS USED TO TREAT PARKINSON DISEASE

Summary: A 66-year-old man is diagnosed with idiopathic Parkinson disease and started on L-dopa and carbidopa therapy.

◆ **Cause of symptoms of idiopathic Parkinson disease:** Degeneration of dopamine-producing neurons in the substantia nigra.

◆ **Mechanism of action of L-dopa:** L-dopa is decarboxylated in prejunctional neurons in the central nervous system (CNS) to restore dopamine (DA) activity in the corpus striatum.

◆ **Reason L-dopa is given with carbidopa:** Carbidopa inhibits peripheral but not central dopa-decarboxylase metabolism of L-dopa. Thus, because a greater fraction enters the CNS, the therapeutic dose can be reduced and certain adverse effects minimized.

CLINICAL CORRELATION

Parkinson disease is a progressive, degenerative movement disorder. Symptoms of idiopathic Parkinson disease are caused by the degeneration of dopamine-producing neurons in the substantia nigra. This causes an imbalance in the actions of dopamine and acetylcholine, which, respectively, inhibit and excite the release of gamma (γ)-aminobutyric acid (GABA) from GABAergic neurons in the corpus striatum. These neurons affect motor activity via pathways leading to the thalamus and cerebral cortex and regulate dopamine output by a feedback loop. The overall physiologic effect is to reduce excitation of the motor neurons of the spinal cord. The clinical effect is the classic parkinsonian movement disorder. These symptoms include a resting tremor, bradykinesia, masked facies, loss of postural reflexes, and rigidity. Replacement of dopamine can help to restore the balance of activity of dopamine and acetylcholine. Dopamine, however, does not cross the blood-brain barrier into the CNS. L-dopa can pass into the CNS where, as its immediate precursor, it is decarboxylated in the CNS to dopamine, which can then interact with postjunctional dopamine D_2 receptors to inhibit GABAergic neuron activity in the striatum. L-dopa, however, is rapidly converted to dopamine in the periphery by the enzyme dopa-decarboxylase. If given by itself, high doses of L-dopa would be needed to provide a beneficial clinical effect in the CNS. **For that reason, L-dopa is given in combination with carbidopa,** which itself **does not cross the blood-brain barrier,** and which **inhibits peripheral, but not CNS, dopa-decarboxylase.** This allows therapeutic levels of L-dopa to enter the CNS at lower doses than would otherwise be necessary, and has the added benefit of reducing the incidence and severity of peripherally mediated adverse effects that would occur with L-dopa alone, such as nausea and vomiting and orthostatic hypotension.

Nevertheless, even with carbidopa, the L-dopa has many clinically important adverse effects. **Involuntary dyskinesias,** perhaps caused by developing dopamine receptor supersensitivity, are common (up to 90% of patients) and often limit the use of this therapy. The end of dose and on-off akinesias may require reducing the dosage intervals or the use of sustained-release preparations. **Behavioral effects are also common, including depression, insomnia, nightmares, and changes in mood. Nausea, vomiting, anorexia,** and **orthostatic hypotension** are not uncommon.

APPROACH TO PHARMACOLOGY OF DRUGS USED TO TREAT PARKINSON DISEASE

Objectives

1. List and explain the mechanisms of action, major adverse effects, and contraindications to the use of L-dopa and carbidopa combination (Sinemet) to treat Parkinson disease.
2. List other drugs or drug classes used to treat Parkinson disease, and describe their mechanism of action, benefits, and adverse effects.

Definitions

Tremor: Rhythmic oscillations of some body part, usually at a joint. In Parkinson disease tremor is present when there is minimal voluntary activity (tremor at rest).
Dyskinesia: Repetitive involuntary choreiform movements of the tongue, limbs, hands, and trunk.
Akinesia: Decreased voluntary movement.
On–off effect: Sudden onset of Parkinsonian symptoms with a usual therapeutic dose of L-dopa that may be the result of progression of the disease with loss of dopamine nerve terminals in the striatum.

DISCUSSION

Class

In addition to L-dopa just described, there are several other drugs or drug classes used to treat Parkinson disease, including the **dopamine agonists, bromocriptine, pergolide, pramipexole, and ropinirole; the selective MAOI, selegiline, the catechol-*O*-methyltransferase (COMT) inhibitors, entacapone and tolcapone; the antiviral drug, amantadine;** and several relatively selective centrally acting muscarinic cholinoreceptor-blocking agents, such as benztropine, biperiden, orphenadrine, procyclidine, and trihexyphenidyl (Table 17-1).

Table 17-1
SELECTIVE LIST OF PARKINSON AGENTS

DRUGS FOR PARKINSON DISEASE	ADVERSE EFFECTS
L-dopa	Dyskinesias, depression, insomnia, nightmares, changes in mood, nausea, vomiting, anorexia, orthostatic hypotension
Dopamine Agonists Bromocriptine Pergolide Pramipexole Ropinirole	Like L-dopa
Selegiline *Rasagiline*	Insomnia, serotonin syndrome (with meperidine, SSRIs, TCAs)
COMT Inhibitors Entacapone Tolcapone	GI disturbances, dyskinesias, sleep disturbances, orange discoloration of the urine, hepatotoxicity (tolcapone)
Amantadine	Restlessness, insomnia, hallucinations, depression, livedo reticularis
Muscarinic cholinoreceptor blockers Benztropine Biperiden Orphenadrine Procyclidine Trihexyphenidyl	Dry mouth, blurred vision, mydriasis, urinary retention, drowsiness, confusion, hallucinations

Dopamine agonists may be used alone or as an adjunct to L-dopa. Alone, there is a lower incidence of dyskinesia and response fluctuations. With L-dopa/carbidopa, dopamine agonists can be used to compensate for the diminishing effect of L-dopa that occurs after 3–5 years, presumably because of progressive destruction of the substantia nigra and loss of dopaminergic neurons. Adverse effects, which are less severe with pramipexole and ropinirole, include GI disturbances, postural hypotension, dyskinesias, and behavioral dysfunction. They are contraindicated in patients with psychosis. Pramipexole and ropinirole are preferred over the ergot deriviitives bromocriptine and pergolide due to their more limited adverse effect profile.

Selegiline, an **antiviral agent** which delays the metabolism of dopamine by monoamine oxidase B in the CNS, is used primarily as adjunctive therapy with L-dopa and carbidopa, generally in the later stages of Parkinson disease. Its adverse effects are minimal, insomnia the most notable. It should not be taken with TCAs, SSRIs, or the opioid meperidine because of potential development of a "serotonin syndrome" with CNS stimulation, hyperpyrexia, and coma.

Entacapone, a COMT inhibitor, is used as an adjunct to L-dopa and carbidopa to **reduce response fluctuations.** It is preferred over tolcapone which is associated with hepatotoxicity. Other adverse effects of this class of drugs include GI disturbances, enhanced dyskinesias that may require a reduction in the dose of L-dopa, sleep disturbances, and an orange discoloration of the urine.

Amantadine may be used early in the therapy of Parkinson disease to ameliorate its symptoms, possibly for only a few weeks before its effects wear off, or as an adjunct to L-dopa and carbidopa. **Adverse effects** include **restlessness, insomnia, hallucinations, depression** and, among many others, **livedo reticularis** (discoloration of the skin).

Muscarinic cholinoreceptor-blocking agents with some selectivity for CNS cholinoreceptors may be used alone to initially **diminish tremor and rigidity** (little effect on bradykinesia). Their adverse effects are those typically described for this class of agents and include dry mouth, blurring of vision, mydriasis, urinary retention, as well as certain behavioral effects including drowsiness, confusion, and hallucinations. **They are to be avoided in patients with angle-closure glaucoma and prostatic hypertrophy** and with other drugs that have muscarinic cholinoreceptor-blocking properties.

Structure

Bromocriptine and pergolide are ergot alkaloid derivatives with activity at both dopamine D_1 and D_2 receptors. Pramipexole and ropinirole are nonergots with greater selectivity for dopamine D_2 receptors.

Mechanism of Action

L-dopa is decarboxylated in the striatum to dopamine which interacts with postjunctional dopamine D_2 receptors to activate inhibitory G-proteins (Gi) and inhibit adenylyl cyclase activity in GABAergic neurons.

Selegiline is a selective monoamine oxidase B inhibitor that delays the metabolism and prolongs the activity of the dopamine.

Entacapone inhibits the peripheral activity of the enzyme COMT to decrease the metabolism of L-dopa and thus increase its bioavailability and transport to the brain and prolong its duration of action. Tolcapone also inhibits COMT in the CNS, which reduces the metabolism of dopamine and prolongs its duration of action. Amantadine's mechanism of action is unsure, but may be related to a change in the metabolism of dopamine that potentiates its action.

Muscarinic cholinoreceptor-blocking agents inhibit the activity of acetylcholine in the striatum thus restoring to some degree the balance of stimulatory activity with the already reduced inhibitory levels of dopamine in patients with Parkinson disease.

Administration

All antiparkinsonian drugs are administered by the oral route.

Pharmacokinetics

The absorption of L-dopa is rapid but is delayed by food and also by certain amino acids that compete for its transport in the GI tract and transport from blood to the brain. The concomitant administration of carbidopa can decrease the peripheral metabolism of L-dopa by up to 80 percent.

COMPREHENSION QUESTIONS

[17.1] Carbidopa reduces which of the following?

A. The activity of dopa-decarboxylase in the CNS
B. The L-dopa dose necessary to achieve a therapeutic effect
C. The severity of L-dopa-associated dyskinesias
D. The time to onset of L-dopa's therapeutic effects

[17.2] Which of the following is the most common limiting adverse effect of L-dopa?

A. Depression
B. Dyskinesia
C. Nausea
D. Orthostatic hypotension

[17.3] Entacapone inhibits which of the following?

A. Dopamine D_2 receptors
B. COMT
C. Monoamine oxidase B
D. Muscarinic cholinoreceptors

Answers

[17.1] **B.** Carbidopa, which does not penetrate the brain, reduces peripheral dopa-decarboxylase activity, and the metabolism of L-dopa. The therapeutic effect of L-dopa can be achieved at a lower dose than would be possible without carbidopa.

[17.2] **B.** The most common limiting adverse effect of L-dopa is dyskinesia that may occur in up to 90 percent of patients. Orthostatic hypotension, depression, and nausea are also adverse effects, but can be more readily managed and tolerated by patients.

[17.3] **B.** Entacapone (and tolcapone) inhibits COMT. Selegiline inhibits monoamine oxidase B. Muscarinic cholinoreceptors are inhibited by biperiden and benztropine among others. Blockade of dopamine D_2 receptors would exacerbate the symptoms of Parkinson disease.

PHARMACOLOGY PEARLS

❖ L-dopa may exacerbate symptoms in psychotic patients.

❖ In the absence of carbidopa, pharmacologic doses of pyridoxine (vitamin B_6) will increase the peripheral metabolism of L-dopa and thereby reduce its therapeutic effect.

❖ Signed patient consent is required for use of tolcapone, as is continuous evaluation of liver function.

REFERENCES

Koller WC, Tolosa E, eds. Current and emerging drug therapies in the management of Parkinson's disease. Neurology 1998;50(suppl 6):51.

Frucht SJ. Parkinson disease: an update. Neurologist 2004;10(4):185–94.

Nutt JG, Wooten GF. Diagnosis and initial management of Parkinson's disease. N Engl J Med 2005;353:1021–7.

An 18-year-old man is brought to the emergency department by paramedics after a series of grand mal seizures. He required repeated doses of IV lorazepam to finally control the episode. A family member with him states that he has had epilepsy since childhood. He is supposed to take phenytoin, but often forgets or refuses. His last seizure was about 3 months ago. In the emergency room he is confused and combative but has an otherwise normal neurologic examination. Blood tests show an undetectable phenytoin level. You give him an IV loading dose of fosphenytoin and restart him on his oral phenytoin.

◆ **What is the mechanism of action of phenytoin?**

◆ **How is phenytoin metabolized?**

ANSWERS TO CASE 18: ANTISEIZURE DRUGS

Summary: An 18-year-old man presents with grand mal seizures and is given phenytoin.

◆ **Mechanism of action of phenytoin:** Blocks sodium channels and inhibits the generation of action potentials.

◆ **Metabolism of phenytoin:** Parahydroxylation and glucuronide conjugation by hepatic microsomal enzymes.

CLINICAL CORRELATION

Phenytoin is one of the most widely used drugs for the treatment of tonic-clonic (grand mal) seizures. It is also a major first-line drug used to treat partial seizures. It works by binding to and prolonging the inactive state of the Na^+ channel thus blocking use-dependent Na^+ conductance and the generation of action potentials. It can be given orally, and its long half-life allows for once-a-day dosing. Phenytoin is metabolized in the liver by microsomal enzymes through parahydroxylation and glucuronide conjugation. Rates of oral absorption and metabolism can vary significantly from one patient to the next. At very low doses elimination is first-order; however, even within the therapeutic range, the liver enzymes responsible for its metabolism is near saturation, resulting in an increase in its half-life. Because of this inability to reach steady state and **phenytoin's low therapeutic index,** dosing of this drug must be individualized and plasma levels closely monitored. **Common side effects include nystagmus, ataxia, confusion, hirsutism, and gingival hyperplasia in children (up to 50%). Idiosyncratic reactions include skin rashes.** Its use should be avoided, if possible, during **pregnancy because it is teratogenic. Phenytoin induces hepatic metabolism by microsomal enzyme induction** and can lower plasma levels of other drugs. Phenytoin's level can be increased by drugs that inhibit its hepatic metabolism. Caution and close monitoring of blood levels of phenytoin must be undertaken when phenytoin is used in combination with other drugs.

APPROACH TO PHARMACOLOGY
OF ANTISEIZURE AGENTS

Objectives

1. List the major antiseizure agents.
2. Describe the mechanism of action of major antiseizure agents.
3. List and discuss the common adverse effects and toxicities of major antiseizure agents.
4. List the therapeutic uses of major antiseizure agents.

Definitions

Seizure: A nonrecurrent abnormal discharge from the brain.

Epilepsy: A chronic dysfunction of recurrent seizures.

Therapeutic index: A measure of the relationship (ratio) between the dose necessary to produce a therapeutic effect, usually expressed as the median effective dose (ED_{50}), and the dose necessary to produce an undesired effect, usually expressed as the median toxic dose (TD_{50}).

First-pass effect: The extensive metabolism of many drugs administered orally that in some instances may limit bioavailability to such an extent that an effective therapeutic dose cannot be achieved.

DISCUSSION

Class

There is some degree of drug specificity relative to seizure type (Table 18-1). In addition to phenytoin, **carbamazepine** is another major first-line antiseizure drug used to treat both partial seizures and generalized tonic-clonic seizures. A number of other available drugs for treating partial and generalized tonic-clonic seizures (e.g., gabapentin, lamotrigine, tiagabine) are also used as second-line or add-on therapeutic agents. First-line drugs available to specifically treat **generalized absence seizures** include **ethosuximide and valproic acid.** These may also be used as second-line or add-on therapeutic agents to treat other seizure types. The **benzodiazepines, diazepam and lorazepam,** also have

Table 18-1
SELECTED ANTISEIZURE AGENTS

Generalized Tonic-Clonic Seizures Phenytoin Carbamazepine
Partial Seizures Phenytoin Carbamazepine
Absence Seizures Ethosuximide Valproic acid
Status Epilepticus Diazepam Lorazepam Phenytoin/Fosphenytoin

important first-line use, along with phenytoin or fosphenytoin, for treating generalized tonic-clonic status epilepticus.

Carbamazepine, a first-line drug for treating partial seizures and generalized tonic-clonic seizures, is also used therapeutically to treat bipolar disorder and trigeminal neuralgia. **Drowsiness, diplopia, and ataxia are common side effects.** GI disturbances, headache, dizziness, and sedation are also not uncommon effects (Table 18-2). **Idiosyncratic reactions include serious skin rash** and rarely a **fatal aplastic anemia.** Carbamazepine may exacerbate or precipitate absence seizures.

Ethosuximide, a first-line drug to treat generalized absence seizures, has generally mild adverse effects related primarily to GI disturbances.

Valproic acid, like ethosuximide, is a first-line drug used to treat generalized **absence** seizures. However, because of the potential for an **idiosyncratic hepatotoxicity,** it is reserved for patients with concomitant generalized tonic-clonic seizures. It is also used to control myoclonic seizures and for the treatment of bipolar disorder and for prophylaxis of migraine headache. Its use in pregnancy is associated with an increased risk of **neural tube defects.**

As for **phenytoin,** the **therapeutic index for these drugs is low.** Thus, serum drug levels need to be carefully monitored.

Mechanism of Action

Carbamazepine acts like phenytoin (see Clinical Correlation—Case 18).

Ethosuximide reduces low threshold T-type Ca^{2+} current in the thalamus that appears to provide pacemaker activity responsible for cortical generation of absence seizures.

Valproic acid may have more than one mechanism of action including an effect on Na^+ channels like phenytoin and carbamazepine, blockade of NMDA receptors, and increased activity of the neurotransmitter (γ)-aminobutyric acid (GABA). The benzodiazepines, diazepam and lorazepam, potentiate GABA neurotransmission.

Table 18-2
SELECTED ANTISEIZURE AGENTS AND ADVERSE EFFECTS

AGENT	SELECTED ADVERSE EFFECTS
Phenytoin	Nystagmus, ataxia, confusion, hirsutism, gingival hyperplasia in children (up to 50%), idiosyncratic reactions (e.g., skin rashes), teratogenicity
Carbamazepine	Drowsiness, diplopia, ataxia, GI disturbances, headache, dizziness, sedation, idiosyncratic reactions (skin rash, aplastic anemia)
Ethosuximide	GI disturbances
Valproic acid	Idiosyncratic hepatotoxicity

Administration

Phenytoin and valproic acid are available for both oral and parenteral (IV) administration. Because phenytoin may precipitate at its site of injection, it has been replaced for intravenous injection by the more water-soluble fosphenytoin which is only available for parenteral administration.

Carbamazepine and ethosuximide are only available for oral administration. Both phenytoin and carbamazepine exist also in extended-release preparations. Valproic acid is hydroscopic and therefore is available for oral administration as a capsule in corn oil or, for pediatric use, in syrup. It is also available as a more patient preferred enteric-coated tablet formulated as divalproex sodium, which is a 1:1 compound of valproic acid and sodium valproic acid. It is also available for parenteral use.

Pharmacokinetics

Because phenytoin's liver metabolic enzymes become saturated at a low dose, relatively small changes in the dose can lead to very large changes in the plasma concentration and, with it, the development of toxicity.

With continuous administration, carbamazepine induces the synthesis of liver microsomal enzymes responsible for its own metabolism resulting in a substantially decreased half-life requiring significant dose adjustment. Through the same induction mechanism, carbamazepine can also alter the metabolism of a number of other drugs. Likewise, there are a number of drugs that can alter the metabolism of carbamazepine by induction of the appropriate microsomal enzymes. Oxcarbamazepine is a closely related anticonvulsant that is less likely to induce microsomal enzyme synthesis.

Valproic acid inhibits its own metabolism and the metabolism of other drugs, including phenytoin. It displaces phenytoin from its binding to plasma proteins.

COMPREHENSION QUESTIONS

[18.1] Blockade of T-type calcium currents is the major mechanism of action for which of the following drugs used to manage seizures?

    A. Carbamazepine
    B. Diazepam
    C. Ethosuximide
    D. Phenytoin

[18.2] Which of the following drugs used to manage seizures requires a significant dose adjustment with continuous administration?

    A. Carbamazepine
    B. Diazepam
    C. Ethosuximide
    D. Phenytoin

[18.3] For which of the following drugs used to manage epilepsy does a small change in its bioavailability result in a disproportionate increase in its blood levels and toxicity?

A. Carbamazepine
B. Diazepam
C. Ethosuximide
D. Phenytoin

Answers

[18.1] **C.** The anticonvulsant activity of ethosuximide when used to treat absence seizures is due to its blockade of T-type calcium currents in the thalamus. Carbamazepine and phenytoin, which are not used to treat absence seizures, block sodium channels. Diazepam, which is not a first-line drug for absence seizures, potentiates GABA neurotransmission.

[18.2] **A.** Carbamazepine induces the synthesis of liver microsomal enzymes responsible for its own metabolism, necessitating a significant dose adjustment with its continued administration.

[18.3] **D.** A small change in the bioavailability of phenytoin may result in a disproportionate increase in its blood level because its metabolic enzymes become saturated even at therapeutic doses.

PHARMACOLOGY PEARLS

 Currently available antiseizure drugs control seizures in about 80 percent of patients with epilepsy.

 Antiseizure drugs increase the risk of congenital malformations, including the "fetal hydantoin syndrome" (phenytoin) and spina bifida (valproic acid).

 The main side effects of phenytoin are nystagmus, ataxia, confusion, hirsutism, and gingival hyperplasia.

 Phenytoin is metabolized by hepatic microsomal enzymes.

REFERENCES

French JA. Efficacy and tolerability of the new antiseizure drugs I: treatment of new onset epilepsy. Neurology 2004;62(8):1252–60.

Levy RH, Mattson R, Meldrum B, et al. Antiseizure Drugs. Philadelphia, PA: Lippincott Williams & Wilkins, 2002.

Lowenstein DH. Seizures and epilepsy. In: Harrison's Principles of Internal Medicine, 15th ed. New York: McGraw Hill, 2000.

An 18-year-old man is brought into the emergency department after being found on the street unresponsive. He is lethargic and does not answer questions. He has been given 1 ampule of Dextrose intravenously without result. On examination, his heart rate is 60 beats per minute, and respiratory rate is 8 per minute and shallow. His pupils are pinpoint and not reactive. There are multiple intravenous track marks on his arms bilaterally. The emergency physician concludes that the patient has had a drug overdose.

◆ **What is the most likely diagnosis?**

◆ **What is the most appropriate medication for this condition?**

◆ **In addition to its therapeutic actions, what other effects might this medication produce?**

ANSWERS TO CASE 19: OPIOID OVERDOSE

Summary: An 18-year-old unresponsive man presents with pinpoint pupils, shallow respirations, and multiple intravenous track marks on his arms bilaterally.

◆ **Most likely diagnosis:** Opioid overdose, likely heroin.

◆ **Most appropriate medication for this condition:** Naloxone.

◆ **Additional effects this medication might produce:** Symptoms of precipitated withdrawal that may include lacrimation, rhinorrhea, sweating, dilated pupils, diarrhea, abdominal cramping, and tremor.

CLINICAL CORRELATION

Opioids are drugs with morphine-like activity that reduce pain and induce **tolerance** and **physical dependence.** Certain individuals seek the euphoria obtained from the intravenous injection of opioids such as heroin. There are three different cell **receptors** specific for opioids: **mu, kappa, and delta** (μ, κ, δ), all of which exist as multiple subtypes. This patient has the classic signs of **opioid overdose: somnolence, respiratory depression, and miosis.** Stimulation of the mu receptor results in analgesia (supraspinal and spinal), respiratory depression, euphoria, and physical dependence. Continuous, heavy use of opioids can result in tolerance, where more drug is required to obtain the same euphoric "high," and also to physical dependence. Naloxone, a competitive antagonist of opioids, is used to treat opioid overdose. Its intravenous administration leads to an almost immediate reversal of all effects of the opioids.

In individuals who are physically dependent, administration of naloxone will immediately precipitate **opioid withdrawal,** which consists of a constellation of signs and symptoms that include nausea and vomiting, muscle aches, lacrimation or rhinorrhea, diarrhea, fever, and dilated pupils. Likewise, when someone physically dependent on opioids ceases its administration there is a more slowly developing (hours or days) constellation of symptoms of opioid withdrawal that includes **sensitivity to touch and light, goose flesh, autonomic hyperactivity, GI distress, joint and muscle aches, yawning, salivation, lacrimation, urination, defecation, and a depressed or anxious mood.** In general, physical dependence induced by opioids with a short half-life tend to result in a rapid severe withdrawal, while physical dependence induced by opioids with a long half-life tends to be associated with a less severe and more gradual course of withdrawal. Although very uncomfortable, opioid withdrawal is **generally not life-threatening.**

The opioid methadone may be administered in a daily dose to individuals physically dependent on opioids, most notably heroin, as a "maintenance therapy" or to ameliorate the symptoms of opioid withdrawal.

APPROACH TO PHARMACOLOGY OF THE OPIOIDS

Objectives

1. Describe the mechanism of action of opioids as analgesics.
2. Explain how opioids reduce pain.
3. List the major opioid agonists and antagonists, their therapeutic uses, and their important pharmacokinetic properties.
4. Describe the adverse effects of opioids.

Definitions

Endogenous opioid peptides: Class of natural endogenous peptides that bind to human mu, delta, and kappa opioid receptors. Four classes of such peptides have been described: (1) the pentapeptide enkephalins (met and leu), (2) the endorphins (β-endorphin), (3) the dynorphins (A, B, C), all of which are proteolytically released from larger precursor molecules, and (4) the endomorphins. Together, they may modulate a number of important functions of the body (e.g., pain, reactions to stress and anxiety).

Fasciculation: Muscular twitching of contiguous groups of muscle fibers

Lacrimation: Secretion of tears from the eyes

Rhinorrhea: Mucous-like material that comes out of the nose

DISCUSSION

Class

Morphine, the prototype opioid, is derived from opium, a crude material obtained from the seed pod of the opium poppy plant. The chemical structure of morphine is shown in Figure 19-1. Many other derivatives of the opium plant (opiates) and other drugs with similar effects (opioids) have been discovered or synthesized. Chemical modifications of the morphine structure results in significant alterations in potency and in the ratio of agonist to antagonist effects (Table 19-1). However, no major improvement in the analgesic effect of this class of opioids has been achieved; morphine is still one of the most widely used opioids. The opioids are classified in several ways: (1) **strength** of **analgesic** effect (strong and weak agents); (2) ratio of **agonist to antagonist effects** (pure agonists, mixed agonist-antagonists, and partial agonists that act both as an opioid agonist and antagonist, and antagonists), and (3) **actions** (analgesic, antitussive, and antidiarrheal drugs).

The major therapeutic application for morphine and other **strong opioids** (e.g., **fentanyl, hydromorphone, methadone**) is the management of moderate to severe pain (e.g., pain associated with trauma, burns, cancer, acute

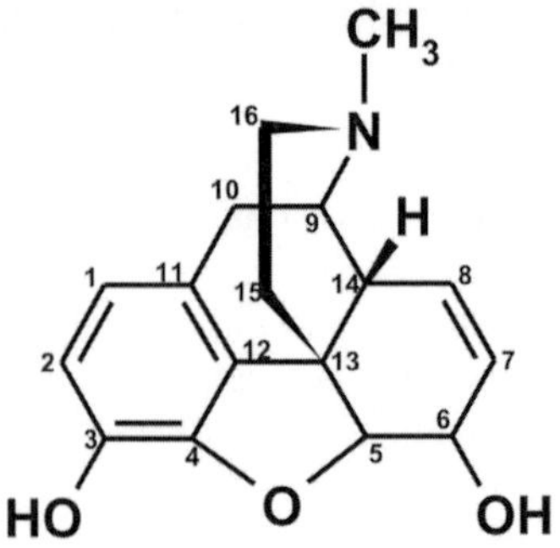

| | Ring Position | | | |
	3[a]	6[b]	17[c]	Substitution
Morphine	$-OH$	$-OH$	$-CH_3$	Prototype
Codeine[d]	$-OCH_3$	$-OH$	$-CH_3$	Methylmorphine
Heroin[e]	$-OCOCH_3$	$-OCOCH_3$	$-CH_3$	Diacetyl morphine
Naloxone[f]	$-OH$	$=O$	$-CH_2CH=CH_2$	Allyl
Thebaine[g]	$-OCH_3$	$-OCH_3$	$-CH_3$	Dimethyl morphine

[a]Substitutions at the C-3 phenolic position and the C-6 hydroxyl position of morphine.
[b]Modification of the methyl group on the nitrogen in the piperidine ring (N-17).
[c]Methyl substitution: decreased first pass effect, increased oral absorption in the brain to morphine.
[d]Allyl substitution: antagonist.
[e]Dimethyl substitution: convulsant.

Figure 19-1. Structure-activity relationships of opioids.

myocardial infarction, and renal or biliary colic). **Weaker opioids** such as **codeine** and **pentazocine** are used to manage mild to moderate pain. Other important therapeutic uses include the management of **diarrhea** (e.g., **codeine, diphenoxylate, loperamide**), dyspnea associated with pulmonary edema secondary to acute left ventricular failure, suppression of the cough reflex (codeine, **dextromethorphan**), and maintenance and withdrawal therapy for opioid dependence (**methadone, buprenorphine**). The antitussive (cough suppressant) action and antidiarrheal action of the opioids are at least partially separable from their analgesic action. Separate drugs have been developed to exploit these effects.

The sites of opioid action include areas in the central nervous system (CNS) where they **raise the threshold to pain** (i.e., decrease the sensation of pain) including (1) the *spinal cord,* where opioids act directly on **receptors** on the **terminals of primary afferent sensory neurons** in the **dorsal horn of the spinal cord** to inhibit release of excitatory transmitters like

Table 19-1
SELECTED OPIOIDS

STRONG OPIOID AGONISTS	NOTES
Morphine (also hydromorphone, oxymorphone, heroin)	See case description Heroin is metabolized to morphine
Methadone	Indications are similar to morphine. Used to treat difficult to manage pain (e.g., cancer, neuropathic pain). Used as an oral opioid substitute to treat opioid dependence. Its long duration of action and slow metabolism result in less severe withdrawal than with other shorter acting opioids.
Fentanyl (also alfentanil, sufentanil, remifentanil)	Has a shorter duration of action than morphine. Available for parenteral use only. Used as a pre-anesthetic medication and for pre- and postoperative pain. Fentanyl (or morphine) is used to supplement the analgesia and sedative-hypnotic effects of nitrous oxide and halothane equals "balanced anesthesia." Rapid IV administration of high doses may cause severe truncal muscle rigidity that can be reversed by naloxone. Available as a transdermal patch and lozenge.
Meperidine	Although still used, in overdose methadone may cause CNS excitation (tremors, delirium, and hyperreflexia) and seizures as a result of formation of an *N*-demethylated metabolite, normeperidine. With MAO inhibitors may cause severe restlessness, excitement, fever, and seizures (serotonin syndrome). It has weak anticholinergic activity that may result in mydriasis (not miosis) and tachycardia. Meperidine has weak or no effect on the cough reflex.
Codeine (also oxycodone, hydrocodone, dihydrocodeine)	Used for moderate pain. Has good bioavailability by the oral route (compared to morphine); 10% converted to morphine. Causes little respiratory depression and less dependence liability than morphine. An overdose may cause seizures. Codeine and other weak opioid agonists are often used in combination with other analgesics such as aspirin (Percodan) or acetaminophen (Percocet).

(continued)

Table 19-1
SELECTED OPIOIDS *(continued)*

WEAK OPIOID AGONISTS	NOTES
Diphenoxylate, Loperamide	Used for the symptomatic treatment of diarrhea. Insolubility of diphenoxylate limits its absorption across the GI tract. Loperamide does not cross the blood-brain barrier. Minimal dependence liability or other centrally mediated opioid effects. To limit its parenteral use, diphenoxylate is only available combined with atropine.
MIXED OPIOID AGONIST-ANTAGONISTS/PARTIAL AGONISTS	
Buprenorphine (also pentazocine, nalbuphine, butorphanol, dezocine, tramadol)	Buprenorphine is a slowly dissociating partial agonist at the μ-opioid receptor. Its agonist actions are resistant to naloxone reversal. It is used primarily for heroin detoxification. It has less dependence liability than morphine. At higher doses it has antagonist activity at the μ-opioid receptor which limits its ability to cause respiratory depression.
OPIOID ANTAGONISTS	
Naloxone and Naltrexone (also nalmefene)	Competitive antagonists at opioid receptors which can precipitate opioid withdrawal. Naloxone is administered IV because of poor oral absorption. It is used to treat acute opioid overdose. Because of its short duration of action, multiple dosing may be necessary. Naltrexone is FDA approved for use in chronic alcoholics to reduce craving for alcohol.
ANTITUSSIVE AGENTS	NOTES
Dextromethorphan	Dextromethorphan, a nonopioid drug, is nearly as effective as codeine as an antitussive agent, but with less constipating effect. It has no or limited analgesic activity or dependence liability. It may cause some dizziness, nausea, or drowsiness. Opioids other than codeine are not commonly used because of their dependence liability.

substance P, (2) the *thalamus,* where opioids act on **ascending pathways** to **directly inhibit pain transmission from the spinal cord to higher centers of the brain** (via the spinothalamic tract and spinoreticular tract), and (3) the *midbrain* periaqueductal gray area and rostral ventral medulla (nucleus raphe magnus) where opioids **activate descending *inhibitory* neurons to the spinal cord,** thus preventing pain transmission. Opioids also act on the cerebral cortex, amygdala, and hippocampus to decrease the emotional reactivity to pain (i.e., decrease the perception of pain). There is also a direct inhibitory effect of opioids on sensory nerve endings. In addition to the CNS, opioids also act on other organs including, notably, the GI tract and kidney.

The most commonly observed effects when the opioids are used for the relief of pain are **sedation, nausea and vomiting, and constipation.** Large doses regularly induce **respiratory depression and euphoria** or mental clouding. The major adverse effects of selected opioids are presented in Table 19-2.

Tolerance to some effects of the opioids (Table 19-3) occurs gradually (days) with repeated administration such that a larger dose is necessary to produce the same initial effect. The tolerance is because of a direct action of opioids on neurons (i.e., cellular tolerance) rather than to an increase in their metabolism (metabolic tolerance). Tolerance does not occur to all the effects of the opioid agonists or to the action of antagonists (see Table 19-3). Tolerance to one opioid agonist can confer tolerance to other opioid agonists, that is, cross-tolerance. However, there is no cross-tolerance between opioid agonists and other nonopioid drugs that act on the CNS such as the benzodiazepines, barbiturates, ethanol, stimulants, etc.

Opioid-induced **respiratory depression** may be potentiated in the presence of sedative-hypnotics agents, antipsychotic agents, or antidepressant agents. Opioids, particularly **meperidine,** may interact with MAOIs (tranylcypromine, phenelzine) to cause a **"serotonin syndrome."**

Structure

Opioids may be full agonists (e.g., morphine, heroin) or partial agonists (e.g., buprenorphine, pentazocine). Morphine is a phenanthrene alkaloid with a phenylmethyl-piperidine ring structure. Simple chemical substitutions can markedly alter its pharmacologic properties (see Figure 19-1).

Mechanism of Action

Opioid agonists bind to G-protein-coupled neural receptors (**mu, delta, kappa**) to **reduce adenylyl cyclase activity,** to reduce prejunctional calcium conductance, which causes a decrease in neurotransmitter release, and to enhance postjunctional potassium conductance, which causes a decrease in cell responsiveness to excitatory neurotransmitters.

Table 19-2

ADVERSE EFFECTS OF OPIOIDS

ADVERSE EFFECT: CAUSE	NOTES
Respiratory depression (major limiting effect) caused by direct inhibition of respiratory center in the brain stem results in decreased sensitivity to hypoxic drive by carbon dioxide.	Occurs at therapeutic doses of morphine. Tolerance develops that parallels tolerance to analgesia. Respiratory depression is generally not a serious clinical problem except in several special circumstances where opioids may be contraindicated: (1) Decreased respiratory reserve (e.g., emphysema, obstructive lung disease); (2) Head injury or CNS tumors; and (3) Pregnancy (to avoid fetal respiratory depression). Respiratory depression is a serious and potentially fatal consequence of opioid overdose.
Sedation/drowsiness	A decreased ability to concentrate. Ambulatory patients and elderly are at risk for accidents. A paradoxical dysphoria and increased anxiety may occur in children and women.
Nausea (30%), vomiting (10%): Caused by direct stimulation of the CTZ in the area postrema of the medulla which activates the vomiting center.	More likely to occur in ambulatory patients. Self-limiting with continued administration because of subsequent direct inhibition by morphine of the vomiting center.
Dependence	See Clinical Correlation, Case 19.
Pneumonia: May result from inhibition of cough reflex.	Increased likelihood in patients whose respiration is already seriously compromised.
Miosis: Stimulation of the Edinger-Westphal nucleus of the oculomotor nerve (III) results in contraction of the pupillary sphincter with constriction of the pupils ("pin-point" pupils).	Occurs at therapeutic doses. Pupils do not dilate, even in the dark. Parasympathetic pathways involve release of ACh in the ciliary ganglion; miosis can be blocked by atropine. Sign of opioid (e.g., heroin) overdose.
Hypotension: Opioids inhibit the (tonically active) vasomotor center in the brain stem to cause some peripheral arterial and venous vasodilation.	Usually not a clinical problem but is a relative contraindication for patients in shock or who have low blood pressure or who are hypovolemic (reduced blood volume). The elderly are particularly susceptible.

Table 19-2

ADVERSE EFFECTS OF OPIOIDS (GENERALLY EXTENSIONS OF PHARMACOLOGIC ACTIVITY) *(continued)*

Constipation (delayed fecal movement/increased absorption of water): Mechanism is uncertain, but probably due to peripheral action on the enteric nervous system to inhibit acetylcholine release. Effect is to increase GI tone with a concomitant decrease in coordinated propulsive activity and motility. Opioids also increase anal sphincter tone and decrease attention to the defecation reflex.	A major complaint of patients receiving opioids for analgesia. There is no clinically significant tolerance in humans. Stool softeners are used to treat (mineral oil/glycerin suppositories).
Urine retention: Opioids decrease urinary output due to decreased renal plasma flow, possible increased release of ADH from pituitary, decreased coordinated contractility of the ureters and bladder, increased urethral sphincter tone, and inattention to the urinary reflex.	Usually not a clinical problem except in patients with enlargement of the prostate. Catheterization may be necessary. More common in elderly. Increased tone of the ureters may result in a paradoxical increase in pain. A similar effect may occur when opioids are used to treat the pain of biliary colic.

Table 19-3

RELATIVE DEVELOPMENT OF TOLERANCE TO OPIOIDS

SUBSTANTIAL	MINIMAL
Analgesia	Constipation
Respiratory depression	Seizures (meperidine, codeine)
Euphoria	Antagonist activity (naloxone, naltrexone)
Sedation	Miosis
Nausea and vomiting	

Administration

Opioids are usually administered orally, but some like morphine can also be administered rectally or parenterally.

Specialized administration

Patient controlled analgesia (PCA): By infusion (morphine/meperidine/hydromorphone).

Regional analgesia: Epidural route is favored because it produces fewer adverse effects. May also be administered into subarachnoid or intrathecal spaces. There may be delayed respiratory depression, nausea, and vomiting that can be reversed with naloxone.

Transdermal fentanyl patch: Used for chronic pain

Buccal fentanyl lozenge/lollipop

Butorphanol nasal spray

Pharmacokinetics

Most opioids are absorbed well. Morphine, given orally, shows variable but significant first-pass metabolism (glucuronide conjugation) with a low oral to parenteral potency ratios (25%). It is usually given parenterally. Codeine and methadone are well absorbed after oral administration (approximately 60%) because of limited first-pass metabolism.

All opioids are metabolized by the liver. Metabolism usually results in more polar metabolites and frequently involves conjugation of the phenolic hydroxyl with glucuronic acid. Excretion is primarily by way of the kidneys. In addition to inactive metabolites, morphine is conjugated in the liver to morphine-3-glucuronide, which has neuroexcitatory properties. Morphine is also metabolized (10%) to morphine-6-glucuronide, which at high levels has analgesic potency greater than morphine itself. Codeine is metabolized, in part, to morphine. Heroin is also metabolized to morphine. Meperidine is metabolized to normeperidine that may be responsible for seizures in patients where it accumulates.

The fetal blood-brain barrier is readily crossed by the opioids, and infants born to mothers given (or self-administering) large doses of opioids may have severe respiratory depression.

COMPREHENSION QUESTIONS

[19.1] Morphine produces analgesia through which of the following actions?

    A. Activation of neuronal adenylyl cyclase

    B. Increased prejunctional neurotransmitter release

    C. Reduction of postjunctional neuronal potassium conductance

    D. Reduction of prejunctional neuronal calcium conductance

[19.2] Which of the following opioid agonists is not metabolized to an active agent with analgesic activity?

A. Morphine
B. Codeine
C. Heroin
D. Meperidine

[19.3] Which of the following is true of the antitussive agent dextromethorphan?

A. It activates mu, delta, and kappa receptors
B. It has analgesic activity in addition to its antitussive activity
C. It has no dependence liability
D. It is more constipating than codeine

Answers

[19.1] **D.** Opioid agonists bind to G-protein-coupled receptors to reduce adenylyl cyclase activity, to reduce prejunctional calcium conductance, which results in a decrease in neurotransmitter release, and to enhance postjunctional potassium conductance, which results in decreased responsiveness to excitatory neurotransmitters.

[19.2] **D.** Meperidine is metabolized to normeperidine that may result in seizures. Morphine is metabolized to morphine-6 glucuronide. Codeine and heroin are metabolized, in part, to morphine.

[19.3] **C.** Dextromethorphan is a nonopioid drug that is nearly as effective as codeine as an antitussive agent but with less constipating effect. It has no analgesic activity or dependence liability.

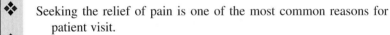

PHARMACOLOGY PEARLS

❖ Seeking the relief of pain is one of the most common reasons for patient visit.

❖ Up to 75 percent of hospitalized patients who receive opioids for their pain still report severe or moderate distress as result of under-dosing, often because clinicians are afraid of causing physical dependence or addiction.

❖ A patient, particularly a terminally ill patient, should never agonize or wish for death because of a physician's reluctance to use adequate doses of opioids!

❖ Seizures may occur in patients with renal failure because of the action of the morphine metabolite morphine-3-glucuronide.

❖ An accentuated action of morphine may occur in patients with renal failure as a consequence of the action of the active morphine metabolite morphine-6-glucuronide.

REFERENCES

Ferrante FM. Principles of opioid pharmacotherapy: practical implications of basic mechanisms. J Pain Symptom Manage 1996;11(5):265–73.

Julius D, Basbaum AI. Molecular mechanisms of nociception. Nature 2001;413(6852):203–10.

Loeser JD, ed. Bonica's Management of Pain. Philadelphia: Lippincott Williams Wilkins, 2001.

McCleane G, Smith HS. Opioids for persistent noncancer pain. Med Clin North Am. 2007;91(2):177–97.

A 22-year-old woman is brought in the emergency department via ambulance because of a suicide attempt. Soon after a "night on the town," she called her boyfriend saying that she took a handful of sleeping tablets. On examination, she appears lethargic, but groans and moves all her extremities to painful stimuli. Her blood pressure is 110/70 mm Hg, heart rate is 80 bpm, and oxygen saturation is 99 percent. Her pupils are of normal size and reactive to light. Her deep tendon reflexes are normal bilaterally. In the field, she was given an intravenous bolus of dextrose and an ampule of naloxone without response. Her boyfriend, with whom she had an argument, brings in the bottle of sleeping medication which reads "lorazepam."

◆ **What is the danger of an overdose with this class of medication?**

◆ **What is the cellular mechanism of action of this class of medication?**

◆ **What pharmacologic agent can be used to treat this patient, and what is its mechanism of action?**

ANSWERS TO CASE 20: BENZODIAZEPINES

Summary: A 22-year-old woman is brought to the emergency department because of a suicide attempt overdose with lorazepam. She is hemodynamically stable, has no focal neurologic deficits, but is lethargic. Intravenous dextrose and naloxone have been given without response.

◆ **Danger of an overdose with this class of medication:** Lorazepam is a benzodiazepine that belongs to a class of agents known as sedative-hypnotics that can depress the activity of the central nervous system (CNS). An overdose of a benzodiazepine, particularly in the presence of another CNS depressant like alcohol, can lead to sedation, hypotension, respiratory depression, coma, and death.

◆ **Cellular mechanism of action of lorazepam:** Binds to a distinct benzodiazepine receptor site on the γ-aminobutyric acid (GABA) receptor-chloride channel complex to allosterically increase the affinity for and frequency of GABA interactions with neuronal $GABA_A$ receptors.

◆ **Pharmacologic agent used to treat benzodiazepine overdose and its mechanism of action:** Flumazenil is a competitive antagonist at benzodiazepine receptors. It is used clinically to reverse the symptoms of benzodiazepine overdose.

CLINICAL CORRELATION

This 22-year-old woman ingested numerous tablets of lorazepam, a benzodiazepine, and exhibits the **classic signs of overdose: drowsiness, confusion, and amnesia.** In general, an overdose of benzodiazepines is not fatal, which is a major advantage over previous classes of drugs used for their sedative-hypnotic properties, such as the barbiturates. Symptoms of benzodiazepine overdose may include **drowsiness, confusion, amnesia, hypotension,** and, in the absence of compromised pulmonary function, **mild respiratory depression.** However, in the presence of other sedative-hypnotic agents like ethanol, which is suspected in this case, there may be **enhanced sedation** and respiratory depression that can result in **coma and even death.**

APPROACH TO BENZODIAZEPINES

Objectives

1. Describe the mechanism of action of benzodiazepines.
2. Study the result of chronic use of benzodiazepines.
3. Identify the withdrawal symptoms of this class of drugs.

Definitions

GABA$_A$ **receptor-chloride channel complex:** A muti-unit protein with which GABA interacts to regulate chloride conductance an action that can be modified by the allosteric interaction of other substrates, such as the benzodiazepines and barbiturates.

Allosteric interaction: A conformational change of a protein (GABA$_A$ receptor-chloride channel complex) caused by non-competitive binding of a substrat (benzodiazepine) at a site other than the active site of that protein.

DISCUSSION

Benzodiazepines are drugs used to treat a variety of disorders including, most notably, anxiety and insomnia, as well as status epilepticus and drug or toxin-induced seizures. They are also used clinically as muscle relaxants, as pre-anesthetic medications, and as amnestic agents for short medical and surgical procedures (Table 20-1).

Chronic use (weeks) of the benzodiazepines (BZ) can result in **tolerance** (a decreased response with continued drug administration) and **physical dependence** with an identifiable **withdrawal syndrome** that includes **severe anxiety and insomnia** and less frequently, as seen with alcohol **withdrawal, tremulousness, tachycardia, hypertension, hallucinations, and seizures** that **can be life threatening.** Withdrawal from shorter acting and intermediate-acting BZ occurs more quickly and is more severe than from longer acting drugs, and is usually managed with tapered dose reduction of the drug. Alternatively, because of the phenomenon of cross-tolerance, benzodiazepines with longer half-lives (e.g., diazepam) can be substituted for shorter acting benzodiazepines or other sedative-hypnotic drugs, like ethanol and the barbiturates, to stabilize the patient and to reduce the severity of the withdrawal syndrome.

Zolpidem, zaleplon, and eszopiclone are structurally different than the benzodiazepines but have a similar mechanism of action. They are widely used for the

Table 20-1
SELECTED CLINICAL USES OF BENZODIAZEPINES

Anxiety disorders
Insomnia
Convulsive disorders
Acute status epilepticus
Presurgical administration to reduce anxiety and for amnestic effects
Spastic disorder or muscle spasm
Involuntary movement disorder (such as restless leg syndrome)
Detoxification from alcohol
Psychiatric conditions (e.g., acute mania, impulse control disorders)

short-term management of insomnia. They have few of the other actions of the benzodiazepines and are less likely to cause physical dependence and drug abuse.

Buspirone is also a nonbenzodiazepine that relieves anxiety selectively. Due to its delayed onset of action, approximately 1 week, it is used primarily to manage chronic generalized anxiety disorder. It has no other benzodiazepine-like effects. Adverse effects include overt stimulation and GI dysfunction.

Flumazenil, a competitive inhibitor at benzodiazepine receptors, will quickly reverse the effects of the benzodiazepines. In dependent individuals it can induce symptoms of withdrawal. It is used to treat significant CNS depression because of benzodiazepine overdose such as in this clinical case.

Mechanism of Action

Like the barbiturates (another class of sedative-hypnotic agents), the benzodiazepines bind to the **GABA$_A$ receptor-chloride channel complex** (Figure 20-1). However, unlike the barbiturates, which increase the *duration* of GABA-mediated chloride channel opening, the benzodiazepines, which bind to a different site, increase the affinity of the complex for GABA and the *frequency* of GABA-stimulated chloride channel opening. This results in **increased chloride**

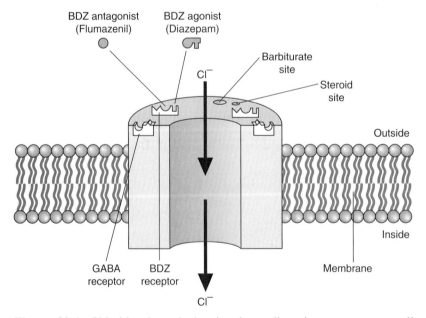

Figure 20-1. Chloride channel showing benzodiazepine receptor on cell membrane. **(Used, with permission, from Toy EC, Klamen DL. Case Files: Psychiatry, 2nd ed. New York: McGraw-Hill, 2007:409.)**

conductance with cell hyperpolarization. Because GABA is the principal inhibitory neurotransmitter of the brain, its increased action, facilitated by a benzodiazepine, will lead to a reduced neuronal stimulation by excitatory neurotransmitters. The outcome, among others, is sedation and hypnosis.

Zolpidem, zaleplon, and eszopiclone act on a subtype of the benzodiazepine receptor (BZ1) and, like the benzodiazepines, reduce chloride conductance in the CNS.

Buspirone is a partial agonist at serotonin 5-HT1A receptors.

Flumazenil competitively inhibits the action of benzodiazepines at their receptors on the GABA receptor–chloride channel complex.

Pharmacokinetics

Benzodiazepines are well absorbed from the GI tract, although clorazepate, a prodrug, is first decarboxylated in gastric juice to the long-acting (>50 hour) **active metabolite *N*-desmethyldiazepam.** Because the lipid solubility of the benzodiazepines varies more than 50-fold, there is considerable variation in their onset of action (diazepam and triazolam > chlordiazepoxide and lorazepam). The **most highly lipid soluble benzodiazepines have a short duration of action** after a low *single dose* because of their rapid redistribution from brain to peripheral tissues (e.g., flurazepam, diazepam, triazolam). However, under most circumstances, the duration of action of the benzodiazepines (Table 20-2) is related to their biotransformation by

Dealkylation to the long acting (>50 hours) active metabolites desmethyldiazepam (e.g., diazepam, chlordiazepoxide) or desalkylflurazepam (flurazepam).

Oxidation to short intermediate-acting metabolites (alprazolam, triazolam).

Rapid conjugation to metabolites with no intrinsic activity (e.g., oxazepam, lorazepam).

Clearance of the benzodiazepines is decreased significantly in the elderly, or in patients with **liver disease.** Thus these populations should, in general, be administered reduced dosages. **Elderly patients** may also be susceptible to **paradoxical agitation** and insomnia. The benzodiazepines should be **avoided in pregnancy** because **neonates may develop withdrawal symptoms.**

Table 20-2
SELECTED BENZODIAZEPINES

BENZODIAZEPINE	ONSET OF ACTION	HALF-LIFE OF PARENT (HOURS)	HALF-LIFE OF METABOLITE (HOURS)	COMPARATIVE ORAL DOSE
Short Acting				
Midazolam (Versed)	Rapid IV	0.5–1	Inactive	None
Triazolam (Halcion)	Intermediate	1–4	Inactive	0.5 mg
Intermediate Acting Alprazolam (Xanax)	Intermediate	6–20	Inactive	0.5 mg
Clonazepam (Klonopin)	Intermediate	20–40	Inactive	0.25 mg
Lorazepam	Intermediate (po) rapid (IV)	10–20	Inactive	1 mg
Oxazepam (Serax)	Slow	10–20	Inactive	15 mg
Temazepam (Restoril)	Slow	10–20	Inactive	30 mg
Long Acting				
Chlordiazepoxide (Librium)	Intermediate (po)	5–30	3–100	10 mg
Diazepam (Valium)	Rapid (po, IV)	20–50	3–100	5 mg
Flurazepam (Dalmane)	Rapid	Inactive	50–100	30 mg

Source: Bosse GM. Benzodiazepines. In: Tintinalli JE, Kelen GD, Stapczynski JS, eds. Emergency Medicine. New York: McGraw-Hill; 2004:1005–57.

COMPREHENSION QUESTIONS

[20.1] An 18-year-old male is having difficulty sleeping because of the death of his grandfather. He is given a benzodiazepine that does which of the following?

A. Binds to serotonin 5-HT$_1$ receptors
B. Binds to GABA$_A$ receptors
C. Is an antagonist at α-adrenoceptors
D. Is an antagonist at dopamine D$_2$ receptors

[20.2] A 22-year-old woman is diagnosed with a generalized anxiety disorder. Which of the following is a contraindication for the use of a benzodiazepine to treat this patient?

A. Cigarette smoking
B. Seizure disorder
C. Diabetes mellitus
D. Sleep apnea

[20.3] A 35-year-old man complains of seeing giant spiders in the hospital room. He is tremulous and agitated, hypertensive, and admits to heavy alcohol use at home. Which of the following actions of the benzodiazepines is the main rationale for their use to manage this patient?

A. Vasodilation
B. Hypnosis
C. Cross-tolerance with alcohol
D. Elevation of mood

[20.4] An 18-year-old man is brought into the emergency department with a seizure that has lasted 15 minutes without resolution. After administering oxygen, which pharmacologic agent is most appropriate to arrest the seizure?

A. Lidocaine
B. Lorazepam
C. Chlordiazepoxide
D. Triazolam

Answers

[20.1] **B.** Benzodiazepines bind to GABA$_A$ receptors to increase chloride influx and to decrease stimulation of neurons by excitatory neurotransmitters.

[20.2] **D.** Sleep apnea is a condition of relaxed soft tissue of the posterior pharynx, which occludes the airway during sleep. Family members usually note loud snoring and episodes of apnea of affected individuals. Sedatives, alcohol, and muscle relaxants are contraindicated in these patients, because severe apnea and death may ensue.

[20.3] **C.** Because there is cross-tolerance between them (they both interact with the $GABA_A$ receptor), a long-acting benzodiazepine can be used to ameliorate the symptoms associated with alcohol withdrawal.

[20.4] **B.** A short-acting benzodiazepine such as lorazepam is usually the best choice in the acute setting to arrest status epilepticus. Triazolam is used as a hypnotic agent.

PHARMACOLOGY PEARLS

❖ Benzodiazepines bind to the $GABA_A$ receptor, increasing chloride influx, rendering the cell less excitable. Because alcohol and barbiturates also bind to the $GABA_A$ receptor complex, there is cross-tolerance among these agents.

❖ Benzodiazepine overdose causes sedation, hypotension, and respiratory depression. Alcohol and barbiturates can potentiate these effects and also lead to coma and death.

❖ Acute benzodiazepine withdrawal can cause tremor, anxiety, tachycardia, hallucinations, and life-threatening seizures.

❖ Flumazenil is a competitive inhibitor of benzodiazepines and will quickly reverse its effects, sometimes inducing withdrawal symptoms.

REFERENCES

Longo LP, Johnson B. Addiction: Part I. Benzodiazepines-side effects, abuse risk and alternatives. Am Fam Physician 2000;61(8):2121–8.

Maczaj M. Pharmacological treatment of insomnia. Drugs 1993;45(1):44–55.

Ninan PT. New insights into the diagnosis and pharmacological management of generalized anxiety disorder. Psychopharmacol Bull 2002;36(2):105–22.

Silber MH. Chronic insomnia. N Engl J Med 2005;353(8):803–10.

A 30-year-old woman presents to the office for treatment of an ingrown toenail. For the past 3 weeks she has had progressively worsening redness,
swelling, and pain from the area around the right great toenail. On examination you find that the distal, medial corner of the right great toenail is ingrow-
ing. The skin on the medial border or the nail is red and tender. There is a
visible purulent drainage as well. You place her on a 1-week course of oral
cephalexin and have her return to the office. On follow-up, the redness is
markedly improved, and there is no further drainage. You surgically correct the
ingrown toenail after achieving local anesthesia with 2 percent lidocaine
injected to infiltrate the digital nerves.

◆ **What is the mechanism of action of lidocaine as an anesthetic
agent?**

◆ **Why does the treatment of infection increase the effectiveness of the
local anesthetic?**

ANSWERS TO CASE 21: LOCAL ANESTHETICS

Summary: A 30-year-old woman with an infected, ingrown toenail receives lidocaine as a local anesthetic.

◆ **Mechanism of action of lidocaine:** Time- and voltage-dependent blockade of the inactivated state of sodium channels on the inner axon membrane, which results in an increased refractory period and threshold for sensory nerve excitation.

◆ **Reason for treating infection prior to use of local anesthetic:** Infection and inflammation lower tissue pH, reducing the diffusion of the agent into the nerve, thus reducing its effectiveness.

CLINICAL CORRELATION

Local anesthetics produce a transient loss of sensation in a defined region of the body without producing a loss of consciousness. They may be used topically, for infiltration, for field block, for intravenous regional block, for nerve block, and for spinal and epidural anesthesia. Lidocaine and related local anesthetics work by inactivating Na^+ channels on axonal membranes, raising the threshold for axonal excitation. Nerves that carry pain and temperature signals are blocked before nerves that perform proprioception or motor functions. Some local anesthetics are effective topically, but most require injection into tissue, around nerves, or into the subarachnoid or epidural space to be effective. Most local anesthetics are weak bases, and at physiologic pH, therefore, a greater proportion will be in their cationic charged form, which is thought to be the active form at their site of action. However, it is the uncharged form that is important for penetration of local anesthetics into biological membranes. When tissue pH is lowered by infection or inflammation, more of the anesthetic is in the cationic form. This reduces its diffusion into the nerve and can reduce its anesthetic effect. Lidocaine and related anesthetics are vasodilators. Local anesthetics are frequently coadministered with dilute solutions of epinephrine, which produces vasoconstriction. This slows the absorption of the anesthetic, which prolongs its effect and lowers the risk of systemic toxicity. Epinephrine administration is contraindicated in areas supplied by end arteries, such as the digits, the tip of the nose, and the penis, as vasoconstriction of end arteries may result in tissue ischemia and necrosis.

APPROACH TO PHARMACOLOGY OF LOCAL ANESTHETICS

Objectives

1. List the drugs used for local anesthesia.
2. Describe the metabolism, adverse effects, and toxicities of local anesthetics.

Definitions

Nystagmus: Rapid, involuntary movement of the eye.
Purulent: Containing, or consisting of pus.
Propioception: Receipt of stimuli originating from internal organs.

DISCUSSION

Class

Depending on their structure, local anesthetics are classified as either **esters or amides** (Table 21-1). The choice of local anesthetic depends on the specific procedure and is usually based on the **desired duration of action** which may be **short** (procaine and chloroprocaine), **intermediate** (mepivacaine, lidocaine, prilocaine), or **long** (bupivacaine, etidocaine, ropivacaine, tetracaine). **Cocaine,** which has its own inherent vasoconstrictor properties, is used primarily for topical local anesthesia of the nose and throat.

Application of **very high levels of local anesthetics,** particularly lidocaine, may result in a **neurotoxicity** referred to as transient radicular irritation. High systemic local anesthetic levels, usually from **accidental intravascular injection, may result in central nervous system (CNS) effects** that may include symptoms ranging from light-headedness and visual disturbances to **nystagmus** and **muscle twitching** to tonic-clonic **seizures, respiratory depression, and death.** Unlike other local anesthetics that may produce hypotension and decreased cardiac conduction, and in rare instances cardiovascular collapse, cocaine overdose produces vasoconstriction and hypertension and may result in cardiac arrhythmias. Bupivacaine, like cocaine, is also notable for being more cardiotoxic than other local anesthetics. **Ester-type local anesthetics** are metabolized to para-aminobenzoic acid derivatives and may result **in allergic reactions** in some patients.

Structure

Local anesthetics generally consist of some ionizable group connected through either an ester or an amide to a lipophilic group.

Table 21-1
LOCAL ANESTETHICS (ROUTE)

ESTERS	AMIDES
Cocaine*	Bupivacaine[†]
Benzocaine*	Lidocaine[†]
Procaine[†]	Mepivacaine[†]
Tetracaine[†,*]	Prilocaine[†]
	Ropivacaine[†]

* topical; [†] parenteral

Administration

Depending on the drug, local anesthetics may be administered by the parenteral route and topically. The extent of systemic absorption of injected local anesthetics from the site of administration, and therefore the duration of their action, is modified by a number of factors. Vasoconstrictor agents like epinephrine are used to decrease local blood flow and thus extend the duration of anesthetic action, and reduce the toxicity, of such local anesthetics as lidocaine, procaine, and mepivacaine. In spinal analgesia, clonidine can also be used concomitantly with local anesthetics to enhance the activation by epinephrine of α_2-adrenoceptors, which reduces sensory nerve firing by inhibition of the release of substance P.

Pharmacokinetics

Ester-type local anesthetics are metabolized rapidly by **nonspecific plasma cholinesterases** and, generally, have **shorter half-lives** than amide-type local anesthetics.

Amide-type local anesthetics are metabolized at various rates by **hepatic microsomal enzymes.** In severe liver disease, toxicity is more likely. Likewise, metabolism may be slowed when amide-type local anesthetics are used with other drugs metabolized by the same enzymes.

COMPREHENSION QUESTIONS

[21.1] Local anesthetic action is a result of blockade of the movement of which of the following ion channels?

A. Calcium
B. Chloride
C. Potassium
D. Sodium

[21.2] An allergic reaction is most likely to occur with which of the following local anesthetics?

A. Bupivacaine
B. Lidocaine
C. Mepivacaine
D. Procaine

[21.3] Which of the following agents is often combined with local anesthetics to prevent its systemic distribution from the site of injection?

A. Acetylcholine
B. Dopamine
C. Epinephrine
D. γ-Aminobutyric acid (GABA)

Answers

[21.1]   **D.** Local anesthetic action is a result of prevention of sodium movement caused by blockade of the inactivated state of neuronal sodium channels.

[21.2]   **D.** An allergic reaction is most likely to occur with ester-type local anesthetics like procaine because of the metabolic formation of the allergen, para-aminobenzoic acid.

[21.3]   **C.** Local anesthetics are often combined with the vasoconstrictor epinephrine to prevent their distribution from the site of injection and thus extend their duration of action and reduce their systemic toxicity.

PHARMACOLOGY PEARLS

 Use of a carbon dioxide–saturated local anesthetic solution ("carbonation") to increase acidity can accelerate onset of anesthetic action.

 Ester-type local anesthetics are metabolized rapidly by nonspecific plasma cholinesterases and generally have shorter half-lives than amide-type local anesthetics.

 High systemic local anesthetic levels, usually from accidental intravascular injection, may result in CNS effects, tonic-clonic seizures, respiratory depression, and death.

REFERENCES

Butterworth JF, Strichartz GR. Molecular mechanisms of local anesthesia: a review. Anesthesiology 1990;72(4):711–34.

Smith C. Pharmacology of local anesthetic agents. Br J Hosp Med 1994;52(9):455–60.

Stoelting RK. Local anesthetics. In: Pharmacology and Physiology in Anesthetic Practice, 3rd ed. New York: Lippincott-Raven, 1999.

White JL, Durieux ME. Clinical pharmacology of local anesthetics. Anesthesiol Clin North America 2005;23(1):73–84.

A 35-year-old man is in the surgical holding area being evaluated prior to a scheduled hernia repair. He asks the anesthesiologist about the type of "anesthetic gas" to be used, because he recalls that his mother developed severe liver problems from general anesthesia for a hysterectomy performed 2 years previously. The patient asks whether nitrous oxide might be used, because he has heard that it was a safe agent. To allay the patient's anxiety, the anesthesiologist proposes spinal anesthetic for the surgery.

◆ **What is the probable general anesthetic agent used for the patient's mother?**

◆ **What is the disadvantage of nitrous oxide as an inhalation anesthetic agent?**

ANSWERS TO CASE 22: INHALATION ANESTHETIC AGENTS

Summary: A 35-year-old man is in the surgical holding area being evaluated prior to a scheduled hernia repair. The patients' mother developed severe liver problems from general anesthesia. The patient asks whether nitrous oxide might be used.

◆ **Probable inhalation anesthetic agent used for the patient's mother:** A halogenated agent, such as halothane.

◆ **Disadvantage of nitrous oxide as an inhalation anesthetic agent:** Lack of anesthetic potency requires large amounts to be used as a single agent, associated with postoperative nausea and vomiting.

CLINICAL CORRELATION

Patients such as the one described in the case are often nervous about "being put to sleep" because of fear about not having sufficient anesthesia and feeling pain, or about "never waking up." However, this is highly unlikely because the expertise in the field of anesthesia and the knowledge of the anesthetic agents is better today than ever before. This patient relates a story of how his mother developed severe liver problems as a result of a general anesthetic agent. Halothane-related mild type I hepatotoxicity is benign, self-limiting, and relatively common, affecting up to 25 percent of individuals, and is characterized by mild, transient increases in serum transaminase and by altered postoperative drug metabolism. However, halothane-related type II hepatotoxicity is associated with massive centrilobular liver cell necrosis often leading to fulminant liver failure. The patient clinically has fever, jaundice, and a grossly elevated serum transaminase level that is probably immune mediated. Approximately 20 percent of halothane is oxidatively metabolized compared to only 2 percent of enflurane and 0.2 percent of isoflurane. Halothane-induced hepatotoxicity may result from the anaerobic formation of reductive reactive intermediates during halothane metabolism, including trifluoroacetic acid (TFA), that cause direct liver damage or initiate an immune response in genetically predisposed individuals. The occurrence of type II hepatotoxicity after enflurane or isoflurane administration is extremely rare, approximately 1 in 35,000 individuals.

APPROACH TO PHARMACOLOGY OF INHALATION ANESTHETIC AGENTS

Objectives

1. List the characteristics of the ideal general anesthetic agent.
2. Describe the pharmacokinetic parameters of inhalation anesthetics that influence the onset of and recovery from anesthesia.

3. List the advantages and disadvantages of the commonly used inhalation anesthetic agents.
4. List the commonly used intravenously administered anesthetic agents and adjunct agents used in a "balanced anesthesia."

Definitions

Minimum alveolar concentration (MAC): Anesthetic dose of an inhalation anesthetic agent at 1 atmosphere, expressed in terms of alveolar tension (mm Hg), which produces immobility in 50 percent of individuals exposed to a noxious stimulus, such as a standardized skin incision.

Blood:gas partition coefficient: The solubility of an inhalation anesthetic in blood relative to air at 37°C (98.6°F).

Second gas effect: The rate of rise of alveolar tension and inflow of an inhalation anesthetic gas can be increased in the presence of high concentrations of another anesthetic gas, usually nitrous oxide.

DISCUSSION

Class

Inhalation anesthetics, as the name implies, are administered via the pulmonary route, often by assisted ventilation. The **ideal anesthetic agent** should be able to induce **unconsciousness, analgesia, amnesia, skeletal muscle relaxation,** and **inhibition of autonomic and sensory reflexes.** However, in practice, a combination of drugs ("balanced anesthesia"), including anesthetic agents that are administered intravenously, is used to provide a more satisfactory anesthesia than is possible with any one anesthetic agent alone, and to minimize their individual adverse effects (Table 22-1).

The **MAC** of an inhalation anesthetic that is necessary to achieve effective anesthetic concentrations is usually expressed as the mole fraction of the gas.

Mole fraction equals partial pressure of anesthetic agent as percentage of total gas pressure (760 mm Hg). For example,

Halothane's MAC = 5.7 mm Hg/760 mm Hg × 100 = 0.75%

MAC is an indicator of anesthetic potency, the **lower the MAC** the **more potent** is the agent (Table 22-2). It is used only as a guide. For example, the anesthesiologist might use either multiples of an inhalation anesthetic agent's MAC or a fraction of an inhalation anesthetic agent's MAC to achieve clinical anesthesia depending on whether or not the agent is used alone (rare for volatile anesthetics), in combination, or with intravenously administered anesthetic agents or preanesthetic agents (Table 22-3).

Most halogenated inhaled anesthetic agents reduce peripheral vascular resistance with the possibility of reflex tachycardia. Halothane is a notable

Table 22-1

ADVANTAGES AND ADVERSE EFFECTS OF INHALATION
ANESTHETIC AGENTS

ANESTHETIC AGENTS*	ADVANTAGES	ADVERSE EFFECTS
Nitrous oxide (N_2O; for minor surgery, used with volatile or intravenous anesthetics)	Odorless rapid induction, minimal cardiovascular effects	Postoperative nausea and vomiting, synergistic respiratory depression with other drugs (opioids, benzodiazepines)
Desflurane (used to maintain anesthesia after induction with another agent)	Very rapid recovery, cardiac output maintained, heart is not sensitized to catecholamines, minimal metabolism to toxic products	Objectionable odor, irritates respiratory tract, decreases blood pressure, tachycardia
Sevoflurane	Pleasant odor, very rapid induction and recovery	Decreases cardiac output, decreases blood pressure, reflex tachycardia
Enflurane	Pleasant odor	Decreases cardiac output, marked decrease in blood pressure, tachycardia, sensitized heart to catecholamine-induced arrhythmias, depresses neuromuscular transmission, can induce seizures
Isoflurane	Rapid induction and recovery, cardiac output maintained, heart is not sensitized to catecholamines, preserves tissue perfusion, very little metabolism to toxic products	Objectionable odor, decreases blood pressure, transient tachycardia, depresses neuromuscular transmission
Halothane† (used primarily in pediatrics)	Pleasant odor, rapid induction, and recovery	Depresses respiratory function, decreases cardiac output and arteria, decreases blood pressure, sensitizes heart to catecholamine-induced arrhythmias, increases cerebral blood flow with increased intracranial pressure, toxic metabolites that may cause hepatotoxicity

*Although available for use, the inhalation anesthetic methoxyflurane is considered obsolete because of potential renal and nephrotoxicity.
†Use is declining.

Table 22-2

MAC VALUES (%)* AND BLOOD: GAS PARTITION COEFFICIENTS
OF SELECTED INHALATION ANESTHETIC AGENTS

ANESTHETIC AGENT	MAC	PARTITION COEFFICIENT
Nitrous oxide	>100.00[†]	0.47
Desflurane	6.00	0.42
Sevoflurane	2.00	0.69
Enflurane	1.70	1.80
Isoflurane	1.40	1.40
Halothane	0.75	2.30

*Expressed as a percentage of lung gases at 1 atmosphere.
[†]MAC values greater than 100 indicate that hyperbaric conditions are necessary to produce anesthesia. MAC = minimum alveolar concentration.

Table 22-3

SELECTED INTRAVENOUS ANESTHETIC AGENTS AND
PREANESTHETIC AGENTS

ANESTHETIC AGENTS	PREANESTHETIC AGENTS
Barbiturates (e.g., thiopental)	Sedative-hypnotics
Benzodiazepines (e.g., diazepam, midazolam, lorazepam)	Opioids Muscle relaxants
Opioids (e.g., fentanyl, sufentanil, alfentanil, remifentanil)	Anticholinergic agents Local anesthetics
Ketamine	
Propofol	
Etomidate	

exception in that it has both vascular constrictor and relaxation activity and blocks reflex sympathetic stimulation of the heart. However, it does sensitize the heart to catecholamine-induced arrhythmias.

Malignant hyperthermia is a **life-threatening, autosomal-dominant disorder** that develops during or after general anesthesia with volatile anesthetics and muscle relaxants (e.g., succinylcholine). Its incidence is 1:10,000. Symptoms include a rapidly occurring hypermetabolic state of **tachycardia, hypertension, severe muscle rigidity, hyperthermia, acidosis, and hyperkalemia.** The biochemical basis of malignant hyperthermia is compromised regulation of calcium flux with increased intracellular concentrations of calcium in skeletal muscle. Treatment includes dantrolene, which prevents release of calcium from the sarcoplasmic reticulum, and supportive measures such as procedures to reduce body temperature and restore electrolyte balance.

Structure

With the exception of nitrous oxide, the major inhalation anesthetic agents in current use today are **halogenated hydrocarbons.** They are either gaseous (nitric oxide) with boiling points below room temperature, or volatile liquids that at room temperature vaporize to the extent necessary to achieve anesthetic concentrations.

Mechanism of Action

The mechanism of action of inhalation anesthetics is not well understood. Current theories suggest that anesthetics directly interact with proteins at hydrophobic sites on ligand-gated ion channels at neural synapses to inhibit the activity of excitatory receptors (e.g., N-methyl-D-aspartic acid [NMDA], nicotinic, serotonin 5-HT_3) or potentiate the activity of inhibitory receptors (e.g., $GABA_A$, glycine).

Pharmacokinetics

The concentration of an inhaled gas in the brain sufficient to achieve anesthesia depends on a number of factors, including the anesthetic agent's concentration in the inspired air, its **solubility** in blood relative to air, the **arteriovenous concentration gradient,** as well as **pulmonary blood flow and pulmonary ventilation rate.**

The concentration (as a percentage) of an inhaled anesthetic in the inspired air directly affects the rate of induction of anesthesia by influencing the rate of transfer of the agent into blood. In clinical practice, an inhaled anesthetic may be administered initially at a relatively high concentration to speed the rate of induction, following which the concentration in the inspired air would be reduced to a level that maintains the anesthetic state.

The solubility of an inhalation anesthetic in blood relative to air at 37°C (98.6°F), as described by its **blood:gas partition coefficient** (see Table 22-2), is an important factor in determining the rate of rise of their arterial tension in the arterial blood, which influences directly the rate of equilibration with the brain and rate of onset of action. For anesthetic agents with low blood solubility, the partial pressure, and therefore the arterial tension, rises relatively quickly. The partial pressure and arterial tension rise more slowly with anesthetic agents of moderate to high solubility.

The greater the difference in the arterial and venous anesthetic concentrations, the more time it will take for an inhaled anesthetic agent to equilibrate with brain tissue and to induce surgical anesthesia. The difference in the arterial and venous anesthetic concentrations is a reflection of the uptake of an anesthetic agent by the tissues, particularly muscle, kidney, liver, and splanchnic bed (which in turn is a reflection of, among other factors, blood flow, and tissue solubility relative to blood).

Pulmonary blood flow also affects the rate of induction of anesthesia. Although counterintuitive, the higher the blood flow (and the higher the cardiac output), the slower the rate of rise of arterial tension, an effect that is most notable for inhaled anesthetics of moderate to high blood solubility. The opposite occurs with a decrease in blood flow, as might occur during shock.

An increase in **pulmonary ventilation rate** (i.e., minute ventilation), for example, by mechanical hyperventilation, increases anesthetic gas tension and the speed of induction, most notably for inhalation anesthetic agents with moderate-to-high blood solubility. Depression of unassisted respiration will have the opposite effect.

The **second gas effect** can also be taken advantage of to increase the rate of rise of alveolar tension of an inhalation anesthetic gas.

Following termination of its administration, recovery from anesthesia depends on the rate of elimination of an anesthetic agent from the brain, which can be influenced by pulmonary blood flow and pulmonary ventilation, and by the tissue solubility and the blood solubility of the anesthetic agent. Clearance by the lungs is the major route of elimination of inhalation anesthetic agents, with perhaps metabolism playing a contributing role for halothane.

COMPREHENSION QUESTIONS

[22.1] Which of the following is most important to quickly achieve a partial pressure of an inhalation anesthetic agent of high blood solubility that is sufficient to induce anesthesia?

    A. A decrease in pulmonary ventilation rate
    B. Coadministration of dantrolene
    C. Low blood and tissue solubility
    D. Low MAC

[22.2] An inhalation agent with a low (1.7) MAC has which of the following?

    A. A rapid onset of action
    B. A low blood:gas partition coefficient
    C. A low oil:gas partition coefficient
    D. A high potency

[22.3] A 34-year-old woman is undergoing general anesthesia for a cholecys-tectomy. After the completion of the case, the anesthesiologist turns off the gas and notes that the patient is recovering from the anesthetic agent very quickly. What are likely properties of this inhalation anesthetic?

A. Associated with decreased pulmonary circulation
B. Associated with an unpleasant odor
C. High MAC
D. High solubility

Answers

[22.1] **C.** The alveolar partial pressure of an inhalation anesthetic with low blood and tissue solubility will rise quickly. Under these conditions, blood and brain will equilibrate, and anesthesia will be induced, rather quickly. An inhalation anesthetic with a low MAC will equilibrate with brain tissue rather slowly. An increase, not decrease, in pul-monary ventilation rate will increase anesthetic gas tension and the speed of induction, particularly for inhalation anesthetic agents with moderate-to-high blood solubility. Dantrolene is not an anesthetic agent. It is used to counter the effects of malignant hyperthermia.

[22.2] **D.** An agent with a low MAC is highly potent, has a high oil:gas par-tition coefficient and high blood:gas partition coefficient, and usually has a slow onset of action.

[22.3] **B.** Agents that have a rapid onset of action and rapid recovery have a low solubility. One such agent is desflurane, which has an unpleasant odor.

PHARMACOLOGY PEARLS

 Modern day inhalation anesthetic agents cause a rapid progression through the classical Guedel stages of anesthesia (analgesia, loss of consciousness, surgical anesthesia, and respiratory and cardio-vascular depression).

 Although independent of gender and weight, MAC may be decreased (increased potency) with age, pregnancy hypothermia, and hypotension.

 MAC may increase (decreased potency) with CNS stimulants.

REFERENCES

Campagna JA, Miller KW, Forman SA. Mechanisms of action of inhaled anesthet-ics. N Engl J Med 2003;348(21):2110–24.
Wiklund RA, Rosenbaum SH. Anesthesiology. N Engl J Med 1997;337(16):1132–41, 1215–9.

A 50-year-old salesman was admitted to the hospital with acute appendicitis. He has no significant medical history, takes no medications, does not smoke cigarettes, and has an alcoholic beverage "once in a while with the boys." He underwent an uncomplicated appendectomy. On the second hospital day, you find him to be quite agitated and sweaty. His temperature, heart rate, and blood pressure are elevated. A short time later he has a grand-mal seizure. You suspect that he is having withdrawal symptoms from chronic alcohol abuse and give IV lorazepam for immediate control of the seizures and plan to start him on oral chlordiazepoxide when he is more stable.

◆ **What are the acute pharmacologic effects of ethanol?**

◆ **What are the chronic pharmacologic effects of ethanol?**

◆ **How is alcohol metabolized?**

◆ **What is the pharmacologic basis for using benzodiazepines to manage alcohol withdrawal?**

ANSWERS TO CASE 23: DRUGS OF ABUSE

Summary: A 50-year-old man is displaying symptoms and signs of acute alcohol withdrawal.

◆ **Symptoms of acute ethanol toxicity:** Disinhibited behavior and judgment, slurred speech, impaired motor function, depressed and impaired mental function, respiratory depression, cutaneous vasodilation, diuresis, gastrointestinal side effects, and impaired myocardial contractility.

◆ **Symptoms of chronic ethanol toxicity:** Alcoholic fatty liver, alcoholic hepatitis, cirrhosis, liver failure, peripheral neuropathy, alcohol amnesic syndrome, pancreatitis, gastritis, fetal alcohol syndrome, nutritional deficiencies, cardiomyopathy, cerebellar degeneration.

◆ **Metabolism of alcohol:** Oxidized primarily in the liver but also in the stomach and other organs to acetaldehyde by the cytosolic enzyme alcohol dehydrogenase (ADH) and by hepatic microsomal enzymes; acetaldehyde is oxidized to acetate by hepatic mitochondrial aldehyde dehydrogenase.

◆ **Benzodiazepines in alcohol withdrawal:** Both alcohol and the benzodiazepines enhance the effect of γ-aminobutyric acid (GABA) on GABA$_A$ neuroreceptors, resulting in decreased overall brain excitability. This cross-reactivity explains why relatively long-acting benzodiazepines (e.g., lorazepam, chlordiazepoxide) can be substituted for alcohol in a detoxification program.

CLINICAL CORRELATION

Ethanol is the most widely used CNS depressant. It is rapidly absorbed from the stomach and small intestine and distributed in total body water. Its exact mechanism of action is not known, but may be related to its generally disruptive effects on cell membrane protein functions throughout the body, including effects on signaling pathways in the CNS. At low doses it is oxidized by cytoplasmic ADH. At higher doses it is also oxidized by liver microsomal enzymes, which may be induced by chronic use. These enzymes are rapidly saturated by the concentrations of alcohol achieved by even one or two alcoholic drinks so that its rate of metabolism becomes independent of plasma concentration. Tolerance to the intoxicating effects of alcohol can develop with chronic use. Cross-tolerance with barbiturates and benzodiazepines may also develop. Because of this cross-tolerance effect, benzodiazepines are the most commonly used agents for the treatment of alcohol withdrawal, a potentially life-threatening syndrome commonly seen 2–3 days after the abrupt cessation of alcohol use by a chronic abuser. A long-acting benzodiazepine can be taken, and gradually tapered, to mitigate this effect. Disulfiram is also used on occasion to manage alcoholism. It is a drug that inhibits aldehyde dehydrogenase that in the presence of alcohol causes an accumulation of acetaldehyde, which results in a highly aversive reaction consisting of flushing, severe headache, nausea and vomiting, and confusion. Naltrexone, an opioid antagonist, is yet another drug used to manage alcoholism.

APPROACH TO PHARMACOLOGY OF ETHANOL

Objectives

1. Define drug abuse, drug tolerance, drug dependence, and drug addiction.
2. List the common drugs of abuse and their properties.
3. List the adverse effects of the common drugs of abuse.

Definitions

Drug abuse: Nonmedical use of a drug taken to alter consciousness or to change body image that is often regarded as unacceptable by society. Not to be confused with drug misuse.

Drug tolerance: Decreased response to a drug with its continued administration that can be overcome by increasing the dose. A cellular tolerance develops to certain drugs of abuse that act on the CNS because of a poorly understood biochemical or homeostatic adaptation of neurons to the continued presence of the drug. Also, in addition to a cellular tolerance, a metabolic tolerance can develop to the effects of some drugs because they increase the synthesis of enzymes responsible for their own metabolism (alcohol, barbiturates).

Drug dependence: Continued need of the user to take a drug. Psychologic dependence is the compulsive behavior of a user to continue to use a drug no matter the personal or medical consequences. Inability to obtain the drug activates a "craving" that is very discomforting. Physical or physiologic dependence is a consequence of drug abstinence after chronic drug use that results in a constellation of signs and symptoms that are often opposite to the initial effects of the drug and to those sought by the user. Psychologic dependence generally precedes physical dependence but, depending on the drug, does not necessarily lead to it. The development of physical dependence, the degree of which varies considerably for different drugs of abuse, is always associated with the development of tolerance, although the exact relationship is unclear.

Drug addiction: A poorly defined, imprecise term with little clinical significance that indicates the presence of psychologic and physical dependence.

Table 23-1
DRUGS OF ABUSE

	NICOTINE	MARIJUANA	COCAINE/AMPHETAMINE
Route of administration	Smoking	Smoking	Smoking, oral IV
Mechanism of action	Mimics action of acetylcholine	Interacts with G-protein-coupled cannabinoid receptors among other actions	Cocaine binds the dopamine reuptake transporter. Amphetamine increases release of neuronal catecholamines, including dopamine
Pharmacologic effects	Stimulant and depressant actions on the CNS and cardiovascular system	Euphoria, uncontrollable laughter, introspection, loss of sense of time, sleepiness, loss of concentration	Euphoria, excitation, increased alertness, an orgasmic-like "rush"
Tolerance and dependence	Tolerance develops rapidly Strong psychologic dependence Withdrawal syndrome indicative of physical dependence	Arguably, some tolerance and very mild physical dependence	Rapid development of tolerance. Withdrawal syndrome characterized by increased appetite, depression, and exhaustion
Therapeutic uses	None	Nausea and vomiting of cancer. Appetite stimulation in AIDS (dronabinol)	Local anesthesia (cocaine). ADHD (methylphenidate). Narcolepsy (modafinil)
Adverse effects	Cancer, obstructive lung disease, cardiovascular disease	Bronchitis, increased pulse rate, reddening of conjunctiva	Paranoid schizophrenia. Amphetamine-specific necrotizing arteritis. Cocaine-related arrhythmias, seizures, respiratory depression, hypertension, stroke, increased fetal mortality, and abnormalities
Treatment of abuse	Nicotine gum and transdermal patch	Behavioral modification	Antipsychotic agents. Antidepressant agents

DISCUSSION

Class

In addition to alcohol, the major drugs of abuse are nicotine, marijuana (Δ9-tetrahydrocannabinol), heroin, and the CNS stimulants, notably cocaine and amphetamine and its derivatives (Table 23-1).

COMPREHENSION QUESTIONS

[23.1] Alcohol is oxidized by which of the following enzymes?

    A. Acetate oxidase
    B. ADH
    C. Aldehyde dehydrogenase
    D. Monoamine oxidase

[23.2] Which of the following is the most common adverse effect resulting from chronic ethanol abuse?

    A. Cirrhosis
    B. Cutaneous vasodilation
    C. Disinhibited judgment
    D. Respiratory depression

[23.3] Which of the following is a drug of abuse that blocks the dopamine uptake transporter?

    A. Alcohol
    B. Cocaine
    C. Marijuana
    D. Nicotine

Answers

[23.1] **B.** Alcohol is oxidized in the liver, stomach, and other organs to acetaldehyde by the cytosolic enzyme ADH and the hepatic microsomal enzymes. Acetaldehyde is oxidized to acetate by mitochondrial hepatic aldehyde dehydrogenase.

[23.2] **A.** Liver cirrhosis is an effect of chronic alcohol use. Disinhibited judgment, respiratory depression, and cutaneous vasodilation are acute effects of alcohol.

[23.3] **B.** Cocaine is a drug of abuse that binds the dopamine reuptake transporter. Ethanol may nonspecifically disrupt cell membrane protein functions. Marijuana interacts with G-protein-coupled cannabinoid receptors. Nicotine mimics the action of acetylcholine.

PHARMACOLOGY PEARLS

 Alcohol is the most widely used drug of abuse.

 Delirium Tremens, a syndrome associated with the abrupt discontinuation of alcohol in a chronic abuser, carries a high mortality rate
  if not promptly identified and treated.

 Withdrawal from other drugs of abuse may cause unpleasant symptoms for the patient, but is rarely life threatening.

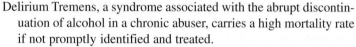 In all hypotheses of addiction, increased concentrations of dopamine
  in the mesolimbic system is considered the neurochemical correlate
  of dependence and addiction.

REFERENCES

Cami J, Farre M. Mechanisms of disease: drug addiction. N Engl J Med 2003;
   349(10):975–86.
Lieber CS. Medical disorders of alcoholism. N Engl J Med 1995;333(16):1058–65.
Saitz R. Unhealthy alcohol use. N Engl J Med 2005;352(6):596–607.
Swift RM. Drug therapy for alcohol dependence. N Engl J Med 1999;340(19):
   1482–90.

An 8-year-old girl is brought in by her mother for evaluation of allergies. Each year in the spring the child develops a runny nose; itchy, watery eyes; and sneezing. She has been treated in the past with diphenhydramine, but the child's teacher says that she is very drowsy during school. She has no other medical problems and is on no chronic medications. Her examination is unremarkable today. You diagnose her with seasonal allergic rhinitis and prescribe fexofenadine.

◆ **What is the mechanism of action of antihistamine medications?**

◆ **What are the common side effects of antihistamine medications?**

◆ **What is the pharmacologic basis of switching to fexofenadine?**

ANSWERS TO CASE 24: ANTIHISTAMINES

Summary: An 8-year-old girl with seasonal allergic rhinitis is switched to fexofenadine because of the sedation caused by diphenhydramine.

◆ **Mechanism of action of antihistamines:** Competitive antagonist of histamine receptors.

◆ **Common side effects:** Sedation, dizziness, nausea, constipation, diarrhea, loss of appetite, anticholinergic effects—dry mouth, dry eyes, blurred vision, urinary retention.

◆ **Rationale for switching to fexofenadine:** Less central nervous system (CNS) penetration and less sedating than earlier antihistamines.

CLINICAL CORRELATION

Histamine is found in many tissues throughout the body. Most histamine is stored in mast cells and basophils. Histamine is released primarily from mast cells via the process of degranulation. Degranulation occurs when immunoglobulin E (IgE) fixates to mast cells, and there is a subsequent exposure to a specific antigen. Complement activation may also induce degranulation. When released, histamine becomes bound to specific membrane-bound histamine receptors. The therapeutic uses of antihistamine medications primarily involve the H_1- and H_2-receptor subtypes. **H_1 receptors are located in the brain, heart, bronchi, gastrointestinal (GI) tract, and vascular smooth muscle.** Their activation increases phospholipase C activity, causing increases in diacylglycerol and intracellular calcium. Activation of H_1 receptors in the brain increases wakefulness. In blood vessels, activation causes vasodilation and increased permeability. H_1-receptor antagonists are competitive inhibitors at this receptor site. H_1-receptor antagonists are frequently used for the treatment of allergic rhinitis, urticaria, and hives. Some are used as prophylaxis for motion sickness and as sleep aids. Older, first-generation, antihistamines cross the blood-brain barrier, contributing to their potentially use-limiting side effect of sedation and can also have significant anticholinergic effects (dry mouth, dry eyes, blurred vision, urinary retention). They must be used with caution in the elderly and in combination with other sedating medications, because the effects can be additive. **Newer, second-generation antihistamines have significantly less penetration into the CNS and reduced anticholinergic activity.** This results in a lower incidence of sedation and fewer anticholinergic side effects. H_2-receptor activity is coupled to cyclic adenosine monophosphate (cAMP). **Activation of H_2 receptors in gastric parietal cells causes an increase in gastric acid production.** Medications that are competitive antagonists of H_2 receptors are used to reduce gastric acid secretion. These are used clinically in the management of peptic ulcer disease, gastroesophageal reflux disease, heartburn, and acid hypersecretory syndromes.

APPROACH TO PHARMACOLOGY OF HISTAMINE AND ANTIHISTAMINES

Objectives

1. Know the synthesis and mechanism of action of histamine.
2. Know the mechanism of action, uses, and adverse effects of antihistamine medications.

Definitions

Allergic rhinitis: An antigen-mediated allergic reaction that causes nasal congestion, sneezing, itchy eyes, and bronchoconstriction; also called hay fever.

DISCUSSION

Class

Histamine, β-aminoethylimidazole, is formed in many tissues by decarboxylation of the amino acid L-histidine by the enzyme histidine decarboxylase. Mast cells and basophils are the principal histamine-containing cells in most tissues. **Histamine is stored in vesicles in a complex with heparin** and **released by either an immunologic trigger** or following a **mechanical or chemical stimulus.** Once released, **histamine produces a number of responses including local vasodilation, transudation of fluid through endothelial cells, and stimulation of nerve ending, producing pain and itching.** In the lung, histamine is a **bronchoconstrictor,** and this action is magnified in patients with asthma. Histamine has actions in the GI tract and causes **contraction of smooth muscle;** it is also a potent secretagogue for gastric acid secretion, pepsin, and intrinsic factor. In the brain, histamine acts as a **neurotransmitter.**

The actions of histamine are mediated by four distinct membrane receptors that are **coupled to G-proteins.** The H_1 receptor, located in smooth muscle cells, endothelium, and brain, is coupled to increased diacylglycerol and Ca^{2+} release. The H_2 receptor is located in gastric mucosa mast cells, immune cells, and brain, and is coupled to increased cAMP. There is no clinical pharmacology yet for H_3 (located in the brain and peripheral neurons) or H_4 (found on eosinophils and neutrophils) receptors, but both of these receptors are targets for therapeutic agents and are under intense investigation. Histamine itself has a variety of untoward effects and is useful only diagnostically to assess bronchial hyperreactivity.

Antihistamines

Compounds that block the active state of histamine H_1 receptors have been used for years and are widely marketed both as prescription and over-the-counter medications. The current group of available drugs can be divided into **first-generation and second-generation agents.** In general, **first-generation agents can cross the blood-brain barrier,** and they have a number of effects in the brain, including sedation and reduction in nausea. Table 24-1 lists some currently used H_1 antagonists.

All of these drugs block the action of H_1 receptors, and they do not possess significant affinity for the H_2 receptor. However, many of the **first-generation**

Table 24-1
CURRENTLY AVAILABLE ANTIHISTAMINES

CHEMICAL CLASS	DRUG	ANTICHOL ACTIVITY	COMMENT
First-Generation Antihistamines			
Ethanolamines	Diphenhydramine Doxylamine Carbinoxamine	+++	I
Ethylamine diamines	Pyrilamine Tripelennamine	+ +	
Piperazines	Cyclizine Meclizine Hydroxyzine	nil nil	I
Alkylamines	Chlorpheniramine Brompheniramine	+ +	I
Phenothiazines	Promethazine Cyproheptadine	+++ +	I
Second-generation Antihistamines			
Piperidines	Fexofenadine Loratadine	nil nil	
Piperazines	Cetirizine Levocetirizine	nil nil	
Alkylamines	Acrivastine	nil	
Phthalazinones	Azelastine	nil	

I = available in an injection preparation; ANTI-CHOL = Anticholinergic

agents have **significant anticholinergic activity,** and this is responsible for a significant degree of their central effects. Second-generation agents are less lipid-soluble and do not penetrate the blood-brain barrier and hence have much fewer central adverse effects.

The major use of H_1-receptor blockers is in the treatment of allergic reactions. Histamine is released by IgE-sensitized cells, especially mast cells and antihistamines can reduce the rhinitis, conjunctivitis, sneezing, and urticaria associated with this reaction. They are most effective in acute allergic reactions with a relatively low antigen burden, and effectiveness diminishes in chronic disorders. Antihistamines are not effective as monotherapy for bronchial asthma. Antihistamines are marketed for treatment of the common cold, but they have very limited effectiveness in this application and their adverse effects (e.g., sedation) outweigh their benefit. Some of the first-generation agents, especially dimenhydrinate, meclizine, cyclizine, and promethazine, are useful for the prophylaxis of motion sickness and vertigo. **Promethazine** is the most potent in this regard but has pronounced sedative activity that limits its usefulness. The sedating action of some antihistamines has been exploited in their use as sleeping aids.

Diphenhydramine is the most commonly used antihistamine in sleeping preparations. The **major adverse effect of the first-generation agents is sedation.** The **anticholinergic activity** produces atropine-like effects including dry mouth, urinary retention, and cough. Second-generation agents avoid these effects but do have adverse effects such as headache, back pain, and in the GI tract cause nausea, loss of appetite, and constipation or diarrhea. Of the presently available second-generation antihistamines, **cetirizine** causes the highest incidence of fatigue and somnolence (approximately 10%); loratadine appears to have the lowest incidence of this effect (approximately 1–2%). These agents may produce cardiovascular adverse effects such as hypotension, bradycardia or tachycardia, and electrocardiograph (ECG) changes.

Administration

All of the agents listed in Table 24-1 are available for oral use, and some of the first-generation agents are available for parenteral use. Topical application of diphenhydramine is useful in the treatment of minor allergic dermatologic reactions. Azelastine is administered by nasal spray.

Pharmacokinetics

Following oral administration, the H_1 antagonists reach peak levels in about 2–3 hours and last 6–24 hours depending on the agent.

H_2-Receptor Antagonists

Histamine is a potent gastric acid secretagogue and this action is mediated by histamine H_2 receptors. Cimetidine, ranitidine, nizatidine, and famotidine are H_2-specific antagonists and are used to treat gastroesophageal reflux disease and peptic ulcers.

COMPREHENSION QUESTIONS

[24.1] The major use of second-generation histamine H_1-receptor blockers is the treatment of which of the following complaints?

A. Cough associated with influenza
B. Hay fever
C. Motion sickness
D. Sleeplessness

[24.2] You see a long-distance truck driver in the clinic who complains of serious allergic rhinitis. Which of the following would be the best antihistamine to prescribe?

A. Diphenhydramine
B. Fexofenadine
C. Meclizine
D. Promethazine

[24.3] Which of the following statements is correct?

A. Antihistamine agents used for allergic rhinitis have antagonistic activity against both H_1 and H_2 receptors.
B. Antihistamine agents are generally useful in the treatment of asthma.
C. Antihistamines are the preferred agent in the treatment of acute anaphylaxis.
D. Second-generation antihistamines have fewer anticholinergic effects than first-generation antihistamines.

Answers

[24.1]   **B.** First-generation agents that cause sedation have been used as sleeping aids, and some have antiemetic effects.

[24.2]   **B.** The other agents are sedating.

[24.3]   **D.** Second-generation antihistamines have less sedating and anticholinergic side effects than first-generation agents.

PHARMACOLOGY PEARLS

 Second-generation antihistamines do not penetrate the blood-brain barrier and have little sedative effect.

 Antihistamines are of little or no benefit in treating the common cold.

REFERENCES

Borish L. Allergic rhinitis: systemic inflammation and implications for management. J Allergy Clin Immunol 2003 Dec;112(6):1021–31.

Quraishi SA, Davies MJ, Craig TJ. Inflammatory responses in allergic rhinitis: traditional approaches and novel treatment strategies. J Am Osteopath Assoc 2004;104(5 suppl 5):S7–15.

Lanier B. Allergic rhinitis: selective comparisons of the pharmaceutical options for management. Allergy Asthma Proc 2007;28:16–9.

A 40-year-old woman presents for evaluation of her chronic migraine headaches. She reports that approximately once a month she has a severe, unilateral headache associated with nausea and extreme photophobia. The headache will last for a full day if not treated. She has had success in reducing the severity of the headaches with opioid pain medications, but usually she is too nauseous to take them. When she is able to tolerate them, she will have to sleep for several hours afterwards. She is missing about a day of work a month because of the headaches. She has no other significant medical history and takes no medications on a regular basis. Her examination today is normal. You decide to prescribe sumatriptan for her to try with her next migraine headache.

◆ **Which receptor is the site of action of sumatriptan?**

◆ **What is the mechanism of action of sumatriptan?**

ANSWERS TO CASE 25: SEROTONIN RECEPTOR AGONISTS AND ANTAGONISTS

Summary: A 40-year-old woman with migraine headaches is treated with sumatriptan.

◆ **Receptor site of action of sumatriptan:** Serotonin 5-HT$_{1D}$ and 5-HT$_{1B}$ receptors

◆ **Mechanism of action of sumatriptan:** Receptor activation inhibits the activity of adenyl cyclase and decreases cAMP accumulation that results in contraction of arterial smooth muscle, especially in carotid and cranial circulation.

CLINICAL CORRELATION

Migraine headaches are common causes of severe symptoms among patients and a leading cause of absenteeism from work and school. Sumatriptan was the first of a class of serotonin (5-HT) agonist medications for the treatment of migraines. Multiple subtypes of 5-HT receptors have been identified. Sumatriptan specifically acts at the 5-HT$_{1D}$ and 5-HT$_{1B}$ receptor subtypes that are coupled to an inhibition of cAMP. Stimulation of these receptors results in vasoconstriction in the carotid circulation that may directly oppose the vasodilation thought to be involved in migraine. At prejunctional sites, activation of these receptors results in decreased transmission of nociceptive signals in the trigeminal nerve. While being fairly specific for the carotid circulation, there can be activity at other vascular sites. Cerebrovascular, peripheral vascular, mesenteric arterial or coronary artery diseases are all contraindications to its use. Vasospastic coronary disease is a contraindication as well.

APPROACH TO PHARMACOLOGY OF SEROTONIN RECEPTOR AGONISTS AND ANTAGONISTS

Objectives

1. Describe the activity of the different classes of serotonin receptors.
2. List the agents which act as serotonin agonists and describe their mechanisms of action and uses.
3. List the agents which act as serotonin antagonists and describe their mechanisms of action and therapeutic uses.

Definitions

Partial agonist: A drug that at full receptor occupancy produces less of a response than a full agonist. Partial agonists can competitively inhibit the response to a full agonist, including the physiologic response to endogenously released hormones and neurotransmitters.

DISCUSSION

Class

Other than the **triptans** (almotriptan, eletriptan, frovatriptan, naratriptan, riza-triptan, sumatriptan, and zolmitriptan), which are the drugs of choice to treat acute, severe migraine headache, there are few clinically important agents that are direct-acting serotonin-receptor agonists. The **ergot alkaloids** (ergotamine [the prototype], dihydroergotamine, ergonovine, methylergonovine) act through the same mechanisms as the triptans and are used **effectively clinically during the prodrome of a migraine attack. Diarrhea, nausea and vomiting, and drowsiness** are their most common adverse effects. **Prolonged vasospasm** resulting from smooth muscle stimulation is a serious consequence of **overdose** that may result in **gangrene and amputation of arms, legs, or digits. Bowel infarction** has also been reported. They are **contraindicated** for patients with **obstructive vascular disease.**

Because of potential serious **cardiac arrhythmias, cisapride,** a $5\text{-}HT_4$ receptor agonist that promotes release of acetylcholine from the myenteric plexus, is used only compassionately to treat gastroesophageal reflux and motility disease. It also causes GI discomfort and diarrhea in a significant number of patients (about 15%).

The major clinical use of **selective serotonin receptor antagonists** is as first-line drugs for **treatment of nausea and vomiting,** resulting from **vagal stimulation that is associated with surgery and cancer chemotherapy.** These agents, the prototype being **ondansetron** (also granisetron, palonosetron, and dolasetron), act on $5\text{-}HT_3$ receptors. Their most common adverse effects are **headache and constipation.** Dolasetron prolongs the QT interval and, therefore, should not be administered to patients with this condition or with other similarly acting drugs.

Alosetron is a $5\text{-}HT_3$ receptor antagonist that is used to treat **IBS with diarrhea.** It is only approved for treatment of women because efficacy has not been documented for men. Its major adverse effects are constipation that may be severe and require discontinuation of therapy. **Ischemic colitis** (incidence about 0.3%), may be **fatal** and therefore precludes the use of alosetron except for patients who have not responded to other therapies.

Mechanism of Action

The **ergot alkaloids** (dihydroergotamine, ergonovine, ergotamine, the prototype, methylergonovine) have **agonist and partial agonist activity at serotonin** ($5\text{-}HT_{1D}$ receptors and $5\text{-}HT_{1A}$ receptors) that, like the triptans (see above), are responsible for their therapeutic action. Their antagonist and agonist and partial agonist activity at α-adrenergic receptors and dopamine receptors are responsible for some adverse actions. Cisapride activation of $5\text{-}HT_4$ receptors on enteric neurons promotes release of acetylcholine that results in increased lower esophageal sphincter pressure. Ondansetron and other selective serotonin antagonists act to inhibit nausea and vomiting through peripheral blockade of serotonin 5-HT$_3$ receptors on intestinal vagal afferent nerves, and through central blockade of serotonin 5-HT$_3$ receptors in the vomiting center and chemoreceptor trigger zone.

Alosetron and palonosetron are highly selective serotonin receptor 5-HT$_3$ antagonists that act peripherally on enteric afferent and cholinergic neurons to reduce intestinal activity and visceral afferent pain. It also acts centrally on the same receptors to inhibit afferent nerve activation of the CNS.

Administration

Sumatriptan may be administered orally, as a subcutaneous injection, or as a nasal spray, making it particularly valuable for migraine patients with nausea and vomiting as symptoms. Ergotamines are available for oral, sublingual rectal, parenteral, and inhaler administration.

Selective serotonin receptor antagonists can be administered orally or IV. They are most effective against nausea and vomiting when administered IV prior to the administration of chemotherapeutic agents.

Pharmacokinetics

Cisapride is metabolized by microsomal enzymes that are inhibited by a wide variety of agents and can lead to large increases in cisapride serum levels and toxicity. Tegaserod is poorly absorbed and should be taken before meals. Severe hepatic or renal disease may significantly reduce its clearance. Ergotamine tartrate may be administered combined with caffeine which facilitates its absorption.

COMPREHENSION QUESTIONS

[25.1] Sumatriptan does which of the following?

    A. Causes vasoconstriction in the carotid and cranial circulation
    B. Increases transmission of nociceptive signals in the trigeminal nerve
    C. Increases adenyl cyclase activity
    D. Is an antagonist at the 5-HT$_{1D}$ receptor subtype

[25.2] The major clinical use of ondansetron is which of the following?

    A. Compassionate treatment of gastroesophageal reflux and motility disease
    B. Major depression
    C. Migraine headache
    D. Nausea and vomiting that is associated with surgery and cancer chemotherapy

[25.3] Prolonged vasospasm is a serious consequence of which of the following?

    A. Alosetron
    B. Cisapride
    C. Ergotamine
    D. Ondansetron

Answers

[25.1] **A.** Sumatriptan, a 5-HT$_{1D}$ receptor agonist, inhibits the activity of adenylyl cyclase and decreases cAMP accumulation that results in contraction of arterial smooth muscle, especially in carotid and cranial circulation.

[25.2] **D.** The major clinical use of ondansetron, a 5-HT$_3$ receptor antagonist, is for treatment of nausea and vomiting that is associated with surgery and cancer chemotherapy. Migraine is treated with triptans and ergot alkaloids. Cisapride, a 5-HT$_4$ receptor agonist, is used only compassionately to treat gastroesophageal reflux and motility disease. Selective serotonin reuptake inhibitors (SSRIs) act to block serotonin transporters and are used to treat major depression.

[25.3] **C.** Prolonged vasospasm caused by smooth muscle stimulation is a serious consequence of overdose with ergotamine. The most common adverse effects of ondansetron are headache and constipation. Serious cardiac arrhythmia is a serious adverse effect of cisapride. The major adverse effect of alosetron, a 5-HT$_3$ receptor antagonist, is constipation.

PHARMACOLOGY PEARLS

 Because the vasoconstrictor activity of ergotamine is long-lasting, its dose and frequency of administration must be limited.

 Ergot alkaloid agents can cause vasoconstriction and should not be used in patients with occlusive vascular disease.

 The effects of selective serotonin receptor antagonists like ondansetron seem to be enhanced with concomitant administration of dexamethasone.

REFERENCES

Lake AE, Saper JR. Chronic headache. New advances in treatment strategies. Neurology 2002;59:S8.

Ramadan NM. Current trends in migraine prophylaxis. Headache 2007;47(suppl 1): S52–7.

You are called to see a 24-year-old G_3P_3 woman who approximately 1 hour ago underwent a vaginal delivery of an 8 lb infant. The nurse is concerned that the patient is continuing to bleed more than would be expected, and that her uterine fundus does not feel firm. A brief history from the nurse reveals that the patient required IV oxytocin augmentation of her labor, but otherwise had an uncomplicated labor and delivery. Her placenta delivered spontaneously and intact. She has no significant medical history. Examination of the patient reveals her to be comfortable and cooperative but she is mildly tachycardic. Her uterine fundus is boggy and nontender on palpation. Vaginal examination shows no cervical or vaginal lacerations, but there is a steady flow of blood from the still-dilated cervix. You diagnose the patient as having a postpartum hemorrhage secondary to uterine atony and order an immediate intramuscular (IM) injection of methylergonovine.

◆ **What is the mechanism of action of methylergonovine?**

◆ **What are the common adverse effects of methylergonovine?**

ANSWERS TO CASE 26: ERGOT ALKALOIDS

Summary: A 24-year-old woman has a postpartum hemorrhage secondary to uterine atony. She is given an IM injection of methylergonovine.

◆ **Mechanism of action of methylergonovine:** α-adrenoceptor agonist with activity on uterine smooth muscle, causing forceful and prolonged uterine contraction.

◆ **Side effects of methylergonovine:** hypertension, headaches, nausea, vomiting.

CLINICAL CORRELATION

Methylergonovine is an amine ergot alkaloid with relatively selective activity at uterine smooth muscle. Ergot alkaloids are structurally similar to norepinephrine, dopamine, and serotonin. They can have agonist or antagonist effects on α-adrenoceptors, dopamine receptors, and serotonin receptors. Methylergonovine acts primarily via α-adrenoceptors and 5-HT$_2$ receptors to cause tetanic uterine contraction. This provides its therapeutic benefit in the treatment of postpartum hemorrhage because of uterine atony. This drug can have other effects mediated by α-adrenoceptors, including acute hypertensive reactions and vasospasm. It is contraindicated in patients with uncontrolled hypertension. Other common side effects include headaches, nausea, and vomiting.

APPROACH TO PHARMACOLOGY OF THE ERGOT ALKALOIDS

Objectives

1. Know the mechanism of action of the ergot alkaloids.
2. Know the therapeutic uses and side effects of ergot alkaloids.

Definitions

Postpartum hemorrhage: Vaginal bleeding exceeding 500 mL after a vaginal delivery or 1000 mL after a cesarean delivery. The most common etiology is uterine atony.

Migraine: A familial disorder marked by periodic, usually unilateral, pulsatile headaches that begin in childhood or early adult life and tend to recur with diminishing frequency in later life. There are two closely related syndromes comprising what is known as migraine. They are classic migraine (migraine with aura) and common migraine (migraine without aura).

DISCUSSION

Class

The ergot alkaloids are produced by the fungi *Claviceps purpurea*. There are two major families of ergots: the peptide ergots and the amine ergots, all contain the tetracyclic ergoline nucleus. The peptide ergots include ergotamine, α-ergocryptine and bromocriptine; the amine ergots include lysergic acid, lysergic acid diethylamide, ergonovine, and methysergide. The ergots have agonist, partial agonist, and antagonist actions at α-adrenergic receptors and serotonin receptors, and agonist or partial agonist actions at central dopamine receptors.

Postpartum Hemorrhage

Ergonovine and its semisynthetic derivative, methylergonovine, cause **powerful contractions of smooth muscle;** the gravid uterus is especially sensitive to this drug. Postpartum hemorrhage is most often treated with oxytocin. In circumstances where oxytocin is not effective, methylergonovine causes forceful contractions of uterine smooth muscle that effectively stops the bleeding. This action appears to be mediated by agonist activity at α_1-adrenergic receptors and agonist action at 5-HT$_2$ receptors. Methylergonovine can be administered orally or IM; effects are seen in 3–5 minutes following IM administration. Acute administration of methylergonovine has few side effects.

Migraine Headache

Dihydroergotamine is useful in the management of migraines. It binds with high affinity to 5-HT$_{1D\alpha}$ and 5-HT$_{1D\beta}$ receptors. It also binds with high affinity to serotonin 5-HT$_{1A}$, 5-HT$_{2A}$, and 5-HT$_{2C}$ receptors, noradrenaline α_{2A}, α_{2B}, and α receptors, and dopamine D$_{2L}$ and D$_3$ receptors. The therapeutic activity of dihydroergotamine in migraine is generally attributed to the agonist effect at 5-HT$_{1D}$ receptors. Two current theories have been proposed to explain the efficacy of 5-HT$_{1D}$ receptor agonists in migraine. One theory suggests that activation of 5-HT$_{1D}$ receptors located on carotid and intracranial blood vessels, including those on arteriovenous anastomoses, leads to vasoconstriction, which correlates with the relief of migraine headache. The alternative hypothesis suggests that activation of 5-HT$_{1D}$ receptors on sensory nerve endings of the trigeminal system results in the inhibition of proinflammatory neuropeptide release. Adverse effects include GI disturbances including diarrhea, vomiting, and vasospasm. The triptans—sumatriptan, rizatriptan, almotriptan, and others—are selective 5-HT$_{1D}$ and 5-HT$_{1B}$ receptor agonists that are also useful for treating an acute migraine headache.

Methysergide is used for **prophylaxis** of migraine. It acts as a 5-HT$_{2A,C}$ antagonist to block 5-HT mediated vasoconstriction in vascular smooth muscle. It is effective in preventing or reducing the frequency of migraines in approximately 60 percent of patients. Chronic use of methysergide is associated with **retroperitoneal fibroplasia and subendocardial fibrosis.** For this reason drug-free periods are recommended if it is used chronically.

Endocrine Abnormalities

Bromocriptine is very effective in reducing the high levels of prolactin production that occur with certain pituitary tumors. It has also been used to suppress lactation. Bromocriptine is a potent dopamine receptor agonist, and its prolactin-suppressive actions are mediated via interaction with this receptor. Side effects are dose related and range from nausea to Parkinson-like syndrome. Bromocriptine has been associated with postpartum cardiovascular toxicity.

COMPREHENSION QUESTIONS

[26.1] Methylergonovine is useful in treating postpartum hemorrhage because it does which of the following?

A. Causes forceful contractions of the myometrium
B. Causes rapid production of thrombin
C. Is a potent vasoconstrictor
D. Stimulates the activity of antithrombin III

[26.2] Which of the following would be the best drug to reduce prolactin levels in a patient with a pituitary tumor?

A. Bromocriptine
B. Ergonovine
C. Ergotamine
D. Methysergide

[26.3] A 35-year-old woman is noted to have dyspnea with exertion. Echocardiography identifies a restrictive cardiomyopathy with decreased flexibility of the heart. The cardiologist notes that one of his medications may be responsible. Which of the following agents is most likely the etiology?

A. Bromocriptine
B. Ergonovine
C. Ergotamine
D. Methysergide

Answers

[26.1]   **A.** Although methylergonovine does cause vasoconstriction, its action in postpartum hemorrhage is mediated by forceful clamping of the myometrium, which restricts blood flow.

[26.2]   **A.** Bromocriptine is a dopamine receptor agonist that is used to treat prolactin-secreting pituitary adenomas.

[26.3]   **D.** Methysergide can induce a fibroelastosis of the heart, which leads to a restrictive cardiomyopathy.

PHARMACOLOGY PEARLS

 Methysergide is useful for prophylaxis of migraine headaches but has no effect on an acute episode.

 Bromocriptine is a dopamine receptor agonist and is used to treat prolactin-secreting pituitary adenomas.

 Methylergonovine is used to treat postpartum hemorrhage caused by uterine atony and causes contraction of the uterine smooth muscle.

REFERENCES

de Groot AN, van Dongen PW, Vree TB, et al. Ergot alkaloids. Current status and review of clinical pharmacology and therapeutic use compared with other oxytocics in obstetrics and gynaecology. Drugs 1998;56(4):523–35.
Schiff PL. Ergot and its alkaloids. Am J Pharm Educ 2006;70:98–108.

A 24-year-old G_3P_3 woman, now 90 minutes after vaginal delivery and having received an injection of methylergonovine, continues to have postpartum bleeding. Her uterus is firmer but still somewhat boggy. Her heart rate remains mildly tachycardic, but her blood pressure has gone up in response to the methylergonovine. Her examination is otherwise unchanged. You now order an IM injection of carboprost tromethamine (prostaglandin $F_{2\alpha}$, or $PGF_{2\alpha}$).

◆ **What is the therapeutic action of $PGF_{2\alpha}$ in postpartum hemorrhage?**

◆ **What is the effect of PGFs on vascular smooth muscle?**

◆ **What is the effect of PGFs on bronchial smooth muscle?**

ANSWERS TO CASE 27: EICOSANOIDS

Summary: A 24-year-old woman has continued postpartum hemorrhage despite ergot alkaloids.

◆ **Therapeutic action of PGF$_{2\alpha}$:** Causes contraction of uterine smooth muscle.

◆ **Effect on vascular smooth muscle:** Arteriolar vasodilation and constriction of superficial veins.

◆ **Effect on bronchial smooth muscle:** Smooth muscle contraction.

CLINICAL CORRELATION

Eicosanoids are a large and varied group of autocoids with effects on most tissues in the body. They are derivatives of eicosanoic acids and are synthesized through-out the body. They typically have short plasma half-lives and are catabolized in the lung. There is no common mechanism of eicosanoid action. Specific cell surface receptors mediate activities of each class of eicosanoid and many different second messenger pathways are involved. Prostaglandin F$_{2\alpha}$ (PGF$_{2\alpha}$) is produced via the prostaglandin H synthase (cyclooxygenase) pathway. It causes arteriolar vasodila-tion, superficial vein constriction, and bronchial smooth muscle contraction and increases the rate of longitudinal muscle contraction in the GI tract. It causes con-traction of uterine smooth muscle in the pregnant uterus. This effect mediates its primary therapeutic use, the treatment of postpartum hemorrhage. Because of the risk of bronchospasm, its use is contraindicated in asthmatics. It can cause nausea, vomiting, diarrhea, and cramps as a result of its effect on the GI tract.

APPROACH TO PHARMACOLOGY
OF THE EICOSANOIDS

Objectives

1. Know the pathways of eicosanoid synthesis.
2. Know the actions of eicosanoids on tissues throughout the body.
3. Know the therapeutic uses, adverse effects, and contraindications to the use of eicosanoids.

Definitions

Eicosanoids: Metabolites of 20-carbon fatty acids.
Prostanoids: Prostaglandins and thromboxanes.
COX: Cyclooxygenase, rate-limiting enzymes (COX-1 and COX-2) in prostaglandin biosynthesis.
HETE: Hydroxyeicosatetraenoic acid.
EET: Epoxyeicosatrienoic acid.

DISCUSSION

Class

The **eicosanoids** are **fatty acid metabolites** that include the **prostaglandins, the thromboxanes,** and the **HETEs** and the **EETs.** These small molecules affect nearly every physiologic system, including blood flow, especially in the kidney, airway diameter, inflammation, ovulation, and uterine smooth muscle tone. The eicosanoids are metabolites of the **20-carbon fatty acid arachidonic acid.** A substrate pool of arachidonic acid is stored as part of the lipids in the plasma membrane. Figure 27-1 outlines the two major biosynthetic routes of eicosanoic metabolites. Most of the free arachidonic acid in cells is liberated from the plasma membrane phospholipid by phospholipase A_2. A minor amount can be liberated from phosphatidylinositides by the action of phospholipase C and diglyceride lipase. The free arachidonic acid is metabolized by either cyclooxygenase to form prostaglandins and thromboxane, or by **lipoxygenases** to form the **HETEs** and **leukotrienes.** There are two isoforms of cyclooxygenases that catalyze the same reaction.

    Cyclooxygenase type 1 (COX-1) is fairly widely distributed in the **stomach, kidneys, and connective tissues.** COX-1 is expressed in a constitutive manner. **COX-2** is also expressed in numerous tissues including the **GI tract, kidneys, ovaries,** and **connective tissues.** Basal cyclooxygenase type 2 (COX-2) expression is very low, but it is highly induced by cytokines, growth factors, and serum factors. The cyclooxygenases perform two catalytic steps: a **cyclooxygenase reaction that introduces oxygen and a peroxidase** reaction that yields PGH_2, the **immediate precursor to all prostaglandins and thromboxane.** PGH_2 is further metabolized to prostaglandins or thromboxane depending on the tissue. **Platelets contain predominantly thromboxane synthase and produce thromboxane A_2; endothelial cells** contain predominantly **prostacyclin synthase and produce PGI_2;** other cells contain specific prostaglandin synthases and produce prostaglandins A–J.

    Lymphocytes and other myeloid cells contain **lipoxygenases** that convert PGH_2 into HETEs or leukotrienes via an unstable HETEs intermediate. Leukocytes express both 5-lipoxygenase and 12-lipoxygenase and produce the corresponding HETEs and the leukotrienes. Platelets express only 12-lipoxygenase and produce 12-HETE.

    Two other metabolic pathways have been shown to produce other arachidonate metabolites. Free arachidonate can be metabolized by members of the P450 family to the EETs that have potent vascular and renal effects. Arachidonate acid intact on a phospholipid can be acted on by free radicals to produce the isoprostanes via a nonenzymatic pathway. The isoprostanes may be important in inflammation but their physiologic role is still under investigation. Eicosanoids have a myriad of effects; only those that are pharmacologically relevant will be discussed here.

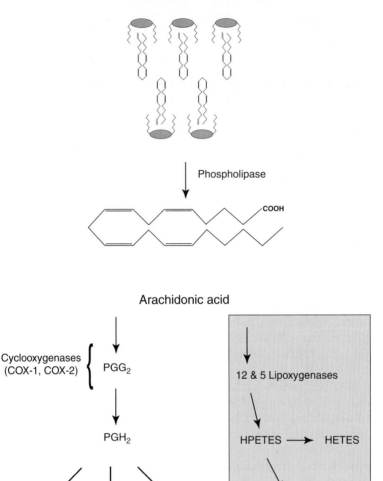

Figure 27-1. Synthesis of eicosanoids.

Vascular System

PGE$_2$ and PGI$_2$ (prostacyclin) are potent vasodilators in most vascular beds. PGI$_2$ is about five times more potent than PGE$_2$ in reducing blood pressure. PGF$_{2\alpha}$ typically causes vasoconstriction especially in pulmonary arteries and veins, and vasoconstricts superficial veins. **Thromboxane A$_2$ is a potent vasoconstrictor** and is a smooth muscle cell mitogen.

Other Smooth Muscle

PGEs relax bronchial and tracheal smooth muscle. The response of the uterine myometrium is complex with low doses of PGE_2 causing contraction and high doses causing relaxation. In the GI tract, PGEs relax circular smooth muscle but the longitudinal muscle is contracted. $PGF_{2\alpha}$, PGD, and TXA_2 cause bronchoconstriction in the airways and contraction of GI smooth muscle.

Gastrointestinal Secretion

PGEs and PGI_2 inhibit gastric acid and pepsin production and increase mucus production; these actions are cytoprotective in the upper GI tract.

Kidney

Prostaglandins are important local regulators of renal blood flow. PGEs and PGI_2 increase renal blood flow and diuresis without changing the glomerular filtration rate. TXA_2 decreases renal blood flow and glomerular filtration rate.

Pharmacologic Uses of Eicosanoids

PGE_1 can be used in neonates to maintain patency of the ductus arteriosus. Infants born with certain congenital heart abnormalities depend on a patent ductus to maintain adequate pulmonary blood flow. **PGE_1** is used to temporarily maintain the patency until surgery can be performed. **PGE_1,** because of its vasodilatory action, can be injected into the corpus cavernosum of the **penis to induce erection.** This use has been largely supplanted by the **phosphodiesterase V inhibitors such as sildenafil. PGE_1 analogs have also been used for cytoprotection of NSAID-induced gastric and peptic ulcers.** This is based on the protective action mediated by the reduction in acid and pepsin production and increased mucus production produced by PGE_1. PGE_1 and PGI_2 and their congeners PGE_2 and PGI_2 have also been used to treat peripheral occlusive vascular disease and have been used for treating Raynaud disease and arteriosclerosis obliterans. Because of its effect to inhibit platelet aggregation and its short half-life, PGI_2 can be used during dialysis instead of heparin. It has also been used to treat pulmonary arterial hypertension.

Uterine contractions are stimulated by 15-methyl-$PGF_{2\alpha}$. It can be used to control persistent postpartum hemorrhage secondary to uterine atony that is unresponsive to other drugs. Besides, 15-methyl-$PGF_{2\alpha}$ can be used in the first and second trimester to induce abortion. PGE_2 congeners are used to facilitate cervical ripening and for the induction of labor. PGE_2 is combined with the antiprogestin RU-486 (mifepristone) to induce first-trimester abortion. Side effects are usually nausea and vomiting. It is contraindicated in asthmatics because of its bronchoconstrictive activities.

Structure

Prostaglandins are derived by metabolism of the 20-carbon fatty acid arachidonic acid.

Mechanism of Action

There are a number of specific membrane receptors that mediate the action of the prostaglandins. There are four prostaglandin E receptors (EP_1–EP_4), two prostaglandin F receptors (FPA and FPB), one prostaglandin I_2 receptor (IP), and two thromboxane receptors (TP_α and TP_β), and two prostaglandin D receptors (DP and $CRTH_2$). These receptors are coupled to increases or decreases in cAMP, and increases in inositol-3 phosphate.

Administration

Most prostaglandins or their analogs are administered by local instillation (e.g., vaginal or cervical gels or suppositories) or continuous infusion. Misoprostol, a PGE_1 analog, is available for oral administration.

Pharmacokinetics

Prostaglandins are rapidly absorbed and inactivated in lung, liver, and kidney. Both the natural prostaglandins and their analogs have a very short half-life (typically minutes).

COMPREHENSION QUESTIONS

[27.1] Which of the following enzymes do leukotrienes require for their biosynthesis?

    A. COX-1
    B. COX-2
    C. 5-Lipoxygenase
    D. 8-Lipoxygenase

[27.2] PGI_2 can be used to achieve which of the following?

    A. Cause peripheral vasoconstriction
    B. Control bleeding from the uterine artery
    C. Facilitate blood clotting
    D. Treat occlusive vascular disease

[27.3] A 38-year-old woman is taking ibuprofen for severe dysmenorrhea but develops epigastric pain. The physician prescribes a medication to prevent gastritis. Which of the following best describes the medication?

A. PGE_1 analog
B. PGE_1 antagonist
C. PGE_2 analog
D. PGE_2 antagonist
E. PGE_2 analog
F. PGE_2 antagonist
G. PGI analog
H. PGI antagonist

Answers

[27.1] **C.** Production of leukotrienes requires 5-lipoxygenase.

[27.2] **D.** PGE_2 and PGI_2 are vasodilators in all vascular beds.

[27.3] **A.** PGE_1 analog, misoprostol, is used to prevent NSAID-associated gastritis.

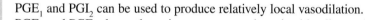

PHARMACOLOGY PEARLS

 PGE_1 and PGI_2 can be used to produce relatively local vasodilation.
 PGE_2 and $PGF_{2\alpha}$ have obstetric uses to control uterine bleeding and to hasten parturition.
 15-methyl-$PGF_{2\alpha}$ stimulates uterine contractions. It can be used to control persistent postpartum hemorrhage.
❖ Thromboxane is a potent vasoconstrictor.

REFERENCES

Rayburn WF. Prostaglandin E2 gel for cervical ripening and induction of labor: a critical analysis. Am J Obstet Gynecol 1989;160:529–34.
Gulmwzoglu A, Forna F, Villar J, et al. Prostaglandins for preventing postpartum haemorrhage. Cochrane Database Syst Rev 2007;18:CD00094.

A 16-year-old female comes to the physician's office because of menstrual cramps. She had menarche at age 13. Her menses lasts for 4–5 days, and she has 28-day cycles. For the first 2–3 days of her menses she states that she has very bad cramping. The cramps have occurred since menarche and seem to have worsened in the past year. They have been so bad at times that she has missed school and has not been able to participate in her after-school sports. She has been taking acetaminophen and over-the-counter "menstrual cramp" pills without adequate relief. She has no significant medical history, takes no medications regularly, and is not sexually active. Her examination is normal. You assess the problem as primary dysmenorrhea and prescribe diclofenac to be used on an as-needed basis.

◆ **What are the therapeutic effects of nonsteroidal anti-inflammatory drugs (NSAIDs)?**

◆ **What is the mechanism of the anti-inflammatory action of NSAIDs?**

ANSWERS TO CASE 28: NONSTEROIDAL ANTI-INFLAMMATORY DRUGS

Summary: A 16-year-old female with dysmenorrhea is prescribed diclofenac [Voltaren-XR].

◆ **Effects of NSAIDs:** Anti-inflammatory, analgesic, and antipyretic.

◆ **Mechanism of action:** Anti-inflammatory effect primarily resulting from inhibition of cyclooxygenase 1 and/or cyclooxygenase 2; may also involve interference with other mediators of inflammation, modulation of T-cell function, stabilization of lysosomal membranes, and inhibition of chemotaxis.

CLINICAL CORRELATION

NSAIDs are widely used for acute and chronic conditions that cause pain, injury, inflammation, or fever. They are available over-the-counter and by prescription. The anti-inflammatory effect is a result of the inhibition of cyclooxygenase (COX), which converts arachidonic acid to prostaglandins. There are two major subtypes of the COX enzyme, with the COX-2 subtype primarily mediating the pain and inflammation responses in tissues throughout the body. COX-1 has significant activity in producing prostaglandins that appear to protect the GI mucosal lining. **Aspirin irreversibly inactivates both COX-1 and COX-2,** whereas all other **NSAIDs are reversible inhibitors of one or both of these enzymes.** The analgesic effect of these medications is thought to be related to the peripheral inhibition of prostaglandin production, but there may be a central inhibition of pain stimuli as well. The antipyretic effect is thought to involve inhibition of IL-1- and IL-6-induced production of prostaglandins in the hypothalamus affecting the thermoregulatory system, resulting in vasodilation and increased heat loss. NSAIDs are metabolized in the liver and excreted by the kidney. They exhibit cross-sensitivity with each other and with aspirin. All NSAIDs can cause non-dose-related episodes of acute renal failure and nephrotic syndrome. They should be used with caution in those with renal insufficiency or in patients taking other potentially nephrotoxic agents. Aspirin and NSAIDs that nonselectively inhibit both COX-1 and COX-2 commonly produce GI disturbances and ulceration. They are contraindicated in persons with known peptic ulcer disease. Newer agents with higher selectivity for COX-2 inhibition have fewer GI side effects and may reduce the rate of NSAID-related gastric ulcers, but have been linked to increased risk of cardiovascular disease.

APPROACH TO PHARMACOLOGY OF NSAIDS

Objectives

1. Know the mechanism of action of aspirin and other NSAIDs.
2. Know the therapeutic uses of NSAIDs.
3. Know the adverse effects, toxicities, and contraindications to NSAID use.

Definitions

Inflammation: A local response to cellular injury that is marked by capillary dilatation, leukocytic infiltration, redness, heat, pain, and swelling.

Familial adenomatous polyposis (FAP): A genetic disorder leading to abnormal growths in the colon.

DISCUSSION

Class

(See Case 27 on eicosanoids for a description of the biosynthesis of the prostaglandins and leukotrienes.) NSAIDs are among the most widely used drugs and are available in various formulations both over-the-counter and by prescription. They are widely used for the relief of pain and fever and to reduce inflammation. There are more than 23 NSAIDs available, and they represent a number of structural classes. Table 28-1 summarizes this class of drugs. They are all small acidic compounds. All are orally active with some pharmacologic differences but they all share the following:

Table 28-1
CLASSES OF NSAIDS

CARBOXYLIC ACIDS			PYRAZOLONES	OXICAMS
Salicylates	Acetic acids	Propionic acids	Phenylbutazone	Piroxicam
Acetylsalicyclic acid	Indomethacin	Ibuprofen	Apazone	Meloxicam
Salicyclic acid	Diclofenac	Naproxen		
	Sulindac	Ketoprofen		
	Tolmetin	Pranoprofen Miroprofen		

Analgesic activity. Effective against pain of low-to-moderate intensity. Lower maximal effects compared to opioids, but no CNS liability.

Anti-inflammatory activity. It is their chief clinical application. They provide symptomatic relief only.

Antipyretic activity.

Gastric and intestinal ulceration. Two mechanisms include local irritation caused by acidic drug, and inhibition of prostaglandins, which exert a cytoprotective effect.

Carboxylic Acids

The salicylates, acetylsalicylic acid (ASA, aspirin), and sodium salicylate have been used for hundreds of years for their analgesic properties. **ASA acts to covalently and irreversibly inhibit both COX-1 and COX-2.** COX-1 becomes acetylated at a serine in the cyclooxygenase-active site, rendering the enzyme inactive. COX-2 is also covalently modified but at a different serine residue. This also eliminates cyclooxygenase activity and alters COX-2 to produce 15-HETE. 15-HETE can be further metabolized to a potent anti-inflammatory compound, 15-epilipoxin A_4. Some of the anti-inflammatory activity of aspirin might be mediated by this metabolite. Inhibition of cyclooxygenase activity of both COX isoforms decreases prostaglandin and thromboxane production, but does not effect the production of eicosanoids through the lipoxygenase pathway. Sodium and magnesium salicylate lack the acetyl group that modifies the COXs and are much weaker anti-inflammatory agents. Their mechanism of action may be to reduce free radical production that is necessary to activate the cyclooxygenases.

Aspirin can be used to reduce pain, temperature, and inflammation. The anti-inflammatory properties make it useful in rheumatoid arthritis (RA), rheumatic fever, and other diseases that produce joint pain.

The **adverse effects of aspirin are dose related. At low doses,** most adverse effects are confined to the **GI tract, commonly gastritis.** At **higher** doses patients suffer **"salicylism," tinnitus, vomiting, and vertigo.** Serious aspirin overdose affects the medulla directly and **depresses respiration.**

Acetic and Propionic Acids

Indomethacin, ibuprofen, diclofenac, and naproxen are other important NSAIDs. Although they reduce prostaglandin production by **inhibiting COX-1 and COX-2,** the mechanism of this inhibition is different from aspirin. These drugs are **reversible inhibitors** of the enzyme and appear to act by interfering with the **binding of arachidonate.** All have been approved for rheumatic disorders, osteoarthritis, localized musculoskeletal pain, dysmenorrhea, and headache. All are readily absorbed from the GI tract. Indomethacin and diclofenac are the most potent of these drugs in inhibiting cyclooxygenase. **Indomethacin also has the highest incidence (35–50%) of adverse effects, most commonly GI. Indomethacin** has been found to produce **ulceration of the upper GI tract.** Naproxen and ibuprofen are also associated with frequent GI adverse effects but are less severe and better tolerated. **All of the NSAIDs can produce renal toxicities including acute renal failure.**

Specific COX-2 Inhibitors

Considerable effort has gone into the development of agents that **specifically inhibit COX-2** compared to COX-1. In theory, such agents would be efficacious for **treating inflammatory states but have fewer adverse effects,** especially in the GI tract because COX-1 would still be able to provide cytoprotection. Two clinical trials support this notion but these drugs still produce adverse effects in the GI tract. Additional studies on total mortality and morbidity will be necessary. **Celecoxib [Celebrex] is the only specific COX-2 inhibitor in the US market. Rofecoxib [Vioxx] and valdecoxib [Bextra] were removed from the market due to an increase in risk of cardiovascular disease and stroke.** It is unclear whether all members of this class are associated with this increase in cardiovascular risk which appears mostly due to myocardial infarction. Celecoxib is useful in treating osteoarthritis, RA, ankylosing spondylitis, dysmenorrhea, acute pain, and pain caused by migraine. **Celecoxib is approved for the treatment of FAP.** Adverse effects are diminished with COX-2-specific inhibitors, but there are still significant side effects. Rare instances of serious stomach and intestinal bleeding have been reported. Hepatotoxicity and acute renal failure have also occurred. Less serious side effects include dyspepsia, diarrhea, peripheral edema, and dizziness.

Other Agents

Acetaminophen is a **non-anti-inflammatory** analgesic agent. It is about as effective at reducing fever and as an analgesic as aspirin, but it lacks anti-inflammatory activity and does not inhibit platelet aggregation. The most important toxicity of acetaminophen is hepatotoxicity. This is caused by the metabolism of the drug to *N*-acetyl-p-benzoquinoneimine (NAPB), which is usually **eliminated by hepatic conjugation with glutathione.** Toxic levels of acetaminophen deplete glutathione and NAPB accumulates to toxic levels. Other adverse effects include skin rash and mild dyspepsia.

COMPREHENSION QUESTIONS

[28.1] Which of the following is the most effective in reducing risk of myocardial infarction?

    A. Acetaminophen
    B. Aspirin
    C. Celecoxib
    D. Ibuprofen

[28.2] Which of the following is the advantage of specific cyclooxygenase-2 (COX-2) inhibitors?

A. Decreased GI side effects
B. Decreased vasoconstrictor activity
C. Increased anti-inflammatory activity
D. Increased inhibition of platelet aggregation

[28.3] A 26-year-old woman takes a "handful" of acetaminophen in a suicide attempt. At the emergency department, it is determined that she has taken enough to be potentially harmful. Which of the following is the best treatment for this patient?

A. Calcium gluconate
B. IgG against acetaminophen
C. N-acetylcysteine
D. Penicillamine

Answers

[28.1] **B.** Aspirin. Because aspirin irreversibly inhibits cyclooxygenase, it effectively eliminates thromboxane production by platelets. It can do this at low doses that do not impair the production of beneficial PGI_2 by endothelial cells.

[28.2] **A.** In theory, inhibition of COX-2 would reduce inflammation and pain while leaving the cytoprotective actions of COX-1 intact. However, the two enzymes appear to overlap in their functions to a considerable degree.

[28.3] **C.** Excess acetaminophen is metabolized in the liver via the mixed function oxidase P450 system to a toxic metabolite, NAPB, which has an extremely short half-life and is rapidly conjugated with glutathione, a sulfhydryl donor, and removed from the system. Under conditions of excessive NAPB formation or reduced glutathione stores, NAPB is free to covalently bind to vital proteins and the lipid bilayer of hepatocytes; this results in hepatocellular death and subsequent centrilobular liver necrosis. The antidote for acetaminophen poisoning is N-acetyl-L-cysteine (NAC), which prevents the formation and accumulation of NAPB, increases glutathione stores, combines directly with NAPB as a glutathione substitute, and enhances sulfate conjugation.

PHARMACOLOGY PEARLS

❖ Aspirin is an irreversible inhibitor of both COX-1 and COX-2.
❖ Acetaminophen does not have anti-inflammatory activity.
❖ The COX-2-specific anti-inflammatory agents may have fewer GI side effects but increase the risk of cardiovascular events.

REFERENCES

Bombardier C, Laine L, Reicin A, et al. Comparison of upper gastrointestinal toxicity of rofecoxib and naproxen in patients with rheumatoid arthritis. VIGOR study group. N Engl J Med 2000;343:1520–28.

Silverstein FE, Faich G, Goldstein JL, et al. Gastrointestinal toxicity with celecoxib vs nonsteroidal antiinflammatory drugs for osteoarthritis and rheumatoid arthritis: the CLASS study: a randomized controlled trial. Celecoxib long-term arthritis safety study. JAMA 2000;284:1247–55.

Solomon DH, Avorn J, Sturmer T, et al. Cardiovascular outcomes in new users of coxibs and nonsteroidal anti-inflammatory drugs: high-risk subgroups and time course of risk. Arthritis Rheum 2006;54:1378–89.

A 58-year-old man presents for follow-up of gout. He has had multiple episodes of gouty arthritis, primarily in the great toe. Each episode has been successfully treated with oral anti-inflammatory medications. He takes no medications regularly and has a normal examination today. Laboratory studies following his last episode showed an elevated uric acid level and normal renal function. A 24-hour urine collection showed normal excretion of uric acid. You prescribe allopurinol to be taken daily in an effort to lower his uric acid level and prevent recurrent gout episodes.

◆ **Which medications are used for the treatment of acute gout?**

◆ **Which medications are used for the treatment of chronic gout?**

◆ **What is the mechanism of action of allopurinol?**

ANSWERS TO CASE 29: MEDICATIONS USED FOR GOUT

Summary: A 58-year-old man with hyperuricemia and recurrent gout is pre-scribed allopurinol.

◆ **Drugs for the treatment of acute gout:** Nonsteroidal anti-inflammatory agents (NSAIDs), colchicine, corticosteroids.

◆ **Drugs for the treatment of recurrent gout:** Probenecid, sulfinpyrazone, allopurinol.

◆ **Mechanism of action of allopurinol:** Inhibition of xanthine oxidase, an enzyme that converts hypoxanthine to xanthine and xanthine to uric acid.

CLINICAL CORRELATION

Allopurinol is the only medication used in clinical practice to **lower uric acid production.** Uric acid is the end product of purine metabolism. The **enzyme xanthine oxidase converts hypoxanthine to xanthine and xan-thine to uric acid.** Allopurinol and its metabolite, alloxanthine, inhibit the synthesis of uric acid by inhibiting xanthine oxidase. Allopurinol may pre-cipitate acute gout when therapy is initiated. Colchicine may be coadmin-istered for the first week of allopurinol therapy to try to reduce the risk of an acute gout flare. Its primary side effects are GI disturbance and rash. There is a very rare, but potentially life-threatening, hypersensitivity reac-tion that may cause fever, bone marrow suppression, hepatic dysfunction, and renal failure.

APPROACH TO MEDICATIONS FOR GOUT

Objectives

1. Know the primary drugs used for gout and their mechanisms of action.
2. Know the adverse effects and contraindications to their usage.

Definitions

Prophylactic: Prevention of a disease or adverse event.
Gout: Condition of painful deposits of urate crystals in the joints and other parts of the body such as the ear pinna.

DISCUSSION

Pharmacology of Class

Allopurinol is a prophylactic drug that reduces the biosynthesis of uric acid. In this manner, **serum uric acid levels are typically reduced,** and the formation of **inflammatory tophi within joints is reduced.** It is a useful **long-term therapy** for patients with chronic gouty arthritis. It is also indicated for the **treatment of hyperuricemia secondary to blood dyscrasias.** Allopurinol can be used to **prevent the progression of uric acid nephropathy,** and for the prophylaxis of both uric acid and calcium oxalate renal stone formation that is typically associated with hyperuricemia. Allopurinol is useful in patients with **recurrent renal stones** or with renal impairment or those that do not respond to probenecid. Patients treated with allopurinol should have adequate renal secretion of uric acid. **Adverse effects include nausea, vomiting, and diarrhea and an allergic skin reaction is reported in 3 percent of patients.** On initial use of allopurinol, uric acid is mobilized from tissues and joints and this may **precipitate an acute gouty attack.**

Structure

Allopurinol is a structural analog of xanthine.

Mechanism of Action

Allopurinol inhibits xanthine oxidase (Figure 29-1) and reduces the biosynthesis of urate. Allopurinol is metabolized to alloxanthine by xanthine oxidase and this metabolite inhibits two steps in the conversion of purines to uric acid.

Allopurinol also increases the reutilization of xanthine and hypoxanthine via hypoxanthine guanine phosphoribosyltransferase (HGPRT) to increase nucleic acid and nucleotide synthesis. This causes a negative feedback that decreases de novo purine biosynthesis. These actions decrease both serum and urine uric acid.

Administration

Allopurinol has good oral bioavailability and its half-life, 1–3 hours and the half-life of its active metabolite alloxanthine, 12–30 hours, permits once-a-day dosing.

Pharmacokinetics

A significant reduction on serum uric acid concentration usually requires 2–3 days, and the reduction of serum urate to normal levels may take 1–3 weeks. Approximately 80 percent of allopurinol is eliminated by the kidney as alloxanthine and the remainder is eliminated in the feces.

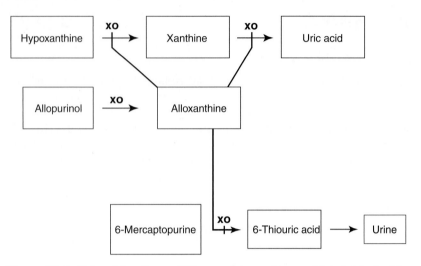

Figure 29-1. Uric acid pathway. XO = xanthine oxidase, which is blocked by alloxanthine, a metabolite of allopurinol.

Other Drugs Used to Treat Gout

Allopurinol is useful in managing gout in patients with normal levels of uric acid excretion. In those patients with gout secondary to impaired renal excretion of uric acid (see Case 8), **probenecid or sulfinpyrazone** is more effective. These **drugs block renal reabsorption of uric acid and thereby increase excretion.**

The pain associated with acute attacks of gout are typically treated with NSAIDs or colchicine. Virtually all NSAIDs have been used successfully to treat the pain associated with gout, but **indomethacin and sulindac remain the most frequently used. Aspirin should not be used to treat gout because it impairs renal excretion of uric acid. Colchicine** is particularly effective in treating gout. Colchicine **binds to microtubules** and impedes cellular movement. This impairs the mobility of leukocytes, which play an important role in the inflammatory process. Colchicine also decreases the production of leukotriene B_4. The most common adverse effects of colchicine are GI with nausea, vomiting, and diarrhea and, rarely, bone marrow depression.

COMPREHENSION QUESTIONS

[29.1] Allopurinol is useful in treating gout because of which of the following property?

    A. It increases the catabolism of uric acid.
    B. It increases the degradation of uric acid.
    C. It decreases the production of uric acid.
    D. It increases renal excretion of uric acid.

[29.2] Colchicine is especially useful in treating an acute attack of gout because it achieves which of the following?

    A. Decreases uric acid deposition
    B. Is potent anti-inflammatory agent
    C. Impairs leukocyte migration
    D. Increases the solubility of uric acid

[29.3] A 44-year-old man is suffering from recurrent gouty arthritis. His serum uric acid level is elevated, and you prescribe allopurinol. Within 1 week of the allopurinol, he develops a painful episode that "feels like gout." Which of the following is the best explanation?

    A. The patient is resistant to the allopurinol and should be placed on another medication.
    B. The patient likely has an arthritis syndrome produced by allopurinol and should have an antinuclear antibody (ANA) drawn.
    C. The patient likely developed acute gout as a result of mobilization of the urate from joints and tissue.
    D. This likely represents a drug-drug interaction, and so the allopurinol should be discontinued.

Answers

[29.1]   **C.** The mechanism of action of allopurinol is to decrease the production of uric acid.

[29.2]   **C.** Impairing leukocyte migration reduces the inflammation associated with a gouty attack.

[29.3]   **C.** The patient likely developed an acute episode of gout as a result of the mobilization of urate from joints and tissue, a phenomenon commonly seen with initiation of allopurinol.

PHARMACOLOGY PEARLS

❖ Allopurinol can precipitate an acute gouty attack. Initial therapy should be combined with an NSAID or colchicine to avoid this effect.

❖ Uric acid is the end product of purine metabolism.

❖ Allopurinol lowers uric acid production, by inhibiting the enzyme xanthine oxidase which converts hypoxanthine to xanthine and xanthine to uric acid.

REFERENCES

Ettinger B, Tang A, Citron JT. Randomized trial of allopurinol in the prevention of calcium oxalate calculi. N Engl J Med 1986;315:1386–9.

Bomalaski JS, Clark MA. Serum uric acid-lowering therapies: where are we heading in management of hyperuricemia and the potential role of uricase. Curr Rheumatol Rep 2004;6:240–7.

A 40-year-old woman has had rheumatoid arthritis (RA) for 5 years. She has been on multiple NSAIDs with some symptomatic relief. On a few occasions she has taken corticosteroids for severe exacerbations. She feels that her disease is getting worse. She has more stiffness and swelling in her wrists and hands. She is currently taking the maximum recommended dosage of ibuprofen, but admits to taking more than she should on bad days. On examination you note active synovitis of both wrists and all of her metacarpophalangeal joints. There is subtle ulnar deviation of all of her fingers. She has several firm, subcutaneous nodules on her arms. You assess her as having an acute exacerbation of RA, along with overall worsening of the disease. You prescribe a short course of oral corticosteroids and start her on methotrexate.

◆ **What is the mechanism of immune suppression mediated by glucocorticoids?**

◆ **What is the mechanism of action of methotrexate?**

ANSWERS TO CASE 30: AGENTS USED
TO TREAT RHEUMATOID ARTHRITIS

Summary: A 40-year-old woman with worsening rheumatoid arthritis (RA) is prescribed corticosteroids and methotrexate.

◆   **Mechanism of immune suppression by glucocorticoids:** Interference with cell cycle of activated lymphoid cells and activation of apoptosis in some lymphoid lines.

◆   **Mechanism of action of methotrexate:** Inhibition of deoxyribonucleic acid (DNA) synthesis by inhibition of dihydrofolate reductase. Inhibits replication and function of T cells and possibly B cells.

CLINICAL CORRELATION

RA is an autoimmune disorder in which the body's immune system attacks its own synovium. This causes joint stiffness, swelling and, if unchecked, joint destruction and disfigurement. Several immunosuppressive agents have been used with success in the treatment of RA. Glucocorticoids are used both for their anti-inflammatory and immunosuppressive effects. They are thought to interfere with the cell cycle of activated lymphoid cells and may activate apoptosis in some lymphoid lines. Its long-term use is limited by multiple side effects and toxicities, including induction of a Cushingoid syndrome, glucose intolerance, and reduction in bone density. Methotrexate is a cancer chemotherapeutic agent that also has immunosuppressive effects. It is a folate analog that interferes with DNA synthesis by inhibition of the dihydrofolate reductase enzyme. Its immunosuppressive effect is mediated through its inhibition of the replication and function of T, and possibly B, lymphocytes. Methotrexate can cause hepatotoxicity, bone marrow suppression, and severe GI side effects.

APPROACH TO PHARMACOLOGY
OF AGENTS USED IN RA

Objectives

1.   Know the agents used for RA and their mechanisms of action.
2.   Know the toxicities and adverse effects of agents used for RA.

Definitions

Rheumatoid arthritis: Chronic disease that is characterized especially by pain, stiffness, inflammation, swelling, and sometimes destruction of joints.

Osteoarthritis: Arthritis characterized by degenerative and sometimes hypertrophic changes in the bone and cartilage of one or more joints and a progressive wearing down of apposing joint surfaces with consequent distortion of joint position usually without bone stiffening.

DISCUSSION

Class

Rheumatoid arthritis is caused by an **inappropriate immune response** that results in **chronic inflammation in and around joints.** The chronic inflammatory process includes the production of a number of **cytokines and inflammatory mediators** that cause **destruction of cartilage within the joint.** Pharmacologic treatment of RA includes **treatment of the acute pain, treatment of the inflammation, and inhibition of the immune system.**

Glucocorticoids such as prednisolone or cortisone are potent anti-inflammatory agents and are also **immunosuppressive.** Glucocorticoids may be administered orally or injected into an affected area. Drugs with an **11-keto group** on the steroid nucleus (cortisone or prednisone) are converted to **11-hydroxyl group** in the liver (to give cortisol and prednisolone). Other synthetic corticosteroids include dexamethasone, betamethasone, and triamcinolone. Various chemical substitutions within these drugs decrease first-pass inactivation by the liver, decrease binding to plasma proteins such as corticosteroid-binding globulin (CBG), and increase the affinity of the drug for its receptor. The actions of glucocorticoids are mediated by a **specific nuclear receptor, the glucocorticoid receptor (GR).** Receptor activation occurs on drug binding, which ultimately leads to increased or decreased transcription of specific genes. The **anti-inflammatory action of the glucocorticoids** is a result, in part, of **induction of annexin-1 (also known as macrocortin),** which is a **specific inhibitor of phospholipase A_2, and inhibits the transmigration of leukocytes.** This **decreases the production of prostaglandins and the inflammatory process.** In addition, the production of a number of cytokines including IL-1, IL-2, IL-6, and TNF-α is decreased by glucocorticoids. This is caused in part by the induction of apoptosis in lymphocytes and leukocytes. Thus the anti-inflammatory and immunosuppressive actions of the glucocorticoids are closely linked. Glucocorticoids are potent inhibitors of cell-mediated immunity but have little effect on humoral immunity.

Glucocorticoids are useful in the management of inflammation in RA, bursitis, lupus erythematosus, nephrotic syndrome, and ulcerative colitis. Glucocorticoids are also used to treat hypersensitivity reactions and allergic reactions and to reduce organ or graft rejection.

The use of **glucocorticoids** is limited by a number of **adverse effects.** Most of these adverse effects are predictable as exaggerated physiologic effects. **Suppression of the pituitary-adrenal axis, hyperglycemia, increased protein metabolism, altered fat metabolism, and increased salt retention (a mineralocorticoid effect)** are frequently seen. **Osteoporosis and peptic ulcers** can be induced by glucocorticoids, and increased susceptibility to **infections** and **poor wound healing** also occur.

Methotrexate is a **folate analog that inhibits dihydrofolate reductase.** This enzyme is responsible for the production of tetrahydrofolate cofactors necessary for purine and thymidylate biosynthesis. Inhibition of the enzyme leads to impaired DNA synthesis, which has the greatest impact on rapidly dividing cells. Methotrexate is **immunosuppressive,** and this activity has led to its use in RA, psoriasis, and other autoimmune disorders. Its use as an **anticancer agent** includes childhood acute lymphoblastic leukemia, lymphoma, and osteogenic sarcoma. Serious adverse effects associated with methotrexate include **myelosuppression,** producing severe leukopenia, bone marrow aplasia, and thrombocytopenia. **GI effects** are common with nausea and vomiting, as well as mouth sores or ulcers. Hepatotoxicity, including acute elevations in transaminase levels, fibrosis, and cirrhosis, has been reported. Pulmonary effects include a nonproductive cough and pneumonitis. Methotrexate is a teratogen and is contraindicated in pregnancy.

More disease-specific approaches in treating RA have led to the development of **disease-modifying agents for rheumatoid disease (DMARDs).**

Recent evidence supports a central role of **tumor necrosis factor alpha** (TNF-α) in the pathogenesis of RA. **TNF-α appears responsible for much of the tissue injury in the disease.** Based on these observations, two new classes of drugs have been developed that specifically target the TNF pathway. One class of drugs is **antibodies specific for human TNF-α.** These antibodies interact with TNF-α and block its ability to interact with TNF-α receptors. **Infliximab** is a chimeric antibody containing a human constant region and murine variable regions. It is administered by infusion approximately once every 8 weeks. Infliximab is also indicated in refractory luminal and fistulizing Crohn's disease. **Adalimumab** is a similar, fully human anti-TNF-α antibody that is self-injected twice weekly. **Etanercept** is a fusion protein created by combining the ligand-binding portion of the human TNF-α receptor with the Fc portion of IgG. The protein acts to bind TNF-α and blocks the association of TNF with its receptor. It is self-injected four times a week. These drugs have proven very effective in patients with RA, and disease progression has been markedly diminished and even reversed in some instances. TNF-α also plays an important role in the body's immune responses, especially to infectious agents. Anakinra is a recombinant protein that mimics the action of IL-1Ra, a natural antagonist of the IL-1 receptor. Anakinra reduces the cartilage degradation and bone resorption caused by IL-1 in RA.

One of the **most serious adverse effects seen with the anti-TNF antibody preparations are severe infections such as tuberculosis.** These drugs should not be administered to patients who have any sign of infection. An increased risk of malignancy has also been reported in patients treated with the anti-TNF antibodies. **Neurologic problems** including dizziness, visual disturbances, and peripheral weakness have also been reported. The adverse effect profile of etanercept is similar with serious infections, neurologic disturbances and a high frequency, 20–30 percent, of injection site reactions.

Other Agents Used to Treat RA

Azathioprine is a **cytotoxic agent that suppresses T-cell activity** to a greater extent than B-cell activity. It is an orally active agent that is metabolized to mercaptopurine, which is also **immunosuppressive.** It is used alone or in combination with corticosteroids in the treatment of RA and other autoimmune disorders such as lupus erythematosus. Adverse effects include bone marrow suppression, leukopenia, and, less frequently, anemia.

Cyclophosphamide is an alkylating agent developed as an anticancer drug. It **suppresses B-cell function** more than T-cell function. It has been used to treat a number of autoimmune disorders including Wegener granulomatosis, RA, and nephrotic syndrome in children. Its anticancer uses include non-Hodgkin lymphoma and Burkitt lymphoma. Myelosuppression, nausea and vomiting, and alopecia are common adverse reactions.

Gold salts have been used to treat patients with progressive RA who have not obtained relief from NSAIDs. Use of gold salts has diminished with the introduction of the DMARDs discussed above. Gold has a **high affinity for sulfur,** and most preparations contain gold attached to a sulfur atom. Aurothioglucose, gold sodium thiomalate, and auranofin all contain a gold atom attached to a sulfur moiety. Gold preparations are injected IM and reach peak concentrations in 2–6 hours. Gold accumulates in organs that are rich in phagocytes and in the lysosomes of synovial cells. **Gold salts decrease the migration and the activity of macrophages,** but its precise mechanism of action is unclear. Gold salts do not have anti-inflammatory activity. The **most common adverse effects** of gold salts are **skin lesions and ulceration in mucus membranes.** Impaired **renal function** and **blood dyscrasias** are also seen in about 10 percent of patients treated with gold salts.

COMPREHENSION QUESTIONS

[30.1] Infliximab is effective in RA because it does which of the following?

    A. Binds to TNF-α and sequesters it from receptors

    B. Is a TNF-α receptor agonist

    C. Is a TNF-α receptor antagonist

    D. Is a synovium-specific anti-inflammatory agent

[30.2] The immunosuppressive effect of methotrexate is a result of its inhibition of which of these?

    A. Dihydrofolate reductase

    B. Leukocyte migration

    C. Microtubule function

    D. Phospholipase A_2

[30.3] A 55-year-old woman is being treated for RA. Her disease has become much worse, and a new medication is added. After 6 months, she notes night sweats, weight loss, chronic cough, and a chest radiograph that indicates a cavitary lesion. Which of the following medications was most likely prescribed for the RA?

    A. Gold salts

    B. Infliximab

    C. Methotrexate

    D. Naprosyn

Answers

[30.1]   **A.** The anti-TNF-α antibodies bind to TNF-α and prevent its association with receptors. They are not direct receptor antagonists.

[30.2]   **A.** Methotrexate inhibits dihydrofolate reductase, which impairs rapidly dividing cells such as lymphocytes and leukocytes.

[30.3]   **B.** The anti-TNF-α immunoglobulin agents are usually well tolerated
and modify the disease process of RA; however, they tend to predis-
pose patients to infections, particularly tuberculosis. The patient in
the question has a typical clinical presentation of tuberculosis.
Diagnosis would be confirmed by sputum culture and acid fast smear,
and therapy started with multiple antituberculosis agents.

PHARMACOLOGY PEARLS

 DMARDS, specifically the anti-TNF-α agents, stop the progression
of RA and may induce remission.

 Methotrexate is a folate analog that inhibits dihydrofolate reductase
and acts as an immunosuppressive agent.

 Glucocorticoid agents act as immunosuppressive agents and anti-
inflammatory agents but have numerous adverse effects.

REFERENCES

Gossec L, Dougados M. Combination therapy in early rheumatoid arthritis. Clin
Exp Rheumatol 2003;21(5 suppl 31):S174–8.

Toussirot E, Wendling D. The use of TNF-alpha blocking agents in rheumatoid
arthritis: an overview. Expert Opin Pharmacother 2004;5:581–94.

Gaffo A, Saag KG, Curtis JR. Treatment of rheumatoid arthritis. Am J Health Syst
Pharm 2006;63:2451–65.

A 67-year-old woman is receiving chemotherapy for metastatic ovarian cancer. She is on her fourth cycle of a multidrug regimen, including cisplatin and doxorubicin. She has developed nausea and vomiting, among other side effects. You decide to premedicate her with intravenous (IV) ondansetron prior to her next dose of chemotherapy and provide oral ondansetron for home use as well.

◆ **What is the mechanism of action of ondansetron?**

◆ **What are the common side effects associated with ondansetron?**

ANSWERS TO CASE 31: ANTIEMETICS

Summary: A 67-year-old woman has chemotherapy-induced nausea and vomiting and is prescribed ondansetron.

◆ **Mechanism of action of ondansetron:** Serotonin (5-HT$_3$)-receptor antagonist in the central nervous system (CNS) and gastrointestinal (GI) tract.

◆ **Side effects of ondansetron:** Headache, diarrhea, dizziness, agitation.

CLINICAL CORRELATION

Nausea and vomiting are frequent side effects of cancer chemotherapy. Control of these symptoms is an important adjunct to chemotherapy. Several agents with varied mechanisms of action are available. The serotonin (5-HT$_3$) receptor system in the CNS and GI tract is felt to be a major trigger of chemotherapy-induced nausea and vomiting. Ondansetron and granisetron are specific 5-HT$_3$-receptor antagonists that are widely used for the treatment of this problem. Granisetron has a higher receptor affinity, is longer acting, and is more potent than ondansetron. Both drugs can be administered intravenously or orally. Metoclopramide, which is primarily a dopamine antagonist, will also antagonize the 5-HT$_3$ receptor when given in high doses. Metoclopramide also blocks receptors in the chemoreceptor trigger zone (CTZ) in the brain that contribute to nausea. Metoclopramide sensitizes the GI tract to acetylcholine (ACh) activity, which increases GI motility and gastric emptying. It is somewhat less effective for chemotherapy-induced vomiting than ondansetron or granisetron and has the potential for extrapyramidal side effects that are seen with dopamine antagonists.

APPROACH TO PHARMACOLOGY
OF ANTIEMETIC AGENTS

Objectives

1. List the therapeutic uses of antiemetic medications.
2. Describe the mechanism of action of the antiemetic medications.
3. Describe the adverse effects of the antiemetic medications.

Definitions

Emesis: Vomiting; a complex reflex that results in emptying of the contents of the small intestine and stomach.

DISCUSSION

Class

Vomiting is a **complex reflex** controlled by the **vomiting center** in the **lateral reticular formation of the medulla.** The vomiting center has **five primary afferents** (see Figure 31-1):

1. The **CTZ** is located outside the blood-brain barrier and is exposed to blood-borne and cerebrospinal fluid emetogenic chemicals. Primary receptors associated with emesis are dopamine D_2, 5-HT_3, and opioid receptors.
2. The **vestibular apparatus** is located in the inner ear, sending afferents pertaining to motion. Primary receptors are histamine H_1 and muscarinic cholinoreceptors.
3. The **pharynx** via the vagus nerve sends afferents of the gag reflex.
4. **Enteric afferents arise** from the GI tract. 5-HT_3 receptors play an important role in these signals.
5. **Cerebral cortical afferents** with information such as stress, anticipation, psychiatric disorders.

Current antiemetic therapy blocks one or more of these afferents to reduce the activity in the vomiting center.

Serotonin 5-HT3 Antagonists

Selective 5-HT_3 antagonists are potent antiemetic agents for emetogenic signals arising in the GI tract and from the CTZ. These agents are especially useful for nausea from **chemotherapeutic agents and for postoperative- or postradiation-**induced vomiting. 5-HT_3 antagonists are not useful for motion sickness or nausea of vertigo. Four agents are currently available: **ondansetron, granisetron, palonosetron, and dolasetron.** They are all

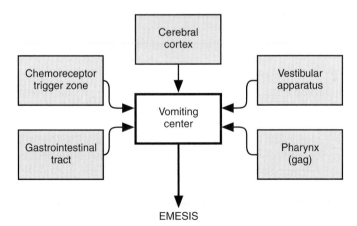

Figure 31-1. Primary afferent components to the vomiting center.

administered intravenously; ondansetron and dolasetron can also be administered orally. These agents are most effective if given 30 minutes prior to chemo- or radiotherapy. Oral agents may be administered once or twice daily.

Dopamine Antagonists

Droperidol is an **antipsychotic butyrophenone** that has significant antiemetic actions. Its antiemetic properties are mediated by **blocking dopamine receptors in the CTZ and in the vomiting center. Droperidol has been associated with a** risk of QT prolongation and torsade de pointes. **Phenothiazines such as promethazine and prochlorperazine block dopamine, histamine, and muscarinic receptors** in the same regions. All are useful for treating nausea and vomiting postoperatively but are very sedating.

Extrapyramidal effects and hypotension have been reported. Droperidol may cause electrocardiogram (ECG) abnormalities such as prolongation of the Q-T interval and ventricular tachycardia.

Metoclopramide is a prokinetic agent that also has antiemetic actions based on its **dopaminergic antagonist activity.** It may be administered orally or parenterally for nausea following chemotherapy or for postoperative nausea. As with the other dopamine antagonists, side effects are rare but may include **extrapyramidal effects: dystonias and Parkinson syndrome** may appear days to months after treatment.

Corticosteroids

Glucocorticoids such as dexamethasone and prednisolone are used to treat nausea and vomiting associated with **chemotherapy.** They are most frequently used in combination with other antiemetics. The molecular basis for the antiemetic action of glucocorticoids is not understood.

Antihistamines

First-generation antihistamines such as cyclizine, diphenhydramine, and dimenhydrinate are useful to treat nausea associated with motion sickness and vertigo. They are **able to penetrate the blood-brain barrier** and their action is most likely to decrease afferents from the vestibular apparatus. The most common adverse effect of these agents is sedation.

Anticholinergic Agents

Scopolamine is the most effective agent for treating nausea associated with **motion sickness or vertigo. It is not effective for nausea of chemotherapy.** It is administered via a **transdermal patch** that delivers drug at a uniform rate for up to 72 hours. By avoiding the peak levels associated with oral administration, incidence of side effects is also reduced. **Scopolamine reduces afferents from the vestibular apparatus** and **decreases the excitability of the labyrinthine receptors.** Side effects, typical of antimuscarinic agents, include **dry mouth, blurred vision, and drowsiness.** It should **not be used in patients with glaucoma or prostatic hypertrophy.**

Other Agents Used as Antiemetics

Benzodiazepines such as lorazepam or diazepam may be used **prior to chemo- or radiotherapy** to reduce the frequency and severity of anticipatory vomiting that occurs in patients who undergo multiple rounds of anticancer therapy. **Dronabinol** is Δ^9-tetrahydrocannabinol, the major active ingredient in marijuana. It is an orally active agent that has been used to stimulate appetite and as an antiemetic. The mechanism of these activities is not known. It is frequently administered in conjunction with a phenothiazine, which reduces the adverse effects of both agents while producing a synergistic antiemetic effect. Adverse effects include euphoria, sedation, dry mouth, and hallucinations.

COMPREHENSION QUESTIONS

[31.1] Droperidol is effective in reducing nausea because it blocks which of the following?

A. ACh receptors in the periphery
B. Dopamine receptors in the CTZ
C. Glucocorticoid receptors in the vomiting center
D. 5-HT$_2$ receptors in the CTZ

[31.2] A patient undergoing chemotherapy with cisplatin has severe nausea. Which of the following would be the drug to use in this patient?

A. Cyclizine
B. Naloxone
C. Ondansetron
D. Scopolamine

[31.3] A fisherman uses a transdermal scopolamine patch to assist with the nausea associated with being on a boat. What is the most likely side effect he will experience?

A. Acute dystonic reaction
B. Euphoria
C. Sedation
D. Tremor

Answers

[31.1] **B.** Droperidol is a dopamine-receptor antagonist that diminishes the activity of the CTZ. It is effective in reducing nausea associated with chemotherapy or radiotherapy.

[31.2] **C.** Ondansetron is a serotonin 5-HT$_3$-receptor antagonist with fewer side effects and greater effectiveness than the other agents in treating patients on chemotherapy.

[31.3] **C.** Sedation is the most common side effect associated with scopolamine patches as a result of stimulation of the muscarinic cholinoreceptor.

PHARMACOLOGY PEARLS

 The scopolamine patch is one of the most effective methods to treat motion sickness.

 Dopaminergic agents such as droperidol and promethazine can lead to extrapyramidal side effects.

 The selective 5-HT$_3$ antagonists are potent antiemetic agents for chemotherapy but are not effective for motion sickness.

REFERENCES

Gralla RJ. New agents, new treatment, and antiemetic therapy. Semin Oncol 2002;29(suppl 2);119–24.

Habib AS, Gan TJ. Evidence-based management of postoperative nausea and vomiting: a review. Can J Anaesth 2004;51:326–41.

Urba S. Radiation-induced nausea and vomiting. J Natl Compr Canc Netw 2007;5:60–5.

A 58-year-old woman with a 20-year history of poorly controlled type II diabetes mellitus comes in for routine follow-up. She has had multiple complications from her diabetes, including retinopathy and peripheral neuropathy. She complains of having several months of feeling as if her stomach is full after eating very little. She is frequently nauseous and bloated. She is on a combination of regular and neutral protamine Hagedorn (NPH) insulin for her diabetes, an angiotensin-converting enzyme (ACE)-inhibitor for her blood pressure, and a 3-hydroxy-3-methylglutaryl-coenzyme A (HMG-CoA) reductase inhibitor for her lipids. Her examination today is unremarkable. A radiographic gastric emptying study shows a prolonged gastric emptying time. You diagnose her with diabetic gastroparesis and prescribe metoclopramide.

◆ **What is the mechanism of action of metoclopramide for gastroparesis?**

◆ **What are some common side effects of metoclopramide?**

ANSWERS TO CASE 32: PROKINETIC AGENTS

Summary: A 58-year-old woman presents with diabetic gastroparesis and is prescribed metoclopramide.

◆ **Mechanism of action of metoclopramide:** Dopamine D_2-receptor antagonist in the GI tract.

◆ **Common side effects:** Sedation, extrapyramidal side effects, increased prolactin secretion.

CLINICAL CORRELATION

Metoclopramide, administered orally or parenterally, works as a prokinetic agent in the GI tract. In the GI tract, dopamine acts to inhibit ACh stimulation of smooth muscle. As a dopamine D_2-receptor antagonist, metoclopramide allows for a greater stimulatory effect of ACh. It may also promote the release of ACh. The increased ACh effect at muscarinic receptors results in increased lower esophageal sphincter pressure and increased gastric emptying. Diabetic gastroparesis is an uncommon complication of poorly controlled diabetes, particularly in diabetics with peripheral neuropathy. In this setting, metoclopramide can promote emptying of the stomach and help to alleviate the symptoms. It is also used clinically in combination with antacids to treat gastroesophageal reflux disease (GERD). Metoclopramide also has central actions. Dopamine D_2-receptor blockade in the CTZ in the CNS is the basis for clinical use of metoclopramide for treatment of nausea and vomiting. Restlessness, anxiety, and insomnia are common adverse effects of metoclopramide and, like other dopamine D_2-receptor antagonists such as haloperidol, metoclopramide at high doses can cause extrapyramidal side effects and tardive dyskinesia, and also increased prolactin secretion that can result in galactorrhea, menstrual dysfunction, gynecomastia, and sexual dysfunction. Other prokinetic agents include cisapride, a $5\text{-}HT_4$-receptor agonist that is only available for compassionate use due to its toxicity, and domperidone (not available in the United States) which is also a dopamine D_2-receptor antagonist, but one that acts only peripherally and, therefore, has few neural adverse effects.

Definitions

Gastroparesis: Slight paralysis of the muscular coat of the stomach.

COMPREHENSION QUESTIONS

[32.1] Metoclopramide is which of the following?

    A. β_1-Adrenoceptor antagonist
    B. Dopamine D_2-receptor antagonist
    C. Muscarinic cholinoreceptor antagonist
    D. Serotonin $5\text{-}HT_1$-receptor antagonist

[32.2] Which of the following is the most likely adverse effect of metoclopramide?

A. Hallucinations
B. Hyperactivity
C. Hyperthyroidism
D. Tardive dyskinesia

[32.3] Metoclopramide acts to achieve which of the following?

A. Increase gastric emptying
B. Decrease transit through the small intestine
C. Decrease lower esophageal sphincter pressure
D. Stimulate vomiting

Answers

[32.1] **B.** Metoclopramide is a dopamine D_2-receptor antagonist.

[32.2] **D.** Adverse effects of metoclopramide include insomnia, tardive dyskinesia, and sexual dysfunction, as well as extrapyramidal side effects
similar to haloperidol and endocrine effects related to increased prolactin secretion (galactorrhea, menstrual dysfunction, gynecomastia).

[32.3] **A.** Metoclopramide increases gastric emptying, increases lower
esophageal sphincter pressure, and inhibits vomiting.

PHARMACOLOGY PEARLS

 Metoclopramide works as a prokinetic agent in the GI tract, acting
as a dopamine antagonist.

 Common side effects of metoclopramide are restlessness and anxiety.
Also, like other dopamine D_2-receptor antagonists such as haloperidol, metoclopramide can cause extrapyramidal side effects and tardive dyskinesia.

 Metoclopramide increases prolactin secretion that can result in
galactorrhea and menstrual irregularities.

REFERENCES

Booth CM, Heyland DK, Paterson WG. Gastrointestinal promotility drugs in the critical care setting: a systematic review of the evidence. Crit Care Med 2002; 30(7):1429–35.

Smith DS, Ferris CD. Current concepts in diabetic gastroparesis. Drugs 2003;63(13):1339–58.

Syed AA, Rattansingh A, Furtado SD. Current perspectives on the management of gastroparesis. J Postgrad Med 2005 Jan–Mar;51(1):54–60

Tonini M, Cipollina L, Poluzzi E, et al. Review article: clinical implications of enteric and central D_2 receptor blockade by antidopaminergic gastrointestinal prokinetics. Aliment Pharmacol Ther 2004;19(4):379–90.

A 48-year-old woman presents for evaluation of abdominal pain. She reports that she gets right upper-abdominal pain after eating. It is worse if she eats fatty or fried food. She has tried over-the-counter antacids without relief. She has no significant medical history, has had no surgeries, and takes no medications on a regular basis. Both her mother and an older sister have had to have their gallbladders removed. On examination, she is moderately obese, but her examination is otherwise normal. An abdominal x-ray is normal. An ultrasound of her abdomen reveals several small gallstones. You diagnose her with cholelithiasis and recommend surgical evaluation. She is adamant in wanting to do anything to avoid surgery, so you prescribe ursodiol.

◆ **What is the mechanism of action of ursodiol?**

◆ **How long does it take to see full effect of this medication?**

◆ **What effect does ursodiol have on low-density lipoprotein (LDL) cholesterol levels?**

ANSWERS TO CASE 33: DRUGS USED
TO DISSOLVE GALLSTONES

Summary: A 48-year-old woman presents with cholelithiasis. She does not desire surgery, and is prescribed ursodiol.

◆ **Mechanism of action of ursodiol:** Reduces cholesterol secretion into bile.

◆ **Length of time to see full effect:** Months to years.

◆ **Effect on LDL cholesterol levels:** No change.

CLINICAL CORRELATION

Gallstones are a common cause of abdominal pain. These often consist of a high proportion of cholesterol, which is excreted from the liver into bile. The bile is taken up in the gallbladder, where the cholesterol may precipitate into stones. Ursodiol is ursodeoxycholic acid, a bile acid. It reduces cholesterol secretion into bile with little change in the secretion of bile acid. It is used in an effort to dissolve cholesterol gallstones in patients who either do not want surgery or are not surgical candidates. The full effect of this medication can take from several months to years. It is also used as an adjunct to shock wave lithotripsy of gallstones. In this treatment, sound waves are used to break gallstones into small fragments. Ursodiol may then be used to attempt to dissolve the fragments. Radiopaque gallstones, which contain calcium, are not effectively dissolved with ursodiol. It is administered orally, and its side effects are primarily GI, with nausea and diarrhea being common. Ursodiol does not alter LDL cholesterol levels in the blood.

APPROACH TO PHARMACOLOGY OF AGENTS USED
TO DISSOLVE GALLSTONES

Objectives

1. Know the drugs used to dissolve gallstones and their mechanism of action.
2. Know the routes of administration and side effects of these drugs.

Definitions

Cholelithiasis: The presence of stones in the gallbladder or common bile duct, or the process of formation of such stones.
Cholecystitis: Inflammation of the gallbladder.
Lithotripsy: Reduction of gallstones using sound waves to small particles that can be excreted from the gallbladder.

DISCUSSION

Class

Gallstones are a major cause of morbidity and mortality, and surgical removal of the gallbladder is among the most common GI surgeries. Although surgical removal is the preferred treatment, other treatments, including **ultrasound lithotripsy** or **pharmacologic dissolution,** are therapeutic options in patients who cannot have surgery. Gallstones can be transported into the duodenum and block the exit of the pancreatic duct, causing pancreatitis. Gallstones can be radiotranslucent, indicating a stone high in cholesterol content, or **radiopaque, indicating a stone with significant mineral** (usually **calcium**) content. **Ursodeoxycholic acid (ursodiol) is a naturally occurring bile acid that is a minor component of bile.** It has been used **successfully to treat** relatively **small, radiotranslucent stones,** especially those within the common bile duct. It decreases the synthesis of bile and reduces the concentration of cholesterol in bile. **Ursodiol solubilizes cholesterol by forming bile acid micelles** and disperses liquid crystals of cholesterol in an aqueous environment. These actions will **slowly cause the dissolution of the gallstone.** Complete dissolution occurs in approximately 30 percent of patients with stones less than 20 mm in diameter. It also decreases the biliary colic that is associated with gallstones in some patients. The prophylactic administration of ursodiol caused a marked reduction in the incidence of gallstones after cardiac surgery. Older approaches to pharmacologic dissolution of gallstones employed organic solvents such as methyl-*tert*-butyl ether (MTBE) or monoglycerides such as monooctanoin. Although rapid dissolution of gallstones could be achieved, leakage of the solvent materials into the lumen of the bowel was associated with serious adverse effects, and these approaches have been largely discontinued. **Adverse effects of ursodiol are minor, typically GI upset and mild diarrhea.**

Structure

Ursodiol is derived from 7β-hydroxycholesterol and is a naturally occurring component in bile.

Administration

Ursodiol is administered orally, two to three times a day, and complete dissolution of stones may require a year. Treatment effectiveness should be monitored by diagnostic ultrasound.

COMPREHENSION QUESTIONS

[33.1] Ursodiol reduces the size of common bile duct gallstones by which of the following mechanisms?

    A. Chelating Ca^{2+} out of the stone
    B. Decreasing the synthesis of bile
    C. Increasing the cholesterol content in bile
    D. Slowly dissolving cholesterol from the stone

[33.2] Complete dissolution of a gallstone by ursodiol typically requires how long?

    A. Several hours
    B. Weeks
    C. Months to years
    D. Several years

[33.3] Ursodiol has been useful to treat which of the following conditions?

    A. Cholestasis of pregnancy
    B. Cirrhosis
    C. Diabetes mellitus
    D. Pancreatitis resulting from trauma

Answers

[33.1]   **D.** Ursodiol is a detergent that slowly causes dissolution of gallstones that are rich in cholesterol. It decreases the amount of cholesterol in bile as well as total bile acid synthesis.

[33.2]   **C.** Ursodiol treatment typically takes months to a year for dissolution of a typical gallstone.

[33.3]   **A.** Ursodeoxycholic acid has been used successfully to treat the symptoms of pruritus associated with cholestasis of pregnancy, a disease thought to be caused by the accumulation of bile salts.

PHARMACOLOGY PEARLS

 Ursodiol is the best nonsurgical therapy for small, radiotranslucent gallstones in patients who are not candidates for surgery.

 Ursodeoxycholic acid has also been used to treat cholestasis of pregnancy.

REFERENCES

Ai T, Azemoto R, Saisho HJ. Prevention of gallstones by ursodeoxycholic acid after cardiac surgery. Gastroenterol 2003;38:1071–6.

Gonzalez-Koch A, Nervi F. Medical management of common bile duct stones. World J Surgery 1998;22:1145–50.

A 45-year-old woman presents with bloating and "gas" after drinking milk. Her symptoms usually start approximately 2 hours after ingesting most dairy products, although she has found that yogurt with active cultures doesn't bother her much. This has been worsening over the past several years. She has learned to avoid dairy products as much as possible, but would like to be able to drink milk or eat ice cream occasionally. She has no significant medical history, takes no medications regularly, and has a normal examination. You diagnose her with lactose intolerance and suggest a trial of lactase when she plans to ingest dairy products.

◆ **What is the cause of lactose intolerance?**

◆ **What is the mechanism of action of lactase?**

ANSWERS TO CASE 34: ENZYME REPLACEMENTS

Summary: A 45-year-old woman with lactose intolerance is prescribed lactase.

◆ **Cause of lactose intolerance:** Insufficient production of lactase by brush border cells of the small intestine.

◆ **Mechanism of action of lactase:** Hydrolyzes lactose to glucose and galactose.

CLINICAL CORRELATION

Lactose intolerance is a very common digestive condition in which there is an underproduction of the natural enzyme lactase by the brush border of the small intestine. Lactase hydrolyzes lactose into the sugars glucose and galactose, which can then be transported from the lumen of the small intestine across cell membranes. A deficiency or absence of lactase results in lactose remaining within the intestinal lumen. The presence of this undigested disaccharide will osmotically attract fluid into the intestinal lumen. As it passes further into the GI tract, lactose will be metabolized by colonic bacteria, which produces bowel gas. The combination of increased amounts of fluid and gas in the intestine contributes to the symptoms of lactose intolerance. Most people with lactose intolerance learn to avoid lactose-containing foods. The low levels of endogenous lactase production in these individuals can be supplemented by lactase given orally with meals containing dairy products. This often reduces, but not completely relieves, the symptoms of gas, bloating, and diarrhea that may occur.

APPROACH TO PHARMACOLOGY OF ENZYME REPLACEMENTS

Objectives

1. Know the conditions for which digestive enzyme replacement can be used.
2. Know the specific digestive enzymes which can be replaced and the therapeutic effects of enzyme replacement.

Definitions

Pancreatin: A preparation of principally amylase, lipase, and proteases.
Pancrelipase: A preparation that is principally lipase that also contains amylase and proteases.

DISCUSSION

Class

Digestive enzymes hydrolyze triglycerides to fatty acids and glycerol, peptides and proteins to amino acids, and **carbohydrates into simple sugars.** Enzyme replacement is used in patients with a congenital lack of enzyme activity as a result of mutation in specific enzymes, or secondary to other disorders that cause deficient pancreatic exocrine secretions such as in **cystic fibrosis, chronic pancreatitis, postpancreatectomy, pancreatic ductal obstruction, and postgastrectomy.** Greater than 90 percent of pancreatic function must be lost before clinically significant effects on digestion are apparent: steatorrhea (from fat malabsorption) and protein malabsorption. **Sucrase** is expressed on the brush border of the small intestine primarily in the distal duodenum and jejunum. It converts sucrose into glucose and fructose. **Isomaltase and maltase** hydrolyze isomaltose and maltose, respectively, into two molecules of glucose. **Lactase** (β-galactosidase) is normally expressed in villus enterocytes in the small intestine. It breaks lactose into the monosaccharides glucose and galactose.

Pancreatic Enzyme Preparations

There are **more than 35 preparations of pancreatin and pancrelipase** currently available. These are **all prepared from porcine pancreas,** but they are not bioequivalent and are not necessarily interchangeable. These agents can prevent malabsorption from the disorders mentioned above and palliation of pain in chronic pancreatitis. Pancreatic enzyme replacements are well tolerated, but can cause GI disturbances such as nausea and diarrhea; allergic reactions to the porcine preparations have also been reported. Very high doses can cause hyperuricemia and hyperuricosuria. The FDA has required that all of these preparations receive FDA approval by 2008.

Pancreatic enzyme replacements are administered orally prior to a meal or snack. They are available in enteric-coated capsule or as noncoated capsules.

Small Intestine Enzyme Preparations

More than 15 percent of adults are lactose intolerant as a result of deficiency in the enzyme lactase. This deficiency leads to **lactose delivery to the colon,** where it osmotically **traps water and it is fermented,** producing **bloating sensations,** discomfort, and intestinal gas. Preparations of lactase for enzyme replacement are prepared from the yeast *Kluyveromyces lactis.* **Lactase is administered orally,** typically taken just prior to ingestion of dairy products. The dosage may be increased until satisfactory results are obtained. Few adverse effects are reported beyond mild GI upset.

Congenital sucrase-isomaltase deficiency (CSID) is a chronic autosomal disease with highly variable levels of enzyme activity. CSID is frequently characterized by nearly complete deficiency in sucrase activity, less severe reductions in isomaltase and maltase activity, and normal lactase activity. In the absence of sucrase activity, unhydrolyzed sucrose and starch are not absorbed from the small intestine, causing osmotic water retention, loose stools, and the typical manifestations of malabsorption.

Sacrosidase is derived from baker's yeast (*Saccharomyces cerevisiae*). It is approved for use in CSID and is effective in improving carbohydrate absorption and alleviating the GI sequelae. It is administered orally just prior to eating food. Adverse effects are rare with one case of hypersensitivity reported to date.

Besides replacing enzymes in the digestive system, enzyme replacement has been useful to correct **genetic deficiencies in lysosomal enzymes. Anderson-Fabry disease** is an **X-linked lysosomal storage disease** that results from a deficiency in **α-galactosidase A.** This enzyme hydrolyses globotriaosylceramide to galactose and lactosylceramide. In patients with the enzyme deficiency, globotriaosylceramide accumulates and is deposited in vascular endothelium, smooth muscle cells, renal glomerular and epithelial cells, myocardial cells and valvular fibrocytes, and neurons. This results in severe pain as a result of damage of small neurons, as well as cardiomyopathy and renal impairment and failure. The disease can be **treated with agalsidase α,** which is a **recombinant α-galactosidase A** produced in vitro in fibroblast cells. A similar replacement enzyme is agalsidase β, which is a recombinant protein produced in a genetically engineered Chinese hamster ovary cell line. Both drugs are given intravenously biweekly, and both drugs reduce the globotriaosylceramide deposits and improve organ function. Both drugs are well tolerated.

COMPREHENSION QUESTIONS

[34.1]   A 17-year-old patient enters your office complaining that every time he drinks a glass of milk he gets GI pain and cramping. Which of the following would be the best choice to treat his condition?

A. Aspirin

B. Lactase

C. Niacin

D. Sucrase

[34.2]   A 9-year-old patient whose main complaint is shooting pain in the arms and legs is seen in your hospital. After careful study you make the diagnosis of Anderson-Fabry disease. Which of the following would be the best course of treatment for this patient?

A. α-Galactosidase A

B. High-dose glucocorticoids

C. Indomethacin

D. Sacrosidase

[34.3] A 45-year-old man has developed chronic pancreatitis as a result of alcohol abuse, and he has been noted to have pancreatic insufficiency. Which of the following circumstances contraindicates the use of pancreatic enzyme replacement in this patient?

A. Allergy to eggs
B. Allergy to pork
C. Diabetes mellitus
D. Pseudogout

Answers

[34.1] **B.** This case of lactose intolerance would be treated with lactase before consumption of dairy products.

[34.2] **A.** Anderson-Fabry disease can be treated successfully with α-galactosidase A.

[34.3] **B.** All pancreatic enzyme replacements are porcine and so an allergy to pork products is a contraindication.

PHARMACOLOGY PEARLS

 Enzyme replacement therapy is effective in treating specific genetic enzyme deficiencies and acquired enzyme deficiencies and is associated with very few adverse effects.

 Lactose deficiency is a common problem and is addressed by avoidance of lactose-containing products or taking lactase orally prior to ingestion of lactose.

 All pancreatic enzyme preparations currently are prepared from porcine pancreas.

REFERENCES

Hauser AC, Lorenz M, Sunder-Plassmann G. The expanding clinical spectrum of Anderson-Fabry disease: a challenge to diagnosis in the novel era of enzyme replacement therapy. J Intern Med 2004;255:629–36.

Sly WS. Enzyme replacement therapy for lysosomal storage disorders: successful transition from concept to clinical practice. Mo Med 2004;101:100–4.

Swagerty DL, Walling AD, Klein RM. Lactose intolerance. Am Fam Physician 2002;65:1845–50, 1855–6.

Martine A. Lipases and lipolysis in the human digestive tract: where do we stand? Curr Opin Clin Nutr Metab 2007:10:256–64.

A 48-year-old man presents for evaluation of heartburn. He reports a burning feeling in his chest after eating. It is worse when he eats spicy foods or tomato sauce. He is sometimes awakened at night with these symptoms. He has tried over-the-counter antacids and histamine H_2 blockers with partial relief. He is on no medications regularly. His examination today is normal. An upper gastrointestinal (GI) x-ray series reveals gastroesophageal reflux. Along with appropriate diet and lifestyle modification recommendations, you prescribe omeprazole.

◆ **What is the mechanism of action of omeprazole?**

◆ **What is the mechanism of action of antacid medications?**

◆ **What is the mechanism of action of histamine H_2-receptor antagonists?**

ANSWERS TO CASE 35: AGENTS FOR UPPER GI DISORDERS

Summary: A 48-year-old man with gastroesophageal reflux disease (GERD) is prescribed omeprazole.

◆ **Mechanism of action of omeprazole:** Irreversible inhibition of the H^+, K^+-ATPase proton pump in parietal cells, reducing transport of acid from the cell into the lumen.

◆ **Mechanism of action of antacids:** Weak bases that directly neutralize gastric acid and reduce pepsin activity.

◆ **Mechanism of action of histamine H_2-receptor antagonists:** Competitive antagonists of histamine at the parietal cell histamine H_2 receptor.

CLINICAL CORRELATION

GERD, a common cause of recurrent heartburn and dyspepsia, is caused by gastric acid irritating the lining of the esophagus. It can be treated by numerous medications. Antacid medications, widely available without a prescription, usually contain aluminum hydroxide, magnesium hydroxide, calcium carbonate, or combinations thereof. They are weak bases that partially neutralize gastric acid. Histamine H_2-receptor antagonists, available over-the-counter or by prescription, competitively antagonize the effect of histamine (released from nearby gastric mucosa enterochromaffin-like [ECL] cells) at the histamine H_2 receptor in gastric parietal cells. Omeprazole was the first medication in a class known as proton pump inhibitors (PPIs). PPIs directly and irreversibly inhibit the action of the H^+, K^+-ATPase that transports H^+ from gastric parietal cells into the lumen of the stomach thus reducing both the basal and stimulated release of gastric acid. PPIs are used for the treatment of refractory GERD, hypersecretory conditions such as Zollinger-Ellison syndrome, for peptic ulcer disease, and as a part of the treatment regimen (in combination with antibiotics) for *Helicobacter pylori* infections. *Helicobacter pylori* is the most common cause of non-drug-induced peptic ulcer disease.

APPROACH TO PHARMACOLOGY OF AGENTS FOR UPPER GI DISORDERS

Objectives

1. List the antacid agents and describe their mechanisms of action, therapeutic uses, and adverse effects.
2. List the histamine H_2-receptor antagonists and PPIs that inhibit gastric acid production and describe their mechanisms of action, therapeutic uses, and adverse effects.

3. List the drugs used therapeutically to promote the defense of the GI tract from the effects of acid, and describe their mechanisms of action, therapeutic uses, and adverse effects.

Definitions

Prodrugs: Inactive compounds that are metabolized in the body to therapeutically active agents.

DISCUSSION

Class

Drugs used to **treat acid-peptic diseases** (Table 35-1) either **reduce gastric acidity** (antacids, histamine H_2-receptor antagonists, and PPIs) or **promote the defense of the GI mucosa** (sucralfate, bismuth subsalicylate, and the prostaglandin analog, misoprostol).

Available **antacid preparations** are used primarily to treat heartburn and dyspepsia. When given concomitantly with other drugs, antacids may reduce their absorption through direct binding or, as a result of an increase in gastric pH, by altering their dissolution or solubility.

Available **histamine H_2-receptor antagonists** are used to treat dyspepsia, GERD, peptic ulcer disease, and stress-induced gastritis.

PPIs are generally considered the first-line drugs for treating acid-peptic disease as a result of their superior efficacy and safety profile. Available PPIs are also used to **treat dyspepsia, GERD, peptic ulcer disease, and stress-induced gastritis, as well as gastrinomas.** For treating peptic ulcer disease caused by *H. pylori*, **PPIs** are used in a multidrug regimen that includes the antibiotics **clarithromycin and amoxicillin and/or metronidazole.**

Sucralfate use has, for the most part, been supplanted by other agents for the treatment of upper GI disorders. It is still used clinically to treat stress-related gastritis.

Misoprostol is used rarely, to **treat nonsteroidal anti-inflammatory drug (NSAID)-induced peptic ulcer disease.**

Bismuth subsalicylate (Pepto-Bismol) is available as a nonprescription agent and is used to treat **dyspepsia, acute diarrhea,** and, as a second-line agent in a multidrug combination, *H. pylori* **infection** where it is thought to inhibit growth of the organism.

Structure

PPIs are substituted benzimidazoles. They resemble histamine H_2-receptor antagonists but have a different mechanism of action. Sucralfate is a complex

Table 35-1
MEDICATIONS FOR PEPTIC ULCERS

ANTACIDS	ADVERSE EFFECTS
Sodium bicarbonate	Bloating, belching, metabolic acidosis as a result of absorbed unreacted alkali at high doses, and fluid retention caused by absorption of sodium chloride that may compromise patients with heart failure and hypertension. Hypercalcemia at high doses when administered with dairy products containing calcium.
Calcium carbonate	Bloating, belching, metabolic acidosis, hypercalcemia.
Magnesium hydroxide	Osmotic diarrhea from unabsorbed magnesium.
Aluminum hydroxide	Constipation from unabsorbed aluminum.
HISTAMINE H$_2$-RECEPTOR ANTAGONIST	ADVERSE EFFECTS
Cimetidine (prototype) *Ranitidine* *Famotidine* *Nizatidine*	Mild diarrhea or constipation, headache, myalgia. Confusion, hallucinations, and excitement, particularly cimetidine, when administered IV to elderly or patients with renal or liver disease.
PROTON PUMP INHIBITORS	ADVERSE EFFECTS
Omeprazole (prototype) *Esomeprazole* *Lansoprazole* *Pantoprazole* *Rabeprazole*	Small increase in incidence of diarrhea and headache. Otherwise, no significant adverse effects documented in humans, although there are theoretical concerns with long-term therapy regarding the development of certain cancers and enteric infections.
GI PROTECTIVE AGENTS	ADVERSE EFFECTS
Sucralfate	Constipation as a consequence of the aluminum salt. It may bind other drugs to limit their absorption (phenytoin, quinoline antibodies).
Bismuth subsalicylate	Black stools and darkening of the tongue.
Misoprostol	Diarrhea and abdominal discomfort. Contraindicated in women unless proved negative for pregnancy.

salt of sucrose sulfate and aluminum hydroxide. Misoprostol is a prostaglandin analog of prostaglandin E_1 (PGE_1). Bismuth subsalicylate is a combination of bismuth and salicylate.

Mechanism of Action

Antacids are weak bases that directly neutralize gastric hydrochloric acid to form a salt and water and to reduce pepsin activity. They may also stimulate the production of prostaglandins and thus increase the defense of the GI mucosa.

Histamine H_2-receptor antagonists are highly specific and selective competitive antagonists of histamine binding to gastric parietal cell histamine H_2 receptors. Thus they prevent activation of adenylyl cyclase and accumulation of cAMP, which mediate acid release into the gastric lumen. Parietal cell acid secretion induced by the secretagogues gastrin and acetylcholine, which act synergistically with histamine, is also inhibited by histamine H_2-receptor antagonists, albeit indirectly. PPIs irreversibly inhibit the H^+, K^+-ATPase proton pump in parietal cells, thus reducing transport of acid from the cell into the lumen of the stomach.

Sucralfate in its viscous form may bind to positively charged proteins to coat epithelial cells and to form a physical barrier in the GI tract that protects the luminal surface and any already formed ulcers from the deleterious effects of gastric acid and pepsin.

Misoprostol, a **PGE_1 analog,** stimulates bicarbonate and mucus secretion and mucosal blood flow, resulting in enhanced neutralization and action of secreted acid. It also binds to parietal cell prostaglandin receptors to modestly inhibit secretagogue-induced acid secretion.

Bismuth subsalicylate, like sucralfate, coats epithelial cells to form a physical barrier in the GI tract and protect it from the deleterious effects of gastric acid and pepsin. It may also stimulate bicarbonate and PGE_2 secretion.

Administration

All antacids, histamine H_2-receptor antagonists, PPIs, sucralfate, misoprostol, and bismuth subsalicylate can be given orally. The PPIs pantoprazole and the histamine H_2-receptor antagonists (cimetidine, famotidine, and ranitidine) are available for parenteral use.

As over-the-counter preparations, magnesium hydroxide, which can cause diarrhea, and aluminum hydroxide, which can cause constipation, are usually administered in combination to balance their effects on the GI tract.

PPIs are inactive, acid-labile, prodrugs that are administered in acid-resistant, enteric-coated preparations to protect them from destruction in the stomach. In the acidic environment of the stomach, sucralfate forms a viscous gel.

Pharmacokinetics

The acid-neutralizing capacity of available antacid preparations varies considerably, being highly influenced by their rate of dissolution, their solubility in water, and the rate of gastric emptying among other factors. Sodium bicarbonate and calcium carbonate react more rapidly with HCl to produce CO_2 and water than do magnesium or aluminum hydroxide and, therefore, may cause bloating and belching.

Histamine H_2-receptor antagonists are absorbed rapidly; however, cimetidine, ranitidine, and famotidine have a bioavailability of only 50 percent. Their clearances can be reduced in the elderly and by renal and hepatic dysfunction. Cimetidine inhibits the activity of several hepatic cytochrome P450 enzymes that can prolong the duration of action of a number of other drugs.

PPI bioavailability is decreased significantly by food. Because maximal inhibition of H^+, K^+-ATPase occurs when proton pumps are actively secreting acid, PPIs are best administered within an hour or so of meals. After dissolution of the enteric-coated PPI capsule in the intestine, the lipophilic prodrug diffuses into the acidic environment of the parietal cell, where it becomes protonated and highly concentrated, and where it is then converted to a reactive sulfonamide cation that irreversibly binds to and inactivates parietal cell H^+, K^+-ATPase through a covalent disulfide linkage. Although their serum half-life is short, PPI inhibition of the proton pump lasts up to 24 hours while synthesis of new H^+, K^+-ATPase occurs. PPIs are metabolized by hepatic P450 microsomal enzymes; however, no clinically significant drug-drug interactions have been documented.

Sucralfate is very insoluble, and therefore it **acts locally** with little systemic absorption from the GI tract.

Misoprostol is absorbed rapidly and is metabolized to an active agent that has a very short serum half-life and short duration of action and therefore must be administered three to four times daily.

Bismuth subsalicylate is rapidly dissociated in the stomach into bismuth, which is eliminated in the stool, and salicylate, which is absorbed systemically.

COMPREHENSION QUESTIONS

[35.1] Which of the following is the most common adverse effect of omeprazole?

    A. Black stools
    B. Constipation
    C. Headache
    D. Vomiting

[35.2] Ranitidine inhibits which of the following?

    A. Gastrin binding to parietal cells
    B. Histamine binding to parietal cells
    C. H^+, K^+-ATPase
    D. Parietal cell prostaglandin receptors

[35.3] Which of the following is true of cimetidine?

    A. It is a prostaglandin analog of PGE₁

    B. It is a prodrug

    C. It is associated with confusion and hallucinations in elderly patients

    D. It reduces the duration of action of other drugs

Answers

[35.1] **C.** The most common adverse effect of omeprazole is headache. Diarrhea, not constipation, is another common adverse effect. Black stools are associated with use of bismuth subsalicylate. Vomiting is not a typical effect.

[35.2] **B.** Ranitidine is a histamine H_2-receptor antagonist that inhibits histamine binding to parietal cells and reduces acid secretion. It indirectly inhibits the synergistic acid secretion stimulated by gastrin binding to parietal cell gastrin receptors. PPIs inhibit parietal cell H^+, K^+-ATPase.

[35.3] **C.** Cimetidine is a histamine H_2-receptor antagonist that uniquely causes confusion and hallucinations, particularly in elderly patients. It also inhibits hepatic microsomal enzymes to increase, not decrease, the duration of action of other drugs. PPIs are prodrugs.

PHARMACOLOGY PEARLS

  Histamine H_2-receptor antagonists cross the blood-brain barrier and placenta, are secreted into breast milk, and therefore should be used judiciously during pregnancy and in nursing mothers.

  Three to four days of PPI administration is necessary to achieve maximal inhibition of acid secretion (up to 98%). Likewise, 3–4 days are needed for acid secretion to return to normal after discontinuation of therapy.

  PPIs are considered first-line agents for peptic ulcer disease and GERD.

REFERENCES

Aihara T, Nakamura K, Amagase K, et al. Pharmacological control of gastric acid secretion for the treatment of acid-related peptic disease: past, present and future. Pharmacol Ther 2003;98(1):109–27.

Chan FK, Leung WK. Peptic-ulcer disease. Lancet 2002;360(9337):933–41.

Suerbaum S, Michetti P. Heliobacter pylori infection. N Engl J Med 2002;347(15):1175–86.

A 22-year-old man presents for the evaluation of abdominal pain and diarrhea. He states that for approximately a month he has had progressively worsening cramping pains. He has had watery diarrhea and, from time to time, has noted blood mixed in with his stool. He has lost approximately 5 lb. He has tried over-the-counter antidiarrheal medications without relief. He is on no medication regularly and has no significant medical history. Examination of his abdomen reveals it to be distended and to have hyperactive bowel sounds. It is diffusely tender with no palpable masses. Rectal examination is very painful and reveals heme-positive watery stool. A blood count shows that he has iron deficiency anemia and an erythrocyte sedimentation rate that is markedly elevated. An office sigmoidoscopy reveals changes consistent with ulcerative colitis. You start him on a short course of corticosteroids and plan to place him on long-term sulfasalazine.

◆ **What is the mechanism of action of sulfasalazine?**

◆ **Sulfasalazine cannot be used by persons allergic to which class of antibiotics?**

ANSWERS TO CASE 36: AGENTS FOR LOWER GI DISORDERS

Summary: A 22-year-old man with ulcerative colitis is started on a short course of corticosteroids and long-term sulfasalazine.

◆ **Mechanism of action of sulfasalazine:** 5-aminosalicylic acid (5-ASA) component of sulfasalazine inhibits leukotriene and prostaglandin production in the colon.

◆ **Sulfasalazine cannot be used by persons allergic to:** Sulfonamides.

CLINICAL CORRELATION

Sulfasalazine is used to achieve and maintain remission in persons with inflammatory bowel disease (IBD: ulcerative colitis and Crohn's disease). It is composed of two constituents—5-ASA bound by an AZO bond (N=N) to sulfapyridine. The AZO bond limits the GI absorption of the inactive, parent compound. However, in the terminal ileum and colon, bacteria break down sulfasalazine into its two components. 5-ASA is the active anti-inflammatory component. Its mechanism of action, while not entirely known, is thought to involve inhibition of the production of inflammatory leukotrienes and prostaglandins in the colon. Its activity is terminated by hepatic acetylation. Sulfapyridine, which is also acetylated, does not appear to play an active role in the reduction of inflammation in the colon. Sulfapyridine mediates the allergic cross-reaction with sulfonamide drugs. 5-ASA can also be administered as mesalamine, balsalazide, and olsalazine, which do not have a sulfa component. Sulfasalazine, balsalazide, and olsalazine are administered orally. Mesalamine has oral, suppository, and enema formulations. The many adverse effects of sulfasalazine, attributable primarily to the systemic actions of sulfapyridine, which for many patients is not tolerated, and which is more common in slow acetylators than fast acetylators, includes severe GI discomfort with nausea, headache, myalgia, bone marrow suppression, possible oligospermia that is reversible, and a hypersensitivity with numerous attendant serious sequelae.

APPROACH TO PHARMACOLOGY OF AGENTS THAT ACT ON THE LOWER GI TRACT

Objectives

1. List drugs used as antidiarrheal agents and describe their mechanisms of action, therapeutic uses, and adverse effects.
2. List drugs used as laxatives and describe their mechanisms of action and adverse effects.
3. List drugs used to treat irritable bowel syndrome (IBS) and IBD.

Definitions

Ulcerative colitis: Inflammatory disease of GI mucosa that is localized in the large intestine.

Crohn's disease: Inflammatory disease of the GI tract that can occur anywhere from the mouth to the anus.

Irritable Bowel Syndrome (IBS): Recurrent abdominal pain with altered bowel movements (constipation or diarrhea), among other symptoms, that is due to alterations in motor and sensory function.

Inflammatory Bowel Disease: Condition with symptoms of chronic GI inflammation.

DISCUSSION

Class

The agents used for **acute treatment of diarrhea of mild-to-moderate severity** (Table 36-1) may also be used for control of **chronic diarrhea** resulting from **IBD and IBS** (Table 36-2). When constipation is predominant, laxatives,

Table 36-1
ANTIDIARRHEAL AGENTS

SELECTED ANTIDIARRHEAL AGENTS	SELECTED LAXATIVES
Opioid agonists Loperamide Diphenoxylate	*Bulk-forming laxatives* Psyllium preparations Methylcellulose Calcium polycarbophil
Kaolin	*Osmotic laxatives* Magnesium citrate Sodium phosphate Magnesium sulfate Sorbitol Lactulose PEG
Pectin	*Stool softeners* Docusate Glycerin Mineral oil
Methylcellulose resins Cholestyramine Colestipol	*Stimulant laxatives* (infrequently used) Aloe, senna, cascara, castor oil
Bismuth subsalicylate	

PEG = polyethylene glycol.

Table 36-2
DRUGS USED TO TREAT BOWEL DISORDERS

DRUGS USED TO TREAT IBS	DRUGS USED TO TREAT IBD
*Alosetron Tegaserod	*Aminosalicylates* Sulfasalazine Balsalazide Olsalazine Mesalamine

Antispasmodic agents
  Calcium channel antagonists,
  anticholinergic agents, opioid
  receptor antagonists
	Glucocorticoids

Tricyclic antidepressants Nortryptiline (e.g.)	Purine analogs Azathioprine 6-Mercaptopurine
	Methotrexate
	Anti-TNF-α agents Infliximab

*Requires physician certification and consent protocol.
IBS = irritable bowel syndrome; IBD = inflammatory bowel disease.

particularly osmotic laxatives (e.g., magnesium oxide), are used as stool softeners (Table 36-1).

Octreotide, an analog of somatostatin, is used primarily to treat diarrhea stemming from **GI tumors, AIDS, short-bowel syndrome, vagotomy, and dumping syndrome.** At low doses (50 mcg subcutaneously), octreotide is used to stimulate intestinal motility in patients with conditions that lead to intestinal obstruction or bacterial overgrowth.

Opioids

Prolonged use of high doses of **diphenoxylate can result in opioid dependence.**

Kaolin-Pectin

When administered concomitantly (within 2 hours of one another) **kaolins and pectins may bind other drugs in the GI tract and reduce their absorption.**

Methylcellulose Resins

Cholestyramine and colestipol may cause **bloating and constipation** and in some patients may result in insufficient absorption of fat. Like kaolin-pectin, the use of **octreotide** may result in constipation and abdominal pain.

The formation of gallstones resulting from reduced gallbladder contractility, and the development of hyperglycemia, and sometime hypoglycemia, as a consequence of an imbalance in the secretions of insulin, glucagons, and growth hormone may also occur with octreotide therapy. **Reduced pancreatic secretions may result in steatorrhea and deficiency of fat-soluble vitamins.**

Bulk-Forming and Osmotic Laxatives

Bulk-forming and osmotic laxatives (except PEG) can cause flatulence and bloating. Osmotic laxatives can result in electrolyte imbalance and should be used cautiously in patients with renal insufficiency or cardiac dysfunction. PEG is used to cleanse the colon prior to endoscopy. If aspirated, mineral oil can cause severe lipid pneumonia and when used chronically can result in decreased fat-soluble vitamin absorption.

Structure

Kaolin is a naturally occurring hydrated magnesium aluminum silicate, whereas pectin is derived from apples.

Octreotide is a more stable, biologically active octapeptide analog of the 14-amino acid regulatory peptide, somatostatin.

PEG is an osmotically active sugar.

Mechanism of Action

Kaolin and **pectin absorb fluids as well as bacteria** and other toxic agents in the GI tract.

The **opioids, loperamide, and diphenoxylate inhibit** the **release of acetylcholine** from cholinergic nerves in the submucosa and myenteric complex to disrupt coordinated colonic motility and to increase water absorption and transit time through the GI tract.

Cholestyramine and colestipol bind excess diarrhea-causing bile salts that may accumulate in Crohn's disease or from resection of the terminal ileum where bile salts are normally absorbed.

Octreotide, like somatostatin, **inhibits the release of numerous GI hormones** (e.g., gastrin, cholecystokinin, serotonin) that results in decreased intestinal fluid secretion and, depending on the subcutaneous dose, increased (50 mcg) or decreased (100–250 mcg) motility among many other effects, including reduced pancreatic secretions.

Bulk-forming laxatives, which are not absorbed from the GI tract, absorb water to form a gel or increase the fluidity of the stools that distends the colon and induces peristalsis. Osmotic laxatives, which are also not absorbed from the GI tract, increase the fluidity of stools. Stool softeners increase the penetration of water and lipids into compacted fecal material (docusate, glycerin) or coat it (mineral oil) to prevent the loss of water.

Administration

Loperamide, administered orally, is a nonprescription opioid agonist. Diphenoxylate is administered orally in combination with low doses of atropine (which also may contribute to the antidiarrheal activity of the preparation) to preclude its self-administration as a drug of abuse.

Octreotide can be administered intravenously or subcutaneously and in a subcutaneous depot formulation.

All laxatives are administered orally except glycerin, which is administered rectally as a suppository.

PEG is administered with an isotonic balanced salt solution to prevent the development of intravascular fluid or electrolyte imbalance.

Pharmacokinetics

Commercial preparations of kaolin and pectin are not absorbed from the GI tract.

Loperamide does not cross the blood-brain barrier and therefore has no analgesic activity or, importantly, potential for abuse that limits the use of other opioids as antidiarrheal agents.

Diphenoxylate, although very insoluble, does penetrate the central nervous system (CNS), and therefore its continuous use can result in opioid dependence.

Octreotide has a serum half-life of 90 minutes, compared with somatostatin, which has a serum half-life of approximately 3 minutes. Its duration of action can be extended up to 12 hours by subcutaneous administration and up to a month by using a depot formulation.

Sorbitol and lactulose are metabolized by colonic bacteria.

COMPREHENSION QUESTIONS

[36.1] Which of the following drugs crosses the blood-brain barrier?

      A. Diphenoxylate
      B. Kaolin
      C. Loperamide
      D. Methylcellulose

[36.2] Which of the following drugs inhibits the release of acetylcholine from cholinergic nerves in the submucosa and myenteric complex?

      A. Cholestyramine
      B. Docusate
      C. Loperamide
      D. Pectin

[36.3] Which of the following drugs shows an allergic cross-reaction with an antibiotic?

    A. Diphenoxylate
    B. Octreotide
    C. Psyllium
    D. Sulfasalazine

Answers

[36.1] **A.** Diphenoxylate can cross the blood-brain barrier and cause dependence. Methylcellulose and kaolin are not absorbed from the GI tract. Loperamide does not cross the blood-brain barrier.

[36.2] **C.** The opioid loperamide inhibits release of acetylcholine from cholinergic nerves in the submucosa and myenteric complex to disrupt coordinated colonic motility and to increase water absorption and transit time through the GI tract. Pectin absorbs fluids in the gastrointestinal tract. Stool softeners like docusate increase the penetration of water and lipids into compacted fecal material.

[36.3] **D.** Sulfasalazine is composed of 5-ASA and sulfapyridine. Sulfapyridine, which does not appear to play an active role in the reduction of inflammation in the colon, mediates an allergic cross-reaction with sulfonamide drugs.

PHARMACOLOGY PEARLS

 Antidiarrheal agents should not be used to treat patients experiencing bloody stools or high fever because of the increased risk of aggravating the underlying condition.

 Cholestyramine and colestipol bind excess diarrhea-causing bile salts.

❖ Many laxatives are commonly overused by the lay public.

REFERENCES

Lesbros-Pantoflickova D, Michetti P, Fried M, et al. Meta-analysis: the treatment of irritable bowel syndrome. Aliment Pharmacol Ther 2004;20:1253–69.

Schiller LR. Review article: the therapy of constipation. Aliment Pharmacol Ther 2001;15(6):749–63.

Stein RB. Medical therapy for inflammatory bowel disease. Gastroenterol Clin North Am 1999;28(2):297–321.

Wald A. Constipation. Med Clin North Am 2000;84(5):1231–46.

Wingate D, Phillips SF, Lewis SJ, et al. Guidelines for adults on self-medication for the treatment of acute diarrhea. Aliment Pharmacol Ther 2001;15(6):773–82.

An 8-year-old boy is brought to your office because of a chronic cough. His mother says that he coughs frequently throughout the day and will have symptoms 2 or 3 nights a month as well. This has been a problem on and off for approximately a year, but seems to be worse in the spring and fall. He also coughs more when he is riding his bike or playing soccer. He has been treated twice in the past year for "bronchitis" with antibiotics and cough suppressants but he never seems to clear up completely. His examination is normal except for his lungs, which reveal expiratory wheezing. You diagnose him with asthma and prescribe an albuterol inhaler.

◆ **What is the mechanism of action of the albuterol?**

◆ **What are the most common side effects of the albuterol?**

◆ **What medications can be used to provide long-term control of the asthma symptoms?**

ANSWERS TO CASE 37: AGENTS USED TO TREAT ASTHMA

Summary: An 8-year-old boy with asthma is prescribed an albuterol inhaler.

◆ **Mechanism of action of albuterol:** β_2-Adrenoceptor agonist in bronchial smooth muscle causes smooth muscle relaxation, inhibits the release of mediators from mast cells, and stimulates mucociliary clearance.

◆ **Most common side effects of albuterol:** Skeletal muscle tremor, tachycardia, and cough.

◆ **Medications for the long-term control of asthma:** Inhaled corticosteroids, long-acting β_2-adrenoceptor agonist, cromolyn or nedocromil; second-line agents include oral theophylline, leukotriene inhibitors, or systemic corticosteroids.

CLINICAL CORRELATION

Asthma is a disease of chronic airway inflammation. This inflammation can cause episodes of wheezing, coughing, and breathlessness, which are reversible either spontaneously or with treatment. The inflammation can also increase bronchial reactivity to certain stimuli, such as allergens, infectious agents, or exercise, which may trigger bronchospasm and symptoms. Inhaled β_2-adrenoceptor agonists (β-agonists) are widely used to treat the acute bronchospastic episodes. They work to relax bronchial smooth muscle via a cyclic adenosine monophosphate (cAMP)-mediated reduction in intracellular calcium concentrations, resulting in relaxation. The increase in cAMP also reduces the release of mediators from mast cells in the airways. Frequent use of these agents can result in a tachyphylaxis. Patients who require frequent dosing with inhaled β-agonists should also be treated with medications to reduce the frequency of bronchospastic events. These include inhaled corticosteroids, long-acting β-agonists, cromolyn or nedocromil, and oral methylxanthines, corticosteroids, or leukotriene modifiers. Inhaled β-agonists commonly cause tremor, tachycardia, and cough.

APPROACH TO PHARMACOLOGY OF DRUGS USED TO TREAT ASTHMA

Objectives

1. Understand the medications used in the treatment of asthma, their mechanisms of action, and adverse effects.
2. Know the difference between short-acting symptomatic treatments and long-acting preventive therapies.
3. List the mediators of airway inflammation involved in asthma.

Definitions

Bronchoconstriction: Constriction of the bronchial air passages, as a result of increased tone in airway smooth muscle cells.

Tachyphylaxis: Rapidly decreasing response to a drug following initial doses.

DISCUSSION

Class

Asthma is characterized by **acute episodes of bronchoconstriction** caused by **underlying airway inflammation.** A common finding in asthmatics is **an increased responsiveness** of the **bronchi and trachea** to **exogenous or endogenous stimuli** that results in **inappropriate contraction of smooth muscle in the airway,** and production of **thick viscid mucus** and **mucosal thickening from edema and cellular infiltration.** Asthma typically occurs with both an **early-phase response** lasting approximately 1–2 hours that is triggered by autocoids and inflammatory mediators such as **histamine, leukotrienes, and prostaglandins.** Immunoglobulin E-sensitized (IgE-sensitized) mast cells play a key role in the early-phase response. The late-phase response that occurs 2–8 hours later is mediated by cytokines from T-helper type 2 (Th2) lymphocytes including granulocyte-macrophage colony-stimulating factor (GM-CSF), and interleukins 4, 5, 9, and 13. These mediators attract and activate eosinophils and increase IgE production by B cells. This leads to the chronic bronchoconstriction, continued mucus production, and cellular infiltration that typify the underlying inflammation in asthma.

There are currently **six classes of drugs** used to treat asthma: **β-adrenoreceptor agonists, acetylcholine antagonists, glucocorticoids, leukotriene modifiers, chromones,** and **anti-IgE monoclonal antibodies.** The National Asthma Education and Prevention Program has revised its 1997 guidelines on the treatment of asthma as illustrated in Table 37-1.

The recommendation for quick relief in all patients regardless of severity is two to four puffs of a **short-acting inhaled β_2-agonist one to three times per occurrence.** Use of short-acting β_2-agonists more than two times a week may indicate the need to initiate long-term therapy. Short-acting β_2-selective drugs for use in asthma include albuterol, terbutaline, metaproterenol, and pirbuterol. These agents bind specifically to the β_2-adrenergic receptor and avoid the cardiovascular effects of β_1-activation. Activation of β_2-receptors causes bronchodilation. Onset of action occurs in minutes and lasts for 4–6 hours. Albuterol and terbutaline can be administered orally; terbutaline is available for subcutaneous injection for emergency treatment. Few side effects of short-term use of β_2-agonist have been reported. Excessive use or the oral preparations may result in cardiovascular effects such as tachycardia.

Long-acting inhaled β_2-agonists, such as salmeterol and formoterol, have a much longer half-life (up to 12 hours). These agents are available in metered-dose

Table 37-1

RECOMMENDATIONS FOR PHARMACOLOGIC MANAGEMENT OF
ASTHMA IN ADULTS AND CHILDREN OLDER THAN 5

ASTHMA SEVERITY	SYMPTOM FREQUENCY	MEDICATIONS
Mild intermittent	<2 days/week, <2 nights/month	None; course of systemic glucocorticoids for occasional, severe exacerbations
Mild persistent	>2 per week but <once per day >2 nights/month	Low-dose inhaled glucocorticoids. Alternate: cromolyn, nedocromil, leukotriene modifier, *or* sustained release theophylline
Moderate persistent	Daily, >1 night/week	Low- to medium-dose glucocorticoids and long-acting inhaled β_2-agonists. Alternate: leukotriene modifier or theophylline
Severe persistent	Continual during day, frequent at night	High-dose glucocorticoids *and* long-acting inhaled β_2-agonist *and* (if needed) systemic glucocorticoids

inhalers that produce fewer side effects than systemic administration. Use of long-acting agents produces the same relaxation in airway smooth muscles and also appears to decrease the release of mediators from mast cells and lymphocytes. The long-acting agents should not be used to reverse an acute attack.

Glucocorticoids are an important treatment for **mild persistent and more severe asthma.** Glucocorticoids are **potent anti-inflammatory agents** and reduce the production of inflammatory mediators and cause apoptosis of leukocytes and decrease vascular permeability. They **do not cause relaxation of bronchial smooth muscle.** The glucocorticoids are used for the prophylactic treatment of asthma; they have no appreciable effect on an acute event. Glucocorticoids administered by **inhalation** provide a high concentration of drug where needed and **minimizes the amount in the systemic circulation.** However, some drug is swallowed during inhalation and some drug is absorbed into the systemic circulation through the lung. Adverse effects are attributable to local effects of the glucocorticoids or the drug entering the systemic circulation. These include **oral candidiasis, increased loss of calcium from bone,** and rarely, **suppression** of the **hypothalamic-pituitary-adrenal axis. Systemic use of glucocorticoids** is recommended in patients with **severe persistent asthma** (see Table 37-1).

Leukotrienes B_4, C_4, and D_4 play an important role in the pathogenesis of asthma. LCB_4 is a potent neutrophile chemoattractant, and LTC_4 and LTD_4 are involved in bronchoconstriction and overproduction of airway mucus. These mediators are derived from arachidonic acid via the enzyme 5-lipoxygenase. Two classes of drugs have been developed that interfere with leukotrienes. **Zileuton** is an **inhibitor of 5-lipoxygenase** and thereby **decreases the biosynthesis of leukotrienes. Zafirlukast** and **montelukast** are **specific, competitive, Cys-LT1 receptor antagonists.** The **Cys-LT1** receptor is responsible for **mediating the bronchoconstrictor activity of all leukotrienes.** The two classes of drugs are equally **effective in the treatment of mild-to-moderate persistent asthma** and appear to be about **as effective as low-dose inhaled glucocorticoids.** All of the leukotriene modifiers are administered orally; the receptor antagonists may be taken once or twice a day, zileuton is taken four times a day. **Zileuton** has been associated with **liver toxicity,** and **monitoring liver enzymes is recommended.**

The **methylxanthines** include theophylline, theobromine, and caffeine; theophylline is used as a **second-line agent to treat asthma.** Theophylline was originally thought to act by **inhibiting cyclic nucleotide phosphodiesterases,** thereby **increasing intracellular cAMP and cyclic guanosine monophosphate (cGMP).** Theophylline is also an **antagonist of adenosine receptors,** and this mechanism of action might be especially important in asthma because **activation of pulmonary adenosine receptors results in bronchoconstriction.** However, the precise mechanism of action of theophylline in the lung remains controversial. Theophylline produces **bronchodilation** and improves long-term control of asthma. Theophylline is available for oral administration, as a suppository, and for parenteral use. Plasma levels of theophylline show considerable variability between patients, and the drug has a **narrow therapeutic window;** blood levels need to be monitored. Infants and neonates have the slowest rates of clearance.

The **chromones, cromolyn and nedocromil,** are unique drugs used for the **prophylaxis** of **mild-to-moderate persistent asthma.** A variety of mechanisms of action have been proposed for these agents including inhibition of mediator release from mast cells and suppression of activation of leukocytes. These various effects are now thought to be mediated by **inhibition of various chloride channels that are responsible for secretion and cellular activation.** They have **no effect on airway smooth muscle tone** and are **ineffective in reversing bronchospasm;** thus they are truly for prevention. Both agents are administered by inhalation and are effective in reducing both antigen and exercise-induced asthma. They are poorly absorbed into the systemic circulation and have mild adverse effects including throat irritation, cough, and nasal congestion. More serious adverse reactions including anaphylaxis, anemia, and pulmonary infiltration are rare.

Inhaled acetylcholine muscarinic cholinoreceptor antagonists have a use in treatment of asthma, but they have been somewhat superseded by other agents. Muscarinic antagonists can effectively block the bronchoconstriction, and the increase in mucus secretion that occurs in response to vagal discharge. **Ipratropium bromide** is a **quaternary ammonium derivative of atropine**

that can be administered by inhalation and that is **poorly absorbed into the systemic circulation.** Ipratropium bromide causes variable degrees of **bronchodilation** in patients; this may reflect the variable degree that parasympathetic stimulation contributes to asthma in individual patients. Ipratropium bromide is useful in patients that are unresponsive or cannot tolerate β_2-receptor agonists and in COPD. In addition, ipratropium bromide increases the bronchodilator activity of albuterol in the treatment of severe acute attacks.

IgE bound to mast cells plays an important role in antigen-induced asthma. A newly developed **monoclonal antibody that targets circulating IgE** and prevents its interaction with mast cells has recently been approved for the treatment of asthma. By decreasing the amount of IgE antibodies available to bind mast cells, IgE cross-linking is less likely and subsequently, the mast cell release of those mediators is decreased. In clinical trials, **omalizumab significantly reduced IgE levels** and reduced the magnitude of both the early- and late-phase responses to antigen. **Omalizumab is indicated for adults and children older than 12 years with moderate-to-severe persistent asthma** who have a **positive skin test or in vitro reactivity to a perennial aeroallergen** and whose **symptoms are inadequately controlled with inhaled corticosteroids.** The **most frequent adverse events included injection site reaction, viral infections, upper respiratory tract infection (20%), sinusitis, headache, and pharyngitis.** These events were observed at similar rates in omalizumab-treated patients and control patients. More serious adverse effects include malignancy (0.5%) and anaphylaxis.

COMPREHENSION QUESTIONS

[37.1] Zileuton is effective in treating asthma because it performs which of the following?

    A. Antagonizes leukotriene receptors

    B. Inhibits cyclooxygenase

    C. Inhibits 5-lipoxygenase

    D. Inhibits mast cell degranulation

[37.2] Which of the following drugs would be best for treatment of an acute attack of asthma?

    A. Inhaled albuterol

    B. Oral albuterol

    C. Oral dexamethasone

    D. Oral salmeterol

Match the following agents (A–H) to the described clinical situation [37.3–37.5].

A. Anticholinergic inhaler
B. β-Agonist inhaler
C. Chromone agent
D. Glucocorticoid inhaler
E. IgE inhibitor
F. Leukotriene receptor antagonist
G. Lipoxygenase inhibitor
H. Methylxanthines

[37.3] A 21-year-old woman with moderately severe asthma on three-drug treatment has elevated liver function tests thought to be caused by one of her medications.

[37.4] A 25-year-old man has bronchospasm that is exercise induced, particularly in the cold weather. He takes his medication 15 minutes prior to anticipated exercise, which will help to prevent the asthmatic attack but does not produce bronchodilation.

[37.5] A 16-year-old female is placed on multiple medications. She has been taking her medications as instructed, but one of the medications is causing her to have tachycardia, nausea, and jitteriness. She has been informed of the need to measure serum levels of this medication.

Answers

[37.1]   **C.** Zileuton diminishes the production of leukotrienes by inhibiting 5-lipoxygenase.

[37.2]   **A.** Inhaled albuterol would provide the fastest acting and most localized therapy for an acute attack.

[37.3]   **G. Zileuton** is an inhibitor of 5-lipoxygenase, thereby decreases the biosynthesis of leukotrienes; it is associated with liver toxicity.

[37.4]   **C.** Chromones are prophylactic agents, useful especially for exercise or cold-induced bronchospasm.

[37.5]   **H.** The methylxanthine agents have a low therapeutic index and often can cause adverse effects.

PHARMACOLOGY PEARLS

 Inhaled corticosteroids are the treatment of choice for the long-term management of persistent asthma.

 Use of short-acting β_2-agonists more than twice weekly indicates inadequate control, and examination of long-term treatment should be considered.

REFERENCES

Lim KG. Management of persistent symptoms in patients with asthma. Mayo Clin Proc 2002;77:1333–8.

Ressel GW, Centers for Disease Control and Prevention, National Asthma Education and Prevention Program. NAEPP updates guidelines for the diagnosis and management of asthma. Am Fam Physician 2003;68:169–70.

Panettieri RA, In the Clinic. Asthma. Ann Internal Med 2007;146:ITC6–16.

A 32-year-old woman comes to your office during the height of the spring pollen season complaining of sneezing and congestion. She gets these symptoms every year. Her nose runs constantly, her eyes water and itch, and she sneezes. She is only getting partial relief from oral antihistamines. She asks if there is anything else that she can do for her allergies. On examination she has red, irritated conjunctiva with clear eye drainage and periorbital discoloration ("allergic shiners"). Her nasal mucosa is boggy and appears congested. You agree with her diagnosis of seasonal allergic rhinitis and prescribe a corticosteroid nasal spray to be used along with her oral antihistamine.

◆ **How long does it take to see the full effect of nasal steroids?**

◆ **What are the common side effects of nasal steroids?**

ANSWERS TO CASE 38: RHINITIS AND COUGH MEDICATIONS

Summary: A 32-year-old woman with seasonal allergic rhinitis is prescribed nasal steroid medication to take together with her antihistamine.

◆ **Length of time until maximal effect of nasal steroids:** 1–2 weeks.

◆ **Common side effects:** Nasal burning, throat irritation, nose bleeds.

CLINICAL CORRELATION

The mechanism of action of nasal steroids for allergic rhinitis is not entirely known. Corticosteroids have a wide range of activity on many inflammatory mediators, including histamine, cytokines and leukotrienes, and cell types such as mast cells, eosinophils, and macrophages, which are involved in allergic symptoms. Nasal steroids are effective at reducing the congestion, rhinitis, and sneezing associated with seasonal and environmental allergies. They require treatment for up to 2 weeks before maximal benefit is seen. For that reason it is recommended that they be used on a daily, not an as needed, basis. The adverse effects of nasal steroids are primarily a result of local effects, because they are not largely systemically absorbed. These include nasal burning and bleeding and throat irritation. Histamine (H_1-receptor) antagonists are also widely used for allergic rhinitis and may be used in combination with nasal steroid medications. H_1-receptors are membrane bound and coupled to G-proteins. Their activation leads to increased phospholipase C activity, with increases in diacylglycerol and intracellular Ca^{2+}. The net effect of this in blood vessels is vasodilation and increased permeability, which clinically contributes to the mucosal swelling and congestion seen in allergic rhinitis.

APPROACH TO PHARMACOLOGY OF DRUGS USED TO TREAT RHINITIS AND COUGH

Objectives

1. Understand the characteristics of rhinitis and cough.
2. List the drugs used for rhinitis, their mechanisms of action, and adverse effects.
3. Know the agents used to treat cough, their mechanisms of action, and adverse effects.

Definitions

Rhinitis: Inflammation of the mucus membranes of the nose.
Allergic conjunctivitis: An inflammatory condition of the conjunctiva secondary to an allergic stimulus. Common symptoms include itchy, red, and tearing eyes.

DISCUSSION

Class

Rhinitis is caused by **increased mucus production, vasodilation, and increased fluid accumulation in mucosal spaces. Inflammatory mediators** including **histamine, leukotrienes, interleukins, prostaglandins, and kinins** are responsible for these effects. Increased production of these mediators can be provoked by an allergic response, or a bacterial or viral infection.

Allergic rhinitis affects 20 percent of the adult population and up to 40 percent of children. **The hallmark of allergic rhinitis is an IgE-mediated inflammatory response.** Antihistamines, anticholinergics, intranasal corticosteroids, and chromones have proven to be useful in treating allergic rhinitis.

Both **first- and second-generation histamine H₁-receptor blockers** (see Case 24) are useful in treating **acute allergic rhinitis,** but their long-term benefits are questionable. First-generation agents, including diphenhydramine, cyclizine, and chlorpheniramine, have been shown to reduce sneezing, nasal congestion, and nasal itching. Second-generation agents, including fexofenadine, cetirizine, and loratadine, have comparable efficacy and significantly fewer adverse effects such as sedation and dry mouth. Second-generation antihistamines effectively reduce all seasonal allergic rhinitis symptoms in children, but dosages must be appropriately reduced. Following oral administration effects are seen with antihistamines in 1–2 hours. The most common adverse effect seen with the second-generation agents are headache, back pain, and cough.

Inhaled nasal corticosteroids such as beclomethasone, budesonide, flunisolide, fluticasone, and triamcinolone acetonide are **useful for long-term management of allergic rhinitis.** This **route of administration reduces the frequent adverse effects associated with systemic administration of corticosteroids.** Corticosteroids are potent anti-inflammatory agents and reduce both the production of inflammatory mediators (cytokines, leukotrienes, and prostaglandins) and cellular components (mast cells, eosinophils, basophils, lymphocytes, macrophages, and neutrophils). The major adverse effects seen with inhaled corticosteroids are **pharyngitis and an increased risk of upper respiratory tract infections.**

The **chromones,** cromolyn and nedocromil, have also been used to treat allergic rhinitis. These agents are administered by inhalation and are poorly absorbed into the systemic circulation. Their major action is to reduce the activity of a number of chloride channels that are important in the release of mediators such as histamine. The major adverse effects of these agents are bronchospasm, cough, and nasal congestion (which can be severe); less frequent adverse effects include anaphylaxis, dizziness, and anemia.

Nasal decongestants are α-adrenoreceptor agonists that **reduce the discomfort** of allergic rhinitis, and to a lesser extent congestion associated with the common cold or flu, by decreasing the volume of nasal mucosa and **causing vasoconstriction of capacitance vessels in the nasal passages.** The most common α-adrenergic agent used as a decongestant is **pseudoephedrine**

(a stereoisomer of ephedrine), which acts directly on α_1-**adrenoreceptors.** Ephedrine has largely been discontinued as a decongestant because it has significant central nervous system (CNS) effects. A major limitation in the use of these agents is rebound hyperemia and worsening of symptoms that often occurs with chronic use or after discontinuation. Nasal decongestants should be used with caution in patients with hypertension.

Cough and Antitussives

Cough is produced by the cough reflex, which is integrated in the cough center in the medulla. The initial stimulus for cough arises in the bronchi where irritation causes bronchoconstriction. Stretch receptors in the trachea and bronchial tree monitor the state of this bronchoconstriction and send vagal afferents to the cough center that trigger the cough reflex. Agents that have antitussive activity act either to relieve the bronchoconstriction or reduce the activity of the cough center.

Codeine and hydrocodone are opioid congeners that are used as antitussives. Cough suppression occurs at lower doses than required for analgesia. The exact mechanism of the antitussive activity of the opioids is unclear because isomers devoid of binding to classic receptors still display antitussive activity. Both codeine and hydrocodone are available as syrups for oral administration.

Dextromethorphan is the d-isomer of the codeine analog methorphan. It has no analgesic or addictive properties and does not act through the classic opioid receptors. Binding sites for dextromethorphan have been identified in membrane preparations from various parts of the brain, but it is still unclear whether they mediate the antitussive actions of the drug.

β-Adrenergic agonists have been shown to reduce cough without having any significant central effects. This **action is likely mediated within the bronchi** and reduces vagal afferent signals to the cough center.

COMPREHENSION QUESTIONS

[38.1]   Pseudoephedrine is used to treat nasal congestion because of which of the following?

A. It is an α_1-adrenergic agonist
B. It is an α_2-adrenergic agonist
C. It inhibits leukotrienes
D. It inhibits the production of IgE

[38.2]   Which of the following would be the best for long-term management of a patient with allergic rhinitis?

A. Diphenhydramine
B. Inhaled glucocorticoids
C. Oral glucocorticoids
D. Oral pseudoephedrine

[38.3] A 24-year-old man is taking two medications to help with the symptoms of allergic rhinitis. He is noted to have a blood pressure of 150/70 mm Hg. The clinician notes that one of the medications may be responsible for the new-onset hypertension. The most likely etiology is which of the following?

A. Inhaled chromone
B. Inhaled glucocorticoids
C. Oral diphenhydramine
D. Oral pseudoephedrine

Answers

[38.1] **A.** Pseudoephedrine is the most common agent used today as a decongestant. It is a directly acting α_1-sympathomimetic agent.

[38.2] **B.** Systemic glucocorticoids cause too many adverse effects; pseudoephedrine acts primarily only on nasal congestion; diphenhydramine is not useful for long-term management.

[38.3] **D.** Pseudoephedrine has activity on the α_1-adrenergic receptor, causing vasoconstriction to the nasal mucosa. Hypertension may also be seen at times.

PHARMACOLOGY PEARLS

❖ The hallmark of allergic rhinitis is an IgE-mediated inflammatory response.

❖ Antihistamines are useful for treating symptoms of acute rhinitis, but their long-term benefit is questionable.

❖ Pseudoephedrine has activity on the α_1-adrenergic receptor, causing vasoconstriction to the nasal mucosa.

REFERENCES

Ressel GW, Agency for Healthcare Research and Quality. AHRQ (agency for healthcare research and quality) releases review of treatments for allergic and nonallergic rhinitis. Am Fam Physician 2002;66:2164, 2167.

Seth D, Secord E, Kamat D. Allergic rhinitis. Clin Pediatr (Phila) 2007;46:401–7.

A 67-year-old man complains of pain in his right hip for the past few weeks. He has had no injury to the area and describes the pain as a "bone ache" that does not radiate. Review of systems is positive only for some weakness of urinary stream and having to get up twice a night to go to the bathroom. His general physical examination is normal. His hip examination is normal with a full range of motion and no tenderness. Examination of his prostate reveals it to be firm, enlarged, and nodular. Blood tests show a markedly elevated prostate-specific antigen (PSA), and biopsy of the prostate shows carcinoma. A bone scan confirms the presence of metastatic disease in the right hip. Along with other adjuvant therapies, a decision is made to start depot leuprolide acetate.

◆ **Leuprolide acetate is an analog of which hypothalamic hormone?**

◆ **What is the mechanism of action of leuprolide acetate?**

◆ **Which pituitary hormones are affected by leuprolide acetate, and how are they affected?**

ANSWERS TO CASE 39: DRUGS ACTIVE ON THE HYPOTHALAMUS AND PITUITARY GLAND

Summary: A 67-year-old man with metastatic prostate cancer is to receive depot leuprolide acetate.

◆ **Leuprolide acetate is an analog of which hypothalamic hormone:** Gonadotropin-releasing hormone (GnRH).

◆ **Mechanism of action of leuprolide acetate:** Chronic administration of GnRH analog results in the reduction of the number of GnRH receptors in the pituitary (downregulation), with resultant decreases in pituitary gonadotropin production.

◆ **Pituitary hormones affected:** Luteinizing hormone (LH) and follicle-stimulating hormone (FSH) production is reduced.

CLINICAL CORRELATION

The hypothalamic-pituitary-gonadal axis is a classic example of a hormonal stimulation-feedback system. The hypothalamus produces GnRH, which binds to specific receptors on pituitary gonadotropic cells. These cells then produce LH and FSH, which act on the gonadal organs. LH and FSH regulate the female menstrual cycle by their effects on the ovarian follicles and the ovarian production of estrogen and progesterone. In males, LH and FSH regulate spermatogenesis and the production of testosterone in the testes. Estrogen, progesterone, and testosterone then function as feedback signals for the hypothalamic production of GnRH. Leuprolide acetate is a synthetic 9-amino acid analog of GnRH. When initially administered, leuprolide acetate results in increases in LH, FSH, and gonadal steroid production because of its action as a GnRH agonist. However, with chronic administration, there is a reduction in the number of GnRH receptors in the pituitary gonadotropic cells. This causes a reduction in FSH or LH and a resultant reduction in gonadal hormone production. In women this effect may be beneficial in conditions such as endometriosis, where estrogen stimulates the growth, and activity of the ectopic endometrial tissue, which causes symptoms. The effect in men is to lower the production of testosterone to near castrate levels. Because prostate cancer is often testosterone dependent, leuprolide acetate can be used as a treatment for prostate cancer in those who are not surgical candidates, do not desire surgery, or have metastatic disease. Leuprolide acetate must be administered parenterally, and it has a depot form, which is active for up to 3 months. It commonly causes "menopausal" side effects, such as hot flashes, as a result of the reduction in gonadal hormone production.

APPROACH TO PHARMACOLOGY
OF NEUROENDOCRINE DRUGS

Objectives

1. Understand the receptors and second messengers involved in the endocrine system.
2. Understand the hypothalamic-pituitary axis and its feedback system.
3. Know the drugs used as agonists and antagonists on the hypothalamic-pituitary axis, their therapeutic uses, mechanisms of action, and adverse effects.

Definitions

Prostate cancer: Common malignancy in men which may be confined to the prostate gland or metastasize to pelvic lymph nodes or bone.

Hormonal therapy: Various malignancies are sensitive to hormones, and thus medications that act as agonists or antagonists are used for therapy.

DISCUSSION

Class of Agents

The **hypothalamic-hypophyseal-end organ system** is a classic negative feedback pathway (Figure 39-1). The multiple steps in this regulatory pathway, and both positive and negative regulation, provide several targets for pharmacologic intervention. The **hypothalamus** secretes a number of **releasing factors,** including **GnRH, corticotropin-releasing hormone (CRH), thyroid-releasing hormone (TRH), and growth hormone-releasing hormone (GHRH),** that are of clinical significance.

These neuroendocrine factors are secreted by the hypothalamus into the hypothalamic-hypophyseal portal circulation, and they act on cognate cell types within the pituitary and cause an increase in the secretion of specific pituitary hormones. For example, **GnRH** produces an increase in the synthesis and release of both **gonadotropins, LH and FSH.** This action is mediated by a specific **seven-transmembrane G-protein coupled receptor** that binds GnRH in cells called gonadotrophs.

FSH acts on the **ovary** to cause **follicular development and maturation;** **LH** causes an increase in the production of **estradiol** and is required for maintenance of the **corpus luteum.** The **LH surge** at midmenstrual cycle triggers **ovulation.** In men, **FSH is required for spermatogenesis, and LH causes an increase in testosterone production.** The actions of the two gonadotropins are also mediated by specific G-protein coupled receptors in the ovary and testis.

17β-Estradiol and testosterone are released into the circulation, and these sex hormones have effects on many tissues. Predominantly **estradiol in**

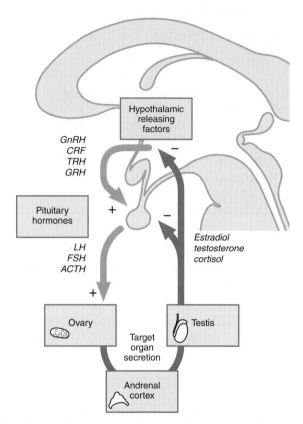

Figure 39-1. Interaction among the hypothalamus, pituitary, and gonad. GnRH = gonadotropic-releasing hormone; CRH = corticotropin-releasing hormone; TRH = thyrotropin-releasing hormone; GHRH = growth hormone-releasing hormone; LH = luteinizing hormone; FSH = follicle-stimulating hormone; ACTH = adrenocorticotropic hormone.

women, and **testosterone and estradiol in men** (produced by peripheral conversion of testosterone to estradiol), act on the hypothalamus and pituitary to decrease the production of the releasing hormone and the gonadotropins, respectively. This closes the negative feedback loop. As in all target tissues, the estrogen and testosterone receptors in the pituitary and hypothalamus are nuclear receptors that modulate the transcription of target genes.

The **adrenal cortex** is regulated in a similar manner. **Corticotropin-releasing factor (CRF)** is released **from the hypothalamus,** and it elicits the synthesis and release of **adrenocorticotropic hormone (ACTH)** from the **pituitary. ACTH acts on the adrenal cortex** and causes an increase in the synthesis of **cortisol from the zona fasciculata** and **adrenal androgens from the zona reticularis.**

The secretion of **growth hormone by the pituitary** is regulated in a different manner. Growth hormone secretion is stimulated by the **hypothalamic hormone GHRH and is inhibited by somatostatin.** Somatostatin acts in a number of tissues besides the pituitary; it inhibits the release of glucagon and insulin from the pancreas and inhibits the secretion of a number of gut peptides. **Prolactin** secretion from the pituitary is also controlled by **positive and negative regulatory factors.** The most important pharmacologically is the **prolactin inhibitory factor (PIF) activity of dopamine agonists.**

APPROACH TO PHARMACOLOGIC USES OF HYPOTHALAMIC PEPTIDES AND ANALOGS

Leuprolide acetate and gonadorelin acetate are synthetic peptide GnRH analogs that are administered either by subcutaneous injection, as a long-acting implant, or by IV infusion. Nafarelin acetate is a comparable peptide analog that can be administered by nasal spray. The frequency of administration is critical to the therapeutic goal. **Acute or pulsatile administration of GnRH analogs increases** production of **LH and FSH** by the pituitary. Used in this manner, GnRH analogs are useful to **stimulate spermatogenesis and testosterone production in men, and to induce ovulation or treat primary hypothalamic amenorrhea in women. Chronic administration,** for example, daily injections or use of depot preparations, **decreases** the production of FSH and LH by the pituitary. This is caused by a **depression in the number of GnRH receptors on gonadotrophs. Chronic leuprolide administration** can be used to achieve maximum androgen blockade (MAB), which **reduces testosterone production by the testis** that is **therapeutically equivalent to orchiectomy.** In men, this is useful to control androgen-dependent hyperproliferation as in **advanced prostate cancer and prostatic hyperplasia.** In women, chronic leuprolide leads to markedly diminished estrogen production which is useful in treating a number of estrogen-dependent hyperproliferative diseases. These include **endometriosis, polycystic ovary disease, and uterine leiomyomas.** Chronic leuprolide has also been used to treat hirsutism in women. The major adverse effect in women is a chemical menopause with vasomotor symptoms and the potential for osteoporosis. In men, leuprolide has been associated with the flare phenomenon, increased cancer growth as a result of transient increase in testosterone production on initiation of therapy. Other adverse effects in men include hot flashes, gynecomastia, and testicular atrophy. A new class of pure GnRH antagonists, including cetrorelix and ganirelix, have been approved for treatment of infertility. These agents do not cause the initial agonist activity seen with leuprolide. Their main advantage is a reduction in the required days of fertility drug therapy per cycle from several weeks (i.e., 3 weeks) to several days. These agents are not approved for use in men.

Somatostatin is unique among the hypothalamic peptides because of its widespread inhibitory activity on secretion and cellular proliferation.

Octreotide is an 8-amino acid cyclopeptide with potent somatostatin agonist activity. Its action to decrease secretion makes it useful to treat hypersecretory states such as VIPomas, chronic pancreatitis, and watery diarrhea from a number of causes including AIDS. Its antiproliferative uses include colorectal cancer and leukemia, and diabetic retinopathy. It is in clinical trials for additional malignancies. It has also been used to treat acute portal hypertension. It is approved for use in the treatment of acromegaly. Adverse effects include nausea, cramps, and increased gallstone formation.

Other hypothalamic peptides are used primarily as diagnostic agents. **GHRH** is a 40-amino acid peptide that can be administered IV for the diagnostic evaluation of idiopathic growth hormone deficiency. Similarly, IV administration of **TRH** is useful in the differential diagnosis of thyroid diseases. **CRH** is a 41-amino acid polypeptide found in the hypothalamus and the gut. CRH is used in cases of ACTH deficiency to distinguish between hypothalamic-pituitary or primary adrenal disease.

The **PIF** activity of **bromocriptine** or **levodopa** can be used to treat states of prolactin excess as in some cases of amenorrhea, galactorrhea, and prolactin-secreting tumors.

COMPREHENSION QUESTIONS

[39.1] Which of the following best describes the action of somatostatin?

    A Inhibition of growth hormone release

    B. Inhibition of prolactin release

    C. Stimulation of insulin release

    D. Stimulation of LH release

[39.2 In the first 2 weeks following a single injection of leuprolide, one would expect which of the following?

    A. Decreased LH production

    B. Decreased testosterone production

    C. Increased LH receptors

    D. Increased testosterone production

[39.3] A 22-year-old woman has severe endometriosis with dysmenorrhea. She is treated with depot leuprolide acetate. One week after her first injection, she notes a marked increase in the dysmenorrhea. What is the explanation?

    A. Direct effect of leuprolide on the endometrial implants

    B. Likely flare with increased gonadotropin effect prior to downregulation of receptors

    C. Probable placebo effect

    D. Resistance of her endometriosis to the leuprolide and probable need for another agent

Answers

[39.1]   **A.** Somatostatin is a major regulator of growth hormone, and its effect is inhibitory of growth hormone release.

[39.2]   **D.** Acute leuprolide will increase FSH/LH and sex steroid production and have little effect on receptor numbers.

[39.3]   **B.** The initial response to GnRH analog is an increase in FSH and estrogen, leading to an exacerbation of the endometriosis. Thereafter, there is a downregulation of GnRH receptors of the pituitary, leading to a decrease in FSH and estrogen.

PHARMACOLOGY PEARLS

 The frequency of administration of leuprolide determines its effect: Acute administration will increase FSH/LH and sex steroids, chronic administration will decrease FSH/LH and sex steroids.

 Chronic leuprolide administration leads to androgen blockade in men, which is useful in treating hormone-dependent cancers such as prostatic carcinoma.

REFERENCES

Holzbeierlein JM, Castle EP, Thrasher JB. Complications of androgen-deprivation therapy for prostate cancer. Clin Prostate Cancer 2003;2:147–52.

Valle RF, Sciarra JJ. Endometriosis: treatment strategies. Ann NY Acad Sci 2003; 97:229–39.

Susini C, Buscail L. Rationale for the use of somatostatin analogs as antitumor agents. Ann Oncol 2006;17:1733–42.

A 28-year-old woman presents for an evaluation of infertility. She and her husband have been attempting to conceive unsuccessfully for a year. She has never been pregnant. She has a history of irregular menstrual cycles, which were treated with oral contraceptive pills for 5 years. She has not taken contraceptives in the past 3 years. She has no other medical history, she takes no medications, and there is no family history of infertility. She does not smoke cigarettes or drink alcohol. Her routine physical and gynecologic examinations are normal. Blood tests were also normal. Basal body temperature charts that she brings in with her show no midcycle temperature elevation, and home urine ovulation prediction tests have all been negative. Her husband has already seen his physician, had a normal examination, and has had a normal semen analysis. She is diagnosed with infertility secondary to anovulation and started on clomiphene citrate.

◆ **What is the mechanism of action of clomiphene?**

◆ **How does clomiphene induce ovulation?**

ANSWERS TO CASE 40: DRUGS ACTIVE ON THE GONADAL AND REPRODUCTIVE SYSTEM

Summary: A 28-year-old woman with infertility and anovulation is treated with clomiphene citrate.

◆ **Mechanism of action of clomiphene:** Competitive antagonist of estrogen receptor.

◆ **Mechanism of induction of ovulation:** Inhibition of estrogen feedback on hypothalamus and pituitary with resultant increase in FSH, which induces follicle production in the ovaries and ovulation.

CLINICAL CORRELATION

The menstrual cycle is regulated by the hypothalamic-pituitary-ovarian axis. GnRH produced in the hypothalamus stimulates the pituitary hormones FSH and LH, which induce the maturation of follicles and release of ova from the ovaries. Estrogen and progesterone produced in the ovaries create a feedback loop on the hypothalamus and pituitary. Clomiphene is a competitive antagonist of the estrogen receptor. It is used for the treatment of infertility in women who have anovulatory menstrual cycles. By antagonizing estrogen receptors in the pituitary gland, clomiphene disrupts the normal negative feedback on the release of FSH. The elevated levels of FSH then help to induce the development of follicles in the ovaries. Potential risks of the use of clomiphene include the stimulation of multiple follicles and release of multiple eggs, with a resultant multiple gestations. It may also cause ovarian enlargement. The antiestrogen effect may precipitate hot flashes and abnormal uterine bleeding.

APPROACH TO PHARMACOLOGY OF GONADAL STEROIDS AND THEIR ANTAGONISTS

Objectives

1. Understand the structures, mechanism of action, and effects of natural gonadal hormones.
2. Know the therapeutic uses and adverse effects of estrogens, progestins, and androgens.
3. List the types, uses, and adverse effects of hormonal contraceptives.
4. Describe the drugs used as antiestrogens, antiprogestins, and antiandrogens, their therapeutic uses, mechanisms of action, and adverse effects.

Definitions

Nuclear receptor: A superfamily of receptor molecules that are activated by steroid hormones, fatty acid derivatives, or products of metabolism such as bile acids. They act by altering the rate of transcription of specific target genes.

ERE: Estrogen-response element. A DNA sequence motif that binds estrogen receptors. The consensus sequence is GGTCANNNTGACC.

SERM: Selective estrogen receptor modulator. A group of drugs that display tissue-specific estrogen agonist or antagonist activity.

DISCUSSION

Class

Estrogens and Progestins

The **gonadotropins and sex steroids** comprise a collection of drugs that have a number of uses including **infertility, contraception, hormone replacement, osteoporosis, and cancer. Antagonists** acting within the system also have uses in treating **hormone-dependent cancers and as abortifacients.**

The **menstrual cycle** is controlled by a complex feedback system between the hypothalamus, pituitary, and ovaries (see Case 39). LH and FSH are released from the pituitary on stimulation by GnRH released from the hypothalamus. **GnRH is released from the hypothalamus in a pulsatile manner under the control of the "pulse generator" in neurons in the arcuate nucleus.** In the proliferative phase of the menstrual cycle, the pulse generator causes release of GnRH at a rate of approximately one pulse per hour, and consequently **release of LH and FSH** from the pituitary is also **pulsatile. The intermittent release of GnRH is a key to controlling the menstrual cycle** because continuous infusion of GnRH results in cessation of release of the pituitary gonadotropins, estrogen, and progesterone, and produces amenorrhea. FSH acts on the graafian follicle to cause maturation of ova and to secrete estrogen. As estrogen levels rise, LH and FSH production is inhibited because of negative feedback that diminishes the *amplitude* of the GnRH pulse; release of FSH is also diminished by inhibin that is released by the ovary. At midcycle, alterations in the responsiveness of the pituitary to gonadotropins occur, and the negative feedback pattern is replaced by a period of positive feedback when estradiol causes an increase in the release of LH and FSH. This change in pituitary responsiveness requires levels of serum estradiol above 150 pg/mL for 36 hours. The positive feedback elicits the midcycle surge of LH and FSH that causes ovulation. After ovulation, the corpus luteum is able to secrete progesterone for its lifetime of 14 days if pregnancy does not occur. Progesterone decreases the frequency of the hypothalamic pulse-generator and inhibits LH and FSH release from the pituitary. A frequent cause of infertility is a disruption in the complex feedback regulatory patterns that results in anovulation.

The **ovary produces a number of estrogens;** the most important are **17β-estradiol and estrone.** 17β-Estradiol and estrone are classical steroid hormones containing a four-ring structure and 18 carbon atoms. **Progesterone** is also a classical steroid composed of **21 carbon atoms.**

The effects of estrogen and progesterone are mediated by **hormone-specific nuclear receptors.** There are **two types of estrogen receptors,** termed ER_α and ER_β. Most tissues express more ER_α, but the relative amounts of the two receptors is tissue and cell dependent. The precise role that each of these receptors plays in mediating the various effects of the estrogens is unclear. 17β-Estradiol has the highest affinity for the ERs; estrone binds to both receptors with a lower affinity. ER_α and ER_β are nuclear receptors that reside within the nucleus bound to the promoters of target genes at estrogen response elements even in the absence of ligand. On binding an estrogen, a conformational change occurs in the receptor such that additional proteins are recruited to the receptor. These proteins, called coactivators, are able to increase the transcription rate of estrogen-dependent target genes. There are also two forms of the progesterone receptor called PRA and PRB. These two isoforms are derived from a single gene by differential use of two promoters within the progesterone receptor gene. Human PRB contains an additional 164 amino acids on the amino terminus of the mature protein; the rest of the PRB is identical to PRA. Both receptors reside within the nucleus bound to PREs and activate gene expression in a fashion similar to ERs, but the target genes are different as a result of differences in the sequence of ERE compared to PRE. In most circumstances, PRA inhibits the action of PRB (and of some other nuclear receptors such as ER_α and ER_β as well). Thus, the amplitude of the effects elicited by progesterone depends on the ratio of the two isoforms.

Estrogens and progesterone have a variety of pharmacologic uses including oral contraception, hormone replacement therapy (HRT) in postmenopausal women, treatment of osteoporosis, and for failure of ovarian development.

Oral Contraceptives

Oral combination contraceptives contain **synthetic estrogens,** most commonly **ethinyl estradiol,** and a **progestin** (for example, norethindrone or norgestrel). Over the past several years the doses of estrogen in combination oral contraceptives have diminished, and the ratio of estrogen to progestin has evolved from a fixed ratio (monophasic) to biphasic and triphasic regimens with varying ratios that attempt to more closely mimic the ratio during the normal menstrual cycle. **The primary mechanism of action of oral contraceptives is prevention of ovulation.** The midcycle LH surge is absent, and endogenous estrogen levels are reduced. Oral contraceptives also alter transport of the ovum down the fallopian tube; increase the viscosity of mucus produced by the cervix, which impairs sperm entry; and create an endometrial environment less favorable to implantation. Several preparations are available for continuous dosing for 84 or 365 days; this reduces the number of bleeding periods per year.

Progestin-only contraceptives may be administered as a daily oral dose, a **depot injection** (medroxyprogesterone acetate), or as a **progestin** (L-norgestrel) **implant.** Their effectiveness approaches combination oral contraceptives, and both the depot injection and the implants have the advantage of a long duration of action (14 weeks for the injection, 5 years for the implants). Progestins alone inhibit ovulation approximately 70 percent of the time, but their effectiveness is increased by effects on the endometrium and cervical mucus production.

Several emergency ("morning-after") contraceptive regimens have been used effectively to prevent pregnancy if used within 72 hours of coitus. The most common regimen consists of two combination oral contraceptive pills containing 50 mcg of ethinyl estradiol and 500 mcg of norgestrel or levonorgestrel immediately and two at 12 hours. Alternative schedules include two doses of 750 mcg of L-norgestrel over 1 day.

Hormone Replacement Therapy

The decline in the production of estrogens that occurs at and following menopause is associated with **increased rates of bone loss** that can result in frank **osteoporosis, vasomotor symptoms** such as hot flashes and night sweats, vaginal dryness and thinning, and genital atrophy. All of these symptoms can be **alleviated by estrogens,** but careful assessment of the risk-benefit ratio for a given patient is essential. The most commonly prescribed oral estrogen preparation for postmenopausal therapy is a complex mixture of natural estrogens (conjugated equine estrogen, Premarin), by mass mostly estrone sulphate and equilin estrogens, and this is usually combined with medroxyprogesterone acetate to avoid unopposed estrogenic stimulation of the endometrium. Other HRT or estrogen replacement therapy (ERT) regimens include oral esterified estrogens, micronized estradiol, and transdermal delivery of estradiol.

Other Uses of Estrogens and Progestins

Estrogens can be used to treat circumstances of inadequate hormone production as in **primary hypogonadism.** This treatment is usually begun early (ages 11–13) to facilitate the development of the secondary sexual organs and to stimulate maximal growth.

Estrogens are also useful in the treatment of **intractable dysmenorrhea** where inhibition of ovulation may be of therapeutic value. Relatively high doses of estrogens have been used to suppress ovarian production of androgens. Both of these therapeutic approaches depend on estrogen-mediated negative feedback inhibition of gonadotropin release.

Adverse Effects of Estrogens and Progestins

Most of the adverse effects associated with estrogens and progestins are extensions of their physiologic actions. **Uterine bleeding** is the most common adverse effect associated with use of estradiol. The **increased risk of cancer** caused by estrogen and progesterone use remains a significant concern. **Unopposed estrogen treatment** has been well documented to cause an approximate threefold increase in the risk of **endometrial cancer.** Addition of a progestin to a treatment regimen essentially eliminates this increased risk. Several recent very large clinical trials examining use of estrogens to treat postmenopausal women have indicated that there is an **increased risk of breast cancer with estrogen** plus progesterone treatment, and further studies suggest that it is the progestin that is likely responsible for this effect. The absolute number of breast cancers that might be attributable to the HRT was very low and appears to be confined to the 60–69-year-old cohort. These studies do also show that estrogens *decrease* the risk of endometrial, ovarian, and colon cancer. The net effect of estrogens and progestins on cancer remains unresolved.

Despite their action to improve serum lipid levels (decreasing low-density lipoprotein [LDL] cholesterol and increase high-density lipoprotein [HDL] cholesterol), and despite a history of anecdotal evidence, data are accumulating that the **most common HRT (Premarin or Prempro), does not reduce the risk of cardiovascular disease in older (60–69 years old) people.** The interpretation of these data has been vigorously debated but it now appears that HRT may be protective in women in the 50–59-year-old cohort who did not experience a long, estrogen-free period. Estrogens do increase the risk of stroke; the underlying mechanism for this increased risk is unclear, but may involve the increased coagulability that is associated with estrogen treatment. Estrogens increase the synthesis of fibrin and coagulation factors II, VII, VIII, IX, and X, and decrease the concentration of antithrombin III. In addition, plasminogen activator inhibitor activity is increased. These changes all contribute to a heightened tendency to form blood clots. This mechanism may also participate in the increased risk of dementia in postmenopausal women treated with estrogens. It must be noted that these serious adverse effects have been documented only with Premarin or Premarin plus progesterone at a fixed dosage, and it is not certain if other dosing regimens or other estrogen preparations cause similar untoward effects. Less serious adverse effects of estrogens include nausea and vomiting and peripheral edema. Some women complain of severe migraine when taking estrogens.

Antiestrogens and SERMs

Two compounds, **clomiphene and fulvestrant, are pure antiestrogens** that **antagonize** the action of estrogen in all tissues examined. Clomiphene is a triphenylethylene consisting of two isomers, *cis*-clomiphene and *trans*-clomiphene. *Cis*-clomiphene is a weak estrogen agonist, whereas *trans*-clomiphene a potent estrogen antagonist. **Clomiphene binds to both ER_α and ER_β, and blocks estrogen activation of these receptors.** The major pharmacologic action of clomiphene is to **block estrogen-mediated negative feedback in the pituitary.** This increases the amplitude of LH and FSH pulses and induces ovulation in women with amenorrhea, Stein-Leventhal syndrome, and dysfunctional bleeding with anovulatory cycles. It does increase the number of ova released, thereby increasing the chances of twinning.

Fulvestrant is a 7α-alkylamide derivative of estradiol that binds to both ER_α **and** ER_β**.** It is administered as a depot injection. The predominant action of fulvestrant is to increase the degradation of ER_α while having little effect on ER_β. This alteration in the ratio of ER_α/ER_β may explain its usefulness in women with tamoxifen-resistant breast cancer. **Adverse effects of the antiestrogens include hot flashes, ovarian enlargement, and nausea.**

The **SERMs,** tamoxifen, raloxifene, and toremifene, are a new class of compounds that display a range of agonist to antagonist activities in a tissue-specific manner. For example, tamoxifen is an estrogen receptor antagonist in the breast but is a weak estrogen agonist in the endometrium. The basis for this tissue specificity is a combination of drug-induced conformational changes in the receptor, and the complement of coactivators expressed in a given cell type. As noted above, when estradiol binds to an ER, a conformational change occurs that facilitates an interaction between coactivator proteins and ER. The SERMs also bind to ER, but they induce a conformation that is different from that caused by estradiol. The configuration of the receptor dictates which coactivator can bind to the receptor; if a cell does not express a coactivator that can bind to the receptor, then the effect of drug binding will be antagonism in that cell type. If the cell does express a coactivator that recognizes a particular configuration, then the drug will have agonist (or partial agonist) activity.

Tamoxifen is a triphenylethylene, is structurally related to diethylstilbestrol, and binds to both ER_α and ER_β. It acts as an **estrogen antagonist in the breast and in the brain,** but it has **weak estrogen agonist activity in the uterus and in bone.** It has mixed action in the liver, decreasing total cholesterol and LDL cholesterol but with no effect on triglycerides. **Tamoxifen is highly efficacious in the treatment of breast cancer.** Tamoxifen has been shown consistently to increase disease-free survival and overall survival; treatment for 5 years has reduced cancer recurrence by approximately 50 percent and death by nearly 30 percent. It is approved for primary prevention of breast cancer in women at high risk, where it causes a 50 percent decrease in the incidence of invasive breast cancer and a 50 percent reduction of noninvasive breast cancer. Because of the development of drug-resistant tumors, treatment should last for no more than 5 years. Adverse effects of tamoxifen include hot flashes, nausea, and vaginal bleeding.

Toremifene also is a triphenylethylene with a chlorine substitution. It is also used for the treatment and prophylaxis of breast cancer.

Raloxifene is a polyhydroxylated nonsteroidal compound with a benzothiophene core. Raloxifene binds with high affinity for both ER_α and ER_β. Raloxifene is an **estrogen agonist in bone**, where it exerts an antiresorptive effect. It reduces total cholesterol and LDL cholesterol. Raloxifene **does not have agonist activity in the uterus.** Its **primary use is the prevention of osteoporosis** in postmenopausal women. Adverse effects include **hot flashes, deep vein thrombosis,** and cramps in the lower extremities.

Aromatase inhibitors include exemestane, anastrazole, and letrozole. These agents act by reducing the peripheral conversion of precursors such as androstenedione and testosterone into estrogens. They significantly suppress serum estradiol levels and offer an alternative to tamoxifen in postmenopausal women with breast cancer.

Antiprogestins

Mifepristone (RU-486) is a 19-nor steroid that has both antiprogestational and antiglucocorticoid effects. It is used most commonly as an **abortifacient in the first trimester** of pregnancy. A single oral dose of mifepristone combined with a vaginal suppository containing prostaglandin E_1 is effective in terminating pregnancy in approximately 95 percent of cases if used in the first 7 weeks of gestation. Adverse effects include nausea, vomiting, and abdominal cramping.

Androgens and Antiandrogens

Testosterone produced by the testes is the major androgen in humans. In many peripheral tissues, testosterone is converted to dihydrotestosterone by the enzyme 5_α-reductase. Most circulating testosterone is bound in the plasma to sex-steroid binding globulin (SSBG). Testicular production of testosterone is regulated by LH released from the pituitary in a manner similar to that of estrogen as previously described. Testosterone has two physiologic actions. As an anabolic agent it promotes linear bone growth, development of internal genitalia, and increases muscle mass. As an androgenic agent, it is responsible for the development of male secondary sexual characteristics. **Dihydrotestosterone** is responsible for the development of external genitalia and hair follicle growth during puberty. Testosterone or dihydrotestosterone bind with high affinity to the androgen receptor (AR), another member of the nuclear receptor family of transcription factors.

There are two distinct chemical classes of androgens: **testosterone and its esters** and the **17-alkyl androgens.** Testosterone esters include testosterone enanthate, testosterone cypionate, and testosterone undecanoate. The 17-alkyl androgens include methyltestosterone, oxandrolone, danazol, and stanozolol. Testosterone and its esters are administered either as depot injections via transdermal patch, or as a gel. The 17-alkyl androgens are orally active.

The **major use of the androgens is the treatment of male hypogonadism,** both in adults and in prepubertal boys who produce low amounts of testosterone. Use in adults has been reported to increase libido, reduce senescence, and reduce the rate of bone resorption. The **major adverse effects of testosterone** and its esters are caused by the **androgenic actions,** which are especially apparent in women and prepubertal children. In women, these adverse effects include hirsutism, acne, amenorrhea, and a thickening of the vocal chords. In **children, androgens can cause premature closure of the epiphyses.** In men, androgens can produce azoospermia, decreased testicle size, and prostatic hyperplasia. The major adverse effects of the 17-alkyl androgens include masculinization and also serious hepatotoxicity. A cholestatic jaundice that is reversible on discontinuation of drug may occur.

Antiandrogens

Abnormal growth of the prostate is usually dependent on androgenic stimulation. This hormonal stimulation can be reduced by orchidectomy or high doses of estrogens, but either of these treatments may be undesirable. **Chemical orchiectomy** can be accomplished with an inhibitor of GnRH synthesis such as **leuprolide** or with **antiandrogens.**

Finasteride and dutasteride are steroid derivatives that competitively inhibit 5_α-reductase type II. Because **prostate growth is dependent on DHT rather than testosterone,** blockade of the enzyme can reduce stimulation of the gland. In clinical trials, finasteride decreased the incidence of prostate cancers but may have led to more aggressive tumors. **Bicalutamide and nilutamide are moderately potent antiandrogens** that antagonize AR. These drugs are usually combined with a GnRH analog such as leuprolide to decrease LH and subsequently testosterone production. **Flutamide is an AR antagonist** that blocks the action of testosterone in target organs. It has been used in the treatment of prostatic carcinoma.

COMPREHENSION QUESTIONS

[40.1] Clomiphene acts to induce ovulation by which of the following mechanisms?

A. Diminishing ER-mediated negative feedback at the pituitary
B. Increasing the action of ER_α in the hypothalamus
C. Increasing the action of ER_α in the ovary
D. Increasing the amount of ER_α

[40.2] Progesterone is added to estrogens in HRT to achieve which of the following effects?

A. Decrease the estrogen action on the breast
B. Decrease the occurrence of endometrial cancers
C. Increase the effectiveness of the estrogens
D. Inhibit bone resorption

[40.3] A 55-year-old woman is noted to be taking tamoxifen to help with breast cancer. She also complains of vaginal bleeding. She asks why she is having vaginal bleeding if the medication blocks estrogen effect in the body. Which of the following is the best explanation?

A. It has estrogen agonist effect of the breast and uterus, thereby leading to endometrial hyperplasia.
B. It is an estrogen antagonist in the breast and uterus, leading to loss of endometrial cells.
C. It has an antagonist effect on the breast but an agonist effect on the uterus.
D. It has no effect on the uterus, and the vaginal bleeding is caused by something else.

Answers

[40.1] **A.** Clomiphene decreases estradiol's negative feedback in the pituitary, and this increases the amplitude of the LH pulse that is responsible for ovulation.

[40.2] **B.** Progestins are added to HRT regimens to decrease the risk of endometrial cancer.

[40.3] **C.** Tamoxifen has an estrogen antagonist effect on the breast but a weak agonist effect on the uterus, leading to endometrial hyperplasia in some women. Endometrial cancer is seen in some patients.

PHARMACOLOGY PEARLS

 Clomiphene is the agent of choice for treatment of infertility as a result of anovulation in women with an intact hypothalamic-pituitary-ovarian axis.

 SERMs are tissue-specific estrogen antagonists that have uses in the treatment of breast cancer and osteoporosis.

 Antiandrogens are used to treat androgen-dependent cancers such as prostate carcinoma.

REFERENCES

Burkman R, Schlesselman JJ, Zieman M. Safety concerns and health benefits associated with oral contraception. Am J Obstet Gynecol 2004;190 (suppl 4): S5–22.

Writing Group for the Women's Health Initiative Investigators. Risks and benefits of estrogen plus progesterone in healthy postmenopausal women. JAMA 2002; 288:321–33.

Rossouw JE, Prentice RL, Manson JE, et al. Postmenopausal hormone therapy and risk of cardiovascular disease by age and years since menopause. JAMA 2007; 297:1465–77.

A 45-year-old man presents for the evaluation of weight gain. He has noticed a 20-lb weight gain in the past few months without any change in his diet or activity level. He has started developing "stretch marks" on his abdomen as well. His wife has noted that even his face seems to be "growing fatter." Review of systems is significant for complaints of fatigue, multiple recent upper respiratory infections, and the development of facial acne. He has no significant medical history and takes no medications. There is a family history of diabetes and hypertension. On examination, his blood pressure is elevated at 165/95 mm Hg, but his other vital signs are normal. His face is plethoric, and he has a small fatty hump developing on his upper back. His abdomen is obese but soft and nontender without masses or fluid. Skin examination is notable for moderate facial acne and multiple violaceous striae on the abdomen. Blood tests show an elevated glucose level of 150 mg/dL, normal electrolytes, and renal function. His thyroid function tests are normal. You suspect idiopathic Cushing disease and order a dexamethasone suppression test to assist with confirming the diagnosis.

◆ **Which pituitary hormone stimulates the release of adrenocortical steroids?**

◆ **What is the major glucocorticoid produced in the adrenal glands?**

◆ **What is the major mineralocorticoid produced in the adrenal glands?**

◆ **What is the major effect of mineralocorticoids?**

ANSWERS TO CASE 41: THE ADRENAL CORTEX

Summary: A 45-year-old man has Cushing disease.

◆ **Pituitary hormonal stimulus of adrenocortical steroid production:** ACTH.

◆ **Primary adrenal glucocorticoid:** Cortisol.

◆ **Primary adrenal mineralocorticoid:** Aldosterone.

◆ **Major mineralocorticoid effects:** Regulation of salt and water balance in the kidney, promote sodium retention, and potassium loss.

CLINICAL CORRELATION

Cushing disease is caused by ACTH-secreting tumors in the pituitary gland. The continuous production of ACTH disrupts the normal circadian production of ACTH and overrides the feedback of adrenal steroids on the hypothalamus and pituitary, resulting in excessive adrenocortical steroid production. Glucocorticoids affect most organs and tissues in the body. Their effects are mediated by specific intracellular glucocorticoid receptors that modulate the transcription rates of specific genes and results in increases or decreases of specific proteins. The major glucocorticoid produced in the adrenal glands is cortisol (hydrocortisone). Glucocorticoids have numerous physiologic effects, including the stimulation of gluconeogenesis, increasing lipolysis, decreasing glucose uptake into fat cells, and redistributing body fat. These effects cause some of the symptoms and signs of Cushing disease, which include glucose intolerance or overt diabetes, weight gain, and increasing truncal obesity. Glucocorticoids also have anti-immune effects, which include decreasing circulating lymphocytes, monocytes, eosinophils, and basophils, increases in circulating neutrophils and atrophy of lymphoid tissue. The excess production of glucocorticoids can therefore lead to immune system suppression and recurrent infections. Under normal physiologic conditions, adrenocortical steroids will exert a negative feedback of ACTH release from the pituitary gland. ACTH release, and subsequent cortisol production, can be suppressed even more by the administration of synthetic steroids such as dexamethasone. ACTH, which is continuously produced by a tumor, will not be suppressed by a feedback mechanism. This formulates the basis for the dexamethasone suppression test, in which a dose of dexamethasone is administered and subsequent cortisol production is measured. Normally this would cause a reduction of circulating cortisol. In Cushing disease the measurement of cortisol will remain at normal, or even elevated, levels.

APPROACH TO PHARMACOLOGY
OF THE GLUCOCORTICOIDS

Objectives

1. Understand the physiologic regulation of the hypothalamic-pituitary-adrenal axis.
2. List the natural and synthetic adrenocortical steroids, their actions, therapeutic uses, and adverse effects.
3. Know the glucocorticoid and mineralocorticoid effects of adrenocortical steroids.
4. Understand the adrenocortical antagonists, their mechanism of action, uses, and adverse effects.

Definitions

Glucocorticoids: In humans the most important glucocorticoid is cortisol. These hormones regulate carbohydrate, protein, and lipid metabolism.
Mineralocorticoids: In humans, aldosterone is the most important mineralocorticoid.
Aldosterone: It regulates Na^+ and K^+ homeostasis.

DISCUSSION

Class

Control of the secretion of glucocorticoids by the adrenal gland is regulated by a classic negative feedback pathway that includes the hypothalamus, pituitary, and the adrenal cortex (see Case 39). The **neuropeptide CRH is a 41-amino acid peptide produced in the hypothalamus** that is **secreted with a circadian rhythm.** Secretion can also be increased by physiologic or psychologic stress. **CRH acts on the pituitary to stimulate the release of ACTH.** ACTH released from the pituitary is transported in the systemic circulation to the **adrenal cortex,** where it acts to stimulate the **zona fasciculata and reticularis to increase the biosynthesis of cortisol and weak androgens** such as **androstenedione** respectively. It also acts on the **zona glomerulosa** to slightly stimulate the production of **aldosterone.** ACTH is a true trophic hormone: it is necessary for the survival of cells of the adrenal cortex, although this effect is somewhat less pronounced in the zona glomerulosa. Cortisol secreted by the adrenal cortex is bound extensively to cortisol-binding globulin (CBG) in the plasma.

Glucocorticoids

Natural and synthetic glucocorticoids play a diverse role in **metabolism, catabolism, and immunity.** Both cortisol, the natural glucocorticoid, and many synthetic glucocorticoids are used therapeutically (Table 41-1). The synthetic

Table 41-1

COMMONLY USED ADRENOCORTICAL AGENTS

AGENT	EQUIVALENT DOSE (MG)	GLUCOCORTICOID POTENCY	MINERALOCORTICOID POTENCY	ANTI-INFLAMMATORY POTENCY
Cortisol	20	100	1	1
Prednisone	5	100	0.4	4
Methylprednisolone	4	100	0.1	4
Triamcinolone	4	100	0.1	5
Dexamethasone	0.75	100	0.05	30
Fludrocortisone	2	100	250	10

glucocorticoids have reduced mineralocorticoid activity and in general increased potency compared to cortisol. Glucocorticoids have a myriad of therapeutic uses. They are potent **anti-inflammatory agents** because they **inhibit prostaglandin production by inhibiting phospholipase A,** the enzyme that yields arachidonic acid from plasma membrane phospholipids. Unlike nonsteroidal anti-inflammatory drugs (NSAIDs), they also **inhibit leukocytes and macrophages that contribute heavily to inflammation.** Glucocorticoids are used to treat joint and bone inflammation, inflammatory bowel disease, bronchial asthma, and dermatitis. Systemic inflammations such as in lupus erythematosus, rheumatoid arthritis, and acute respiratory distress syndrome are also treated with glucocorticoids. Glucocorticoids are potent immunosuppressive agents and are used either alone or in conjunction with other immunosuppressive agents to suppress organ rejection following transplant, and to reduce the severity of allergic reactions including contact dermatitis, serum sickness, and allergic rhinitis. Other uses include prevention of respiratory distress syndrome in infants (by induction of surfactant), prevention of nephrotic syndrome, and at high doses to reduce cerebral edema. Adrenal insufficiency either acute or congenital is treated with glucocorticoids. Finally glucocorticoids are useful diagnostically as in the dexamethasone suppression test described above.

Although they are highly efficacious agents, the **adverse effect profile** of glucocorticoids limits their use typically to short (approximately 2 weeks) periods. **Chronic use of glucocorticoids** beyond this duration produces **adrenal suppression** and can cause iatrogenic Cushing syndrome. The metabolic sequelae of **Cushing syndrome** include **fat redistribution (buffalo hump and moon facies), hyperglycemia,** and **elevations in insulin secretion leading to frank diabetes.** Continued protein degradation can cause **myopathy** and **muscle wasting,** and **thinning of the skin** that becomes prone to **bruising and striae. Immunosuppression** leads to susceptibility to infection and poor wound healing. **Peptic ulcers and osteoporosis** are other potential consequences of glucocorticoid use. **Adrenal suppression** occurs with chronic glucocorticoid use as a result of continuous suppression of ACTH production by the pituitary. The absence of the trophic hormone leads to adrenal atrophy and an inability to respond to stress, which can be life-threatening. Neurological adverse effects include **hypomania, acute psychosis, and depression.** At sufficient doses, all glucocorticoids have some mineralocorticoid activity that can lead to **electrolyte imbalances and water retention.**

Mineralocorticoids

Aldosterone is the naturally occurring mineralocorticoid. It is secreted by the **zona glomerulosa of the adrenal cortex. Secretion of aldosterone is increased by angiotensin II and K^+, especially when serum Na^+ is low.** The physiologic action of aldosterone is to **increase Na^+ reabsorption** in the distal convoluted tubule and cortical collecting tubule via the amiloride-sensitive Na^+ channel. As Na^+ is reabsorbed, K^+ or H^+ is secreted into the urine and water is retained. Aldosterone also causes Na^+ reabsorption in the salivary and sweat glands and the mucosa of the gastrointestinal (GI) tract. Aldosterone is not useful as an oral agent because of a nearly 100 percent first-pass effect by the liver. **Fludrocortisone** (see Table 41-1) has both glucocorticoid and mineralocorticoid activity. An alternative to fludrocortisone is **deoxycorticosterone (DOC)** which is a potent mineralocorticoid.

Structure

Synthetic glucocorticoids are all analogs of the natural occurring cortisol. Various modifications of the steroid nucleus have important pharmacokinetic effects to increase glucocorticoid potency relative to mineralocorticoid potency, to decrease first-pass effect and increase half-life, and to decrease binding to CBG. Aldosterone has a unique epoxide structure in the "D" ring that prevents its inactivation.

Mechanism of Action

Both the **glucocorticoids and the mineralocorticoids** bind to **specific nuclear receptors within target cells.** The **glucocorticoid receptor** is in an inactive state in the cytoplasm of target cells bound to a variety of heat-shock proteins, especially HSP 90. On binding a glucocorticoid, the heat-shock proteins dissociate, the GR forms a homodimer and **translocates to the nucleus** and binds to the **promoter region of specific target genes.** Via the process of coactivator or corepressor recruitment, transcription of these specific target genes is either increased or decreased. The mineralocorticoid receptor (MR) is expressed in the kidney, salivary glands, and GI tract. It binds aldosterone with high affinity but also binds cortisol with nearly the same affinity. Cortisol is prevented from binding to MR by rapid inactivation to cortisone by the enzyme hydroxysteroid dehydrogenase type II which is expressed in mineralocorticoid target tissues.

Administration

Glucocorticoids can be administered orally, by injection, by inhalation (especially for use in asthma), rectally, and topically. Patients taking glucocorticoids for longer than 2 weeks must be slowly tapered off the drug so that adrenal function can be restored.

Pharmacokinetics

The half-life and duration of action of glucocorticoids depends on the route of administration and the particular agent. In general, glucocorticoid effects are seen within 4–6 hours. Most corticosteroids are metabolized in the liver to sterol ketones or hydroxides and eliminated by the kidney.

Glucocorticoid and Mineralocorticoid Antagonists

There are some clinical circumstances such as inoperable adrenal tumors, prior to surgery and for diagnostic use, where **inhibition of glucocorticoid action** is desirable. **Metyrapone is a specific inhibitor of 11-hydroxylation,** and can thereby inhibit **the synthesis of corticosterone and cortisol.** In the presence of normal pituitary function there is a **compensatory increase in 11-deoxycortisol production. Metyrapone is also useful in the assessment of adrenal function.** Following metyrapone administration, urinary 17-hydroxysteroids, metabolites of adrenal glucocorticoid synthesis, typically double if the adrenals are functioning normally. **Chronic metyrapone can cause hirsutism, nausea, sedation, and rash.**

Aminoglutheamide blocks the conversion of cholesterol to pregnenolone. This **inhibits the synthesis of all hormonally active steroids.** It has been used to reduce glucocorticoid levels in patients with Cushing syndrome because of adrenal tumors or excessive ectopic production of ACTH. It has also been used to treat estrogen-dependent breast cancer and prostate cancer. Adverse effects are common and include GI upset and neurologic disturbances.

Ketoconazole is an **antifungal agent;** at high doses it **nonspecifically blocks several enzymes, especially P450 enzymes** that are involved in adrenal and gonadal steroidogenesis. It is the most effective inhibitor of steroid hormone biosynthesis available in patients with Cushing disease. **Adverse effects include hepatic dysfunction with increased transaminases and liver failure.**

Mifepristone is a 19-nor steroid that is a potent antagonist of both the glucocorticoid and progesterone receptors. It has been used to reduce the activity of glucocorticoids in patients with ectopic ACTH production or adrenal carcinoma. The main use of mifepristone is as an antiprogestin (Case 40) as an abortifacient when combined with prostaglandin E_1.

Two mineralocorticoid antagonists are available, spironolactone and eplerenone. Spironolactone antagonizes the mineralocorticoid and the androgen receptor (AR). It is used to treat hypertension (see Case 12) usually in combination with a thiazide or a loop diuretic. It can be used diagnostically to restore potassium levels to normal in patients with hypokalemia secondary to hyperaldosteronism. Based on its **antiandrogen activity,** it has been **used to treat hirsutism in women.** Adverse effects include **hyperkalemia, sedation, cardiac arrhythmias, gynecomastia, sedation, headache, and GI upset.**

Eplerenone is a **new generation, aldosterone receptor–specific antagonist.** It is approved for use in **congestive heart failure, post-myocardial infarction, and hypertension.** It **avoids the antiandrogen activity of spironolactone. Adverse effects** include mild **hyperkalemia,** but clinical experience is limited.

COMPREHENSION QUESTIONS

[41.1] Which of the following best describes appropriate protocols for with-
        drawal of glucocorticoids from a patient who has been taking large
        doses for 6 months?

     A. Maintain dose of glucocorticoids and add metyrapone
     B. Maintain dose of glucocorticoids and add spironolactone
     C. An alternate-day dosage regimen of glucocorticoids should be
        begun
     D. Slow reduction of the glucocorticoid dose over 1–2 weeks

[41.2] A patient with severe shoulder pain resulting from inflammation is not
        responding to treatment with naproxen. You elect to begin a course of
        treatment with oral dexamethasone. What is the basis that the gluco-
        corticoid will be more effective as an anti-inflammatory agent?

     A. Glucocorticoids inhibit both prostaglandin production and inflam-
        matory cells
     B. Glucocorticoids are more potent inhibitors of cyclooxygenase than
        naproxen
     C. Glucocorticoids inhibit biosynthesis of both COX-1 and COX-2
     D. Glucocorticoids will reduce the edema in the inflamed area

[41.3   A 32-year-old woman is prescribed a pill for excessive hair on her face
        and arms. She notes that she has been going to the bathroom at night
        more often. What is the most likely explanation for the nocturia?

     A. Diabetes insipidus effect of the medication
     B. Osmotic load to the kidney from the medication delivery system
     C. Distal renal tubule effect of the medication
     D. Hyperglycemic effect from the medication

Answers

[41.1] **D.** Long-term use of glucocorticoids results in adrenal suppression
        and atrophy. A slow "weaning" from the drug is necessary so that the
        adrenals can recover.

[41.2] **A.** Glucocorticoids reduce prostaglandin production like NSAIDs
        and they also inhibit most of the cells that are involved in the inflam-
        matory process.

[41.3] **C.** The medication is probably spironolactone, which is a competitive
        inhibitor of androgens at the receptor level, and also an antimineral-
        corticoid effect at the distal tubule, inhibiting free water resorption.
        As such, it is a potassium-sparing diuretic agent.

PHARMACOLOGY PEARLS

❖ Adverse effects, especially adrenal suppression, seriously limit the use of glucocorticoids to 2 weeks or less.
❖ Spironolactone antagonizes the mineralocorticoid and the AR. Adverse effects include hyperkalemia, sedation, cardiac arrhythmias, gynecomastia, sedation, headache, and GI upset.
❖ Eplerenone is a new generation, aldosterone receptor–specific antagonist without the antiandrogen component.
❖ Metyrapone is a specific inhibitor of 11-hydroxylation that inhibits the synthesis of corticosterone and cortisol.

REFERENCES

Boers M. Glucocorticoids in rheumatoid arthritis: a senescent research agenda on the brink of rejuvenation? Best Pract Res Clin Rheumatol 2004;18:21–9.
Trence DL. Management of patients on chronic glucocorticoid therapy: an endocrine perspective. Prim Care 2003;30:593–605.

A 44-year-old woman presents to the office because of fatigue. She has felt sluggish for months and thinks she may be anemic. She has started taking iron pills but isn't feeling any better. She has been sleeping well and doesn't feel depressed. She has noticed some thinning of her hair and feels as if her skin is dry. She takes a multivitamin and iron supplement, otherwise no medications. She has smoked a pack of cigarettes a day for approximately 20 years, occasionally drinks alcohol, and doesn't exercise. Her mother takes some kind of thyroid pill and has diabetes. On examination, her blood pressure and pulse are normal. Her hair is thinned but there are no focal patches of alopecia or scarring of the scalp. Her skin is diffusely dry. Her thyroid gland feels diffusely enlarged, is nontender, and has no nodules. The remainder of her examination is unremarkable. Lab tests show a normal complete blood count (CBC), glucose, and electrolytes. Her thyroid-stimulating hormone (TSH) level is elevated, and T_4 level is reduced. You diagnose her with hypothyroidism and start her on oral levothyroxine sodium.

◆ **What is levothyroxine sodium?**

◆ **How is triiodothyronine (T_3) produced in the body?**

◆ **What is the mechanism of action of thyroid hormones?**

ANSWERS TO CASE 42: THYROID HORMONES

Summary: A 44-year-old woman is diagnosed with hypothyroidism and pre-scribed levothyroxine.

◆ **Levothyroxine sodium:** Synthetic sodium salt of thyroxine (T_4).

◆ **Derivation of T_3 in the body:** Approximately 75 percent from the deiodination of T_4; also produced by the coupling of monoiodotyrosine (MIT) and diiodotyrosine (DIT).

◆ **Mechanism of action of thyroid hormones:** Bind with receptors in nuclei of target cells and alter synthesis rates of specific messenger ribonucleoprotein acids (mRNAs), increasing production of certain proteins including Na^+, K^+-ATPase.

CLINICAL CORRELATION

Thyroid hormones have wide-ranging effects of tissues throughout the body. They are involved primarily in the regulation of metabolism. The hypothalamic-pituitary-thyroid axis regulates release of active hormone from the thyroid via a feedback loop. Thyrotropin-releasing hormone (TRH) is pro-duced in the hypothalamus and stimulates the release of TSH from the ante-rior pituitary. TSH binds to membrane receptors in the thyroid and stimulates the production and release of T_4 and T_3 via a cyclic adenosine monophosphate (cAMP)-mediated system. Synthesis of T_4 exceeds T_3 by approximately four-fold; most circulating T_3 comes from the deiodination of T_4. T_4 and T_3 are almost entirely protein bound, mostly to thyroxine-binding globulin (TBG) and albumin. Unbound thyroid hormone binds to receptors located in the nuclei of target cells. This alters the rate of synthesis of specific mRNAs which lead to the increased production of proteins, including Na^+, K^+-ATPase. This results in a net increase in ATP and oxygen consumption, raising the metabolic rate. Hypothyroidism occurs when there is inadequate thyroid hormone pro-duction and release to meet the body's metabolic demands. In primary hypothyroidism the thyroid gland is unable to synthesize adequate amounts of thyroid hormone. The pituitary releases increasing amounts of TSH to try to stimulate production, leading to the characteristic laboratory findings of low circulating levels of thyroid hormones with an elevated TSH. Conversely, pri-mary hyperthyroidism is diagnosed by the presence of elevated thyroid hor-mone levels and a suppressed level of TSH. Hypothyroidism is most often treated by the oral administration of synthetic T_4 in the form of levothyroxine sodium. This replaces both T_4 and, by deiodination, T_3.

APPROACH TO PHARMACOLOGY OF THYROID DRUGS

Objectives

1. List the hormones involved in the hypothalamic-pituitary-thyroid axis and the synthesis of thyroid hormones.
2. Know the actions of thyroid hormones.
3. List the thyroid hormone preparations, their therapeutic uses, actions, and adverse effects.
4. Describe the antithyroid agents, their mechanisms of action, therapeutic uses, and adverse effects.

Definitions

Myxedema: Serious hypothyroidism.
Thyrotoxicosis: Hyperthyroidism.

DISCUSSION

Class

Thyroid Agonists

Thyroid hormones are required for optimum development, growth, and maintenance of function of virtually every tissue of the body. Either hypo- or hyperthyroidism leads to untoward symptoms that need to be treated. The thyroid gland produces both thyroxine (T_4) and triiodothyronine (T_3). Adequate dietary intake of sufficient **iodide (I^-) is essential** to maintain normal biosynthesis of thyroid hormones. **Iodide is transported into the thyroid cell by a sodium-iodide symporter (NIS)** and then transported through the **apical plasma membrane into the colloid of the thyroid** gland. Within the colloid, **iodide is oxidized to iodine by thyroidal peroxidase.** The process called organification involves the iodination of tyrosine residues of the colloidal protein thyroglobulin to form **MIT and DIT.** The coupling of two molecules of DIT forms T_4 and the coupling of one molecule of MIT, and one molecule of DIT forms T_3. Under normal circumstances and sufficient iodide, the ratio of T_4 to T_3 is 4:1. T_3 can also be formed by the removal of an iodide molecule from T_4 by the action of 5′-deiodinase, which is present within the thyroid gland and in peripheral tissues.

Iodinated thyroglobulin undergoes endocytosis at the apical border and then extensively degraded within the thyroid cells by proteolysis prior to secretion of T_4 and T_3. Although T_3 is produced with the thyroid, approximately **80 percent of circulating levels of T_3 are produced by the action of 5′-deiodinase in the periphery,** especially the **liver.** Alternatively T_4 can be *degraded* by the action of deiodinase to reverse T_3, which is an inactive metabolite. Normally approximately 40 percent of T_4 is converted to T_3, 38 percent is converted to rT_3, and the remainder is degraded by other, typically hepatic pathways. Greater than 99 percent of both T_4 and T_3 are bound in the plasma to TBG; T_4 binds to TBG much more avidly. **Only the unbound "free" hormone exerts physiologic effects.**

Secretion of thyroid hormones is regulated by a **classical hypothalamus-pituitary-thyroid negative feedback loop. TRH is produced within hypo-thalamus.** It acts on **thyrotrophs in the pituitary to cause the release of thyrotropin (TSH),** which in turn stimulates all steps in the **biosynthesis and secretion of thyroid hormones.** Circulating levels of thyroid hormone decrease the amount of TRH that is released from the hypothalamus, completing the feedback loop.

Thyroid hormone is critical for normal brain development. The **absence of normal thyroid hormone function in the first months of the infant leads to irreversible cretinism.** Thyroid hormone induces myelin basic protein, and hypothyroidism leads to decreased production of this protein and defective neuronal myelination. Thyroid hormones have an important effect on oxygen consumption in many tissues including heart, skeletal muscle, kidney, and liver; brain gonads, and spleen are not affected. This calorigenic effect is important to normal thermogenesis. Thyroid hormones also increase lipolysis.

Thyroid hormone has direct actions on the heart and vascular system. Hyperthyroidism leads to tachycardia, increased stroke volume, increased pulse pressure, and decreased vascular resistance. Hypothyroidism leads to bradycardia, and reversal of the above effects. Thyroid hormones increase the conversion of cholesterol to bile and increase LDL uptake by the liver and thereby reduce plasma cholesterol concentrations.

Hypothyroidism can be treated effectively by hormone replacement. Common causes of hypothyroidism include **autoimmune destruction** of the thyroid gland **(Hashimoto disease), congenital hypothyroidism, or impaired pituitary or hypothalamic function.** Thyroid hormones are indicated for the treatment and prophylaxis of goiter by suppressing abnormal growth of the thyroid gland. Thyroid hormones are also useful in the treatment of TSH-dependent thyroid cancers. Adverse effects of thyroid hormones are a hyperthyroid state with increased calorigenesis and oxygen demand, tachycardia, and increased cardiac workload.

Structure

Synthetic preparations of T_4 (levothyroxine), T_3 (liothyronine), and a 4:1 mixture of T_4/T_3 (liotrix) are preferable to desiccated preparations of thyroid prepared from animals that are more variable in biologic activity.

Mechanism of Action

The actions of the thyroid hormones are mediated by nuclear thyroid receptors that act by increasing or decreasing transcription of target genes. There are three major thyroid receptors: $TR\beta_1$, $TR\beta_2$, and $TR\alpha_1$. Whereas $TR\beta_1$ and $TR\alpha_1$ are expressed in virtually every tissue, $TR_{\beta2}$ is expressed exclusively in the anterior pituitary. These receptors bind T_3 in the nucleus. T_4 can bind to the receptors but at much lower affinity and with much less, if any, effect on transcription. Thyroid receptors are bound in the absence of ligand to the promoters of target genes, and in some cases the nonliganded receptor exerts a potent inhibition of basal transcription. T_3 binding to TR results in recruitment of coactivators and subsequent disinhibition and increased rates of transcription.

All the above preparations of thyroid hormone can be administered orally. Levothyroxine and liothyronine are also available for parenteral administration. Doses are individualized and monitored by measuring the level of circulating TSH.

Pharmacokinetics

T_4 has a very long half-life (7 days), in large part because of its extensive binding to TBG. The half-life of T_4 is lengthened to 9–10 days in hypothyroidism and decreased to 3–4 days in hyperthyroidism. Thyroid hormones are degraded mostly by the liver and excreted in the bile.

Thyroid Antagonists

Hyperthyroidism can be treated with agents that **decrease the biosynthesis of thyroid hormones** that **decrease cellular response to thyroid hormones,** or **destruction** of the **thyroid gland with radioactive isotopes** of thyroid hormones or surgery. The **thioamides, methimazole and propylthiouracil,** are the major drugs for treating hyperthyroidism. These drugs act by **inhibiting peroxidation of iodide and organification of thyroglobulin. Propylthiouracil** also acts to **inhibit the coupling reaction that forms MIT and DIT.** Adverse effects of **thioamides** include a **maculopapular rash, and less commonly arthralgia, skin rashes, hepatoxicity, cholestatic jaundice, and a lupus-like syndrome.** Potentially life-threatening **agranulocytosis** has occurred with their use.

Historically, iodides were the major antithyroid agents. Large oral doses of iodide inhibit organification and the secretion of thyroid hormones. **Iodide is useful in treating acute thyrotoxicosis (thyroid storm),** and to reduce the size, vascularity, and fragility of a hyperplastic thyroid preoperatively. Most patients will escape the blocking effects of iodide in 2–8 weeks.

Monovalent anions such as perchlorate (CIO_4^-), thiocyanate (SCN^-), and pertechnetate (TCO_4^-) are competitive inhibitors of the iodide transport mechanism, rarely used compared to thioamides due to adverse effects.

Radioactive 131 iodine is rapidly trapped and concentrated in the colloid of the thyroid gland exactly as occurs with the stable ^{127}I. Radiation is nearly exclusively delivered to the parenchymal cells of the thyroid and leads to a dose-dependent destruction of part or the entire gland. In many circumstances it is considered the treatment of choice for chronic hyperthyroidism. It should not be used in patients who are pregnant because of its action on the thyroid of the fetus.

COMPREHENSION QUESTIONS

[42.1] A woman enters your clinic with an enlarged thyroid and you suspect simple adenomatous goiter. Which of the following would be the best treatment for this condition?

    A. IV infusion of TSH
    B. Levothyroxine
    C. Propylthiouracil
    D. Thyroid ablation with ^{131}I

[42.2] The mechanism by which thiocyanate reduces synthesis of thyroid hormones is by inhibition of which of the following?

    A. Iodine oxidation
    B. Iodide transport
    C. TSH biosynthesis
    D. TRβ

[42.3] A 33-year-old man is noted to have tachycardia, heat intolerance, weight loss, and an enlarged thyroid gland. Which of the following is the probable ultimate treatment for this patient?

    A. Long-term corticosteroid therapy
    B. Propranolol therapy
    C. Radioactive iodine
    D. Surgical resection

Answers

[42.1]   **B.** Goiter is an indication for thyroid hormone replacement.

[42.2]   **B.** Anions such as perchlorate and thiocyanate inhibit the transport of iodide into thyroid cells.

[42.3]   **C.** This patient likely has Graves disease, the most common cause of hyperthyroidism in the United States, typically presenting with a painless goiter and symptoms of hyperthyroidism. The treatment of choice is radioactive iodine.

PHARMACOLOGY PEARLS

 Levothyroxine is the drug of choice for treatment of hypothyroidism.

 The free, unbound thyroid hormone is the active component.

❖ The thioamides, methimazole and propylthiouracil, are the major drugs for treating hyperthyroidism, and act by inhibiting peroxidation of iodide and organification of thyroglobulin. Propylthiouracil also acts to inhibit the coupling reaction that forms MIT and DIT.

REFERENCES

Klein I, Danzi S. Evaluation of the therapeutic efficacy of different levothyroxine preparations in the treatment of human thyroid disease. Thyroid 2003;13: 1127–32.

Wiersinga WM. Thyroid hormone replacement therapy. Horm Res 2001;56(suppl 1): 74–81.

Nayak B, Burman K. Thyrotoxicosis and thyroid storm. Endocrinol Metab Clin North Am 2006;35:663–86.

A 12-year-old boy is brought to the office by his parents because of abdominal pain for the past day. Prior to this, the parents noted that he was drinking a lot of water and going to the bathroom frequently. He said that his mouth was very dry and he was very thirsty. Until the past day or two he was eating more than usual but was losing weight. He has no significant medical history, and the family history is unremarkable. On examination, he appears moderately ill, and his blood pressure is normal, but he is tachycardic. His mucous membranes are dry. His abdomen is diffusely tender but without rebound or guarding. A urine dipstick test in the office reveals the presence of large ketones and glucose. A glucose measurement from a drop of blood obtained by fingerstick is markedly elevated at 550 mg/dL. You immediately admit the patient to the hospital for newly diagnosed type I diabetes mellitus in ketoacidosis and start an infusion of IV fluids and regular insulin.

◆ **What is the structure of natural human insulin?**

◆ **What effect does insulin have on potassium?**

◆ **What is the effect of α-adrenergic stimulation on insulin secretion?**

◆ **What is the effect of β-adrenergic stimulation on insulin secretion?**

ANSWERS TO CASE 43: THE PANCREAS AND GLUCOSE HOMEOSTASIS

Summary: A 12-year-old with newly diagnosed type I diabetes mellitus has ketoacidosis.

◆ **Structure of human insulin:** A 51-amino acid polypeptide that consists of two chains linked by two disulfide bridges.

◆ **Effect of insulin on potassium:** Promotes cellular K^+ uptake.

◆ **Effect of α-adrenergic stimulation:** Inhibition of insulin secretion.

◆ **Effect of β-adrenergic stimulation:** Increased insulin secretion.

CLINICAL CORRELATION

Insulin is a 51-amino acid polypeptide that is produced in pancreatic β-cells and stored as a complex with Zn^{2+}. The primary stimulus for insulin release is glucose, but amino acids, fatty acids, and ketone bodies may stimulate its release. Glucagon and somatostatin also may modulate its secretion. α-Adrenergic stimulation is a predominant inhibitory mechanism, whereas β-adrenergic stimulation increases its release. Insulin acts by binding to specific membrane receptors that have tyrosine kinase activity. Tyrosine in the receptor becomes phosphorylated and the receptor in turn phosphorylates a number of intracellular substrates that lead to increased glucose uptake. In muscle and adipose tissue, glucose transport is mediated by the recruitment of hexose transport molecules into the plasma membrane. Among its many actions, insulin increases glucose transport, glycogen synthesis and deposition, lipogenesis, and protein synthesis. It decreases intracellular lipolysis and hepatic gluconeogenesis. Insulin also stimulates cellular potassium uptake. Type I diabetes mellitus is a disease in which pancreatic β-cells fail to produce adequate amounts of insulin. Insulin must then be supplemented. Currently used insulin preparations are human insulin produced by recombinant deoxyribonucleic acid (DNA) techniques. There are short-, intermediate-, and long-acting insulin preparations available. The most widely used insulin products must be given by injection or inhalation, usually requiring 1–4 subcutaneous injections a day or continuous subcutaneous infusion with an insulin pump. Regular insulin can also be given intravenously in the setting of diabetic ketoacidosis. A new insulin product is available for inhalation use. Insulin injections are also used in type II diabetics, who cannot achieve adequate control with oral agents. The most significant risk of insulin therapy is the induction of hypoglycemia. Hypoglycemia may produce tachycardia, sweating, and confusion. In severe cases, hypoglycemia may progress to coma, seizures, or even death.

APPROACH TO PHARMACOLOGY OF INSULIN AND ORAL HYPOGLYCEMIC AGENTS

Objectives

1. List the structure and function of endogenous insulin.
2. Know the characteristics, therapeutic uses, and adverse effects of insulin preparations.
3. Understand the mechanisms of action, uses, and adverse effects of oral hypoglycemic agents.
4. Understand the mechanisms of action, uses, and adverse effects of agents used to raise blood sugar levels.

Definitions

Type I diabetes: Historically called juvenile onset diabetes or insulin-dependent diabetes mellitus (IDDM), it is a hyperglycemic condition caused by inadequate production of insulin by B cells of the pancreas.

Type II diabetes: A condition of hyperglycemia caused by resistance to circulating levels of insulin. Also called non-insulin-dependent diabetes mellitus (NIDDM). The incidence of this condition is increasing markedly in the United States and is especially prevalent in the Hispanic population.

DISCUSSION

Pharmacology of Class

Insulin is secreted by the B cells of the pancreas. The islet of Langerhans within the pancreas is made of four cell types, each secretes a distinct polypeptide. The **B (or β) cells secrete insulin, the A (or α) cells secrete glucagon, the D (or δ) cells secrete somatostatin,** and the PP or F cells secrete pancreatic polypeptide. **Human insulin comprises two chains, the A and B chains,** that are produced by the formation of **one intrapeptide and two interpeptide disulfide bonds** from a 110-amino acid precursor called **preproinsulin.** This precursor is cleaved within the endoplasmic reticulum and Golgi complex to form mature insulin and C-peptide. Insulin secretion is a tightly regulated process that normally maintains a stable concentration of plasma glucose through both postprandial periods and periods of fasting. **Glucose is the most important stimulus to insulin secretion in humans.** Insulin secretion is also stimulated by GI inhibitory polypeptide 1, glucagon-like peptide 1, gastrin, secretin, cholecystokinin, vasoactive intestinal polypeptide, gastrin-releasing peptide, and enteroglucagon. Neural input via catecholamines also regulate insulin secretion as stated above. **Glucose enters the pancreas via a specific**

transporter, **GLUT-2,** and is **rapidly phosphorylated by glucokinase.** Glucokinase is considered to be the glucose sensor within the B cell and its activity ultimately leads to increased intracellular Ca^{2+} within the B cell and this causes insulin secretion. Insulin promotes the uptake of carbohydrates, proteins, and fats in most tissues. It influences metabolism by stimulating protein and free fatty acid biosynthesis and inhibits the release of fatty acids from adipose cells. Insulin stimulates the production of glycogen and triglycerides.

Insulin is the mainstay for the treatment of virtually all type I diabetics and many type II diabetics. There are several principal types available that differ in their onset and duration of action (Table 43-1).

The **goal of insulin therapy is to control plasma glucose levels as tightly as possible.** Most of the sequelae of diabetes such as **retinopathy, renal damage, and neuropathy** are caused by the **hyperglycemic condition** rather than the absence of insulin. Current regimens generally use an intermediate or long-acting preparation supplemented with injections of short- or rapid-acting preparations to meet postprandial needs. Premixed mixtures of different types of insulins are also available. An insulin powder for inhalation [Exubera] is approved for use in patients with type I and type II diabetes mellitus. Inhaled insulin uses a device similar to an asthma inhaler for fixed insulin dosage prior to meals. The most common adverse effect of insulin administration is **hypoglycemia.**

Table 43-1
INSULIN PREPARATIONS

AGENT	TIME TO ONSET	DURATION OF ACTION (HOURS)
Rapid acting (lispro, aspart, glulisine)	5–15 minutes	3–5
Short acting (regular insulin)	30 minutes	5–8
NPH insulin	1–2 hours	18–24
Long acting (detemir, glargine)	4–6 hours	20–36
Insulin glargine	2–6 hours No peak action	24+
Exubera (inhaled insulin)	10 minutes	6

Structure

Human insulin derived by recombinant technology in bacteria or yeast has supplanted the use of bovine or pork insulins.

Mechanism of Action

All of insulin's activities are mediated by the insulin receptor which is expressed in most tissue types. The insulin receptor consists of an extracellular α-subunit that forms the insulin-binding site and a transmembrane β-subunit that possesses tyrosine kinase activity. The mature insulin receptor is a dimer composed of 2 α- and 2 β-subunits. Insulin binds its receptor in the picomolar range within a binding pocket formed by the two α-subunits. Binding produces conformational changes in the receptor that activate intrinsic tyrosine kinase activity that results in autophosphorylation of one β-subunit by the other. This autophosphorylation increases the tyrosine kinase activity of the receptor toward other substrates, especially the docking proteins insulin-receptor substrate 1 (IRS-1) and IRS-2. Phosphorylation of IRS-1 and IRS-2 results in further downstream phosphorylation and activation of MAP kinase and phosphatidylinositol-3-kinase. This network of phosphorylation ultimately leads to translocation of glucose transporters, especially GLUT-4, to the plasma membrane. This results in an increase in glucose transport into muscle and adipose tissue. Phosphorylation of various substrates in this insulin pathway also increases glycogen synthesis, lipogenesis, protein synthesis, and activation of transcription factors that mediate effects on cell growth and division.

Administration

Most currently available preparations are injected subcutaneously, inhaled, or delivered by continuous infusion. Short-acting soluble insulin is the only form that should be administered IV. A recently approved dry powder insulin product is available for inhalation use.

Oral Hypoglycemic Agents

Oral hypoglycemic agents increase the secretion of insulin by the pancreas or alter tissue sensitivity to insulin. These agents are typically used to control hyperglycemia in patients with type II diabetes (Table 43-2).

Sulfonylureas

Sulfonylureas act to **increase the release of insulin from the pancreas. First-generation sulfonylureas** include tolbutamide, chlorpropamide, tolazamide, and acetohexamide. **Second-generation agents** include glyburide, glipizide, gliclazide, and glimepiride, which are considerably **more potent** than the earlier agents. All are **substituted arylsulfonylureas** with different substitutions on the benzene ring and at one nitrogen residue of the urea moiety.

Table 43-2

COMMON AGENTS FOR DIABETES

MEDICATION	MECHANISM OF ACTION/INDICATIONS	SPECIAL CONSIDERATIONS	COST
Insulin	Supplement patient's own insulin production	Must check blood glucose frequently to monitor therapy and prevent complications	$–$$$
Sulfonylurea	Augments patient's own insulin production, works at the pancreatic B-cells	Can cause hypoglycemia, can accumulate in renal insufficiency and cause prolonged hypoglycemia. Best for young patients with FPG <300mg/dL	$
Metformin	Increases glucose uptake by muscle, decreases gluconeogensis in the liver, decreases insulin resistance	In patients with renal insufficiency, or liver dysfunction, may cause lactic acidosis	$
α-Glucosidase	Inhibits breakdown of complex carbohydrates in the GI tract.	Can cause GI distress, and must be taken TID with meals. Dose-dependent hepatotoxicity	$$
Pioglitazone	Promote skeletal muscle glucose uptake, decrease insulin resistance	Hepatoxicity, edema	$$$–$$$$
Repaglinide, Nateglinide	Nonsulfonylureas—but works in a similar manner—rapid onset of action. Monotherapy or in combination with metformin	Caution in elderly, renal, or hepatic insufficiency. Must dose TID with meals	$$

With permission, from Case Files: Internal Medicine, 2004.

Sulfonylureas are used to control glucose levels in type II diabetics who cannot achieve adequate control with diet alone. A limitation in the use of the sulfonylureas is secondary failure, that is, failure to maintain glucose levels with chronic use. **Adverse effects of sulfonylureas include hypoglycemia, nausea and vomiting, anemia, and dermatologic reactions.**

Mechanism of Action

Sulfonylureas bind to a high-affinity sulfonylurea receptor on B cells that inhibits a K^+-efflux channel. This leads to **depolarization of the cell with an increase in Ca^{2+} entry** through voltage-gated Ca^{2+} channels. The increased intracellular Ca^{2+} causes an increase in insulin secretion. Sulfonylureas **also stimulate the release of pancreatic somatostatin,** which can reduce the secretion of glucagon.

Administration

All of the sulfonylureas are administered orally.

Pharmacokinetics

First-generation sulfonylureas have relatively long half-lives: Chlorpropamide is 32 hours, tolazamide is 7 hours, tolbutamide is 5 hours. The second-generation agents tend to have shorter half-lives (approximately 4 hours) which makes them less prone to causing hypoglycemia.

Other Insulin Secretagogues

Two relatively new insulin secretagogues, repaglinide and nateglinide, are approved for use in **type II diabetics.** Both of these agents act by **decreasing the activity of K^+ channels as described for the sulfonylureas.** This increases insulin release. Chemically, **repaglinide is a meglitinide, nateglinide is a D-phenylalanine derivative.** Repaglinide has a half-life of approximately 1 hour and a very rapid onset of action that makes it well suited to control postprandial increases in plasma glucose. It should be taken approximately 10 minutes before a meal. It is metabolized in the kidney and should be used cautiously in patients with renal impairment. Nateglinide is also used to control plasma glucose after meals. It should be taken 1–10 minutes prior to eating. Both these drugs can cause hypoglycemia but nateglinide has the lowest incidence of this adverse effect.

Insulin Sensitizers

Thiazolidinediones

A **hallmark of type II diabetes is insulin resistance.** The hormone is present at significant plasma concentrations but is ineffective in reducing plasma glucose. **Thiazolidinediones (TZDs) act to increase tissue sensitivity to insulin.** TZDs appear to **increase glucose uptake in adipose and muscle tissues.** Two TZDs are approved for use: **pioglitazone and rosiglitazone.**

The effects of the TZDs are mediated by agonist activity at the peroxisomal proliferator-activated receptor γ (PPAR-γ). PPARs are members of the nuclear receptor family that are present in the nucleus of cells tethered to the promoters of target genes. PPARs bind a rather diverse group of ligands including fibrates and TZDs. There are three members of PPAR receptors, PPARα, PPARβ, and PPARγ; the latter mediates the effects of the TZDs. TZDs are effective in approximately 70 percent of type II diabetics. TZDs alter plasma lipid levels by reducing triglycerides, high-density lipoprotein (HDL) and low-density lipoprotein (LDL) cholesterol.

Biguanides

Metformin lowers plasma glucose levels in the absence of functioning B cells, it does not increase insulin secretion but **decreases insulin resistance** by increasing glucose uptake and decreasing glucose production. These actions are mediated by increasing the activity of AMP kinase. It is useful in patients with type II diabetes and **does not cause weight gain** or provoke hypoglycemia as do the sulfonylureas. Biguanides are frequently used in combination with TZDs or insulin secretagogues when monotherapy has not provided adequate glycemic control.

Common adverse effects include nausea, vomiting, diarrhea, and abdominal pain. Biguanides are **cleared by the kidney** and are **contraindicated in patients with renal disease.**

Polypeptide Analogs

Pramlintide is a synthetic analog of amylin which is produced by the pancreas in concert with insulin. It decreases postprandial hyperglycemia and improves glucose control when administered with insulin. It is injected subcutaneously and is approved for treatment of both type 1 and type II diabetes.

Exenatide is a synthetic analog of glucagon-like-polypeptide-1 (GLP-1), originally isolated from the saliva of the Gila monster, and is classified as an "incretin mimetic." The incretin include GLP-1 and glucose-dependant insulinotropic polypeptide (GIP) and are potent stimulators of insulin release and inhibitors of glucagon release. Exenatide mimics the enhancement of glucose-dependent insulin secretion and other antihyperglycemic actions of incretins. Several clinical trials have demonstrated the effectiveness of exenatide either with metformin or in combination with metformin and a sulfonylurea. It also appears to reduce food intake.

Enzyme Inhibitors

Monosaccharides such as **glucose and fructose** can be absorbed across the intestine and into the portal circulation. Complex disaccharides, starches, and disaccharides that comprise a significant percentage of the carbohydrates ingested, must be broken into monosaccharides before they can be absorbed. Pancreatic α-amylase and α-glucosidases are primarily responsible for this hydrolysis of more complex carbohydrates. **Inhibitors of α-glucosidase such**

as acarbose and miglitol inhibit the intestinal breakdown of complex carbohydrates. Acarbose inhibits the α-glucosidases, sucrase, maltase, glu-
coamylase, dextranase. It weakly inhibits α-amylase. **Miglitol** is 5–6 times
more potent than acarbose and inhibits the same α-glucosidase, as well as isomaltase and β-glucosidases (responsible for hydrolysis of lactose) as well.
Inhibition of these digestive enzymes reduces postprandial absorption of complex carbohydrates and thereby reduces plasma glucose levels. They are
approved for treatment of type II diabetes as monotherapy or combined with a
sulfonylurea if additional hypoglycemic effect is needed. **Adverse effects
include flatulence, diarrhea, and abdominal pain,** most likely caused by the
increase in carbohydrates in the distal small intestine and colon. α-Glucosidase
inhibitors prevent the progression from a prediabetic state into new cases of
type II diabetes and this may become a new indication for these drugs.

Agents That Increase Plasma Glucose

Glucagon is useful for the **emergency treatment of severe hypoglycemia**
when **unconsciousness prevents oral administration of nutrients and IV
glucose is unavailable.** Glucagon binds to specific receptors in the **liver** that
increase cAMP and promote the catabolism of glycogen into glucose.
Glucagon must be administered parenterally.

COMPREHENSION QUESTIONS

[43.1] Which of the following is the goal of insulin therapy?

    A. Control serum glucose as tightly as possible
    B. Control triglyceride biosynthesis
    C. Maintain adequate hepatic glycogen stores
    D. Maintain serum K^+ homeostasis

[43.2] The thiazolidinediones are useful in treating type II diabetes because
they have which of the following effects?

    A. Decrease the degradation of insulin
    B. Increase insulin release
    C. Increase glucose utilization
    D. Increase glucose uptake in muscle cells

[43.3] A 42-year-old man is diagnosed with diabetes mellitus. He has tried
diet and exercise without success. A second-generation sulfonylurea
agent is prescribed. Which of the following is the most likely side
effect he will experience?

    A. Agranulocytosis
    B. Hypoglycemia
    C. Lactic acidosis
    D. Myositis

Answers

[43.1] **A.** The goal in treating diabetes is tight control of serum glucose to avoid the complications of hyperglycemia.

[43.2] **D.** The TZDs are insulin sensitizers; they do not alter insulin secretion or degradation but act to increase glucose uptake in adipose and muscle.

[43.3] **B.** In general, the most common adverse effect of the agents for diabetes is hypoglycemia.

PHARMACOLOGY PEARLS

❖ The goal in treating diabetes is tight glucose control to prevent the micro- and macrovascular complications.

❖ Human recombinant insulin is preferable to either bovine or porcine insulin.

❖ Biguanides such as metformin are cleared by the kidney and are contraindicated in patients with renal disease.

❖ Glucagon is useful for the emergency treatment of severe hypoglycemia when unconsciousness prevents oral administration of nutrients and IV glucose in unavailable.

REFERENCES

Inzucchi SE. Oral antihyperglycemic therapy for type 2 diabetes: scientific review. JAMA 2002;287:360–72.

Quinn L. Type 2 diabetes: epidemiology, pathophysiology, and diagnosis. Nurs Clin North Am 2001;36:175–92.

Cohen A, Horton ES. Progress in the treatment of type 2 diabetes: new pharmacologic approaches to improve glycemic control. Curr Med Res Opin 2007;23: 905–17.

A 66-year-old woman presents for an annual health maintenance visit. She is generally feeling well and has no specific complaints. She takes hydrochlorothiazide for hypertension, levothyroxine sodium for hypothyroidism, and a multivitamin. She went through menopause at age 48 and never took hormone replacement therapy. She is a former cigarette smoker, having a 30 pack-year history and having quit 20 years ago. She occasionally has a glass of wine with dinner and walks three or four times a week for exercise. On examination you note that her height is 1 inch less than it was 3 years ago. Her vital signs are normal. She has a prominent kyphoscoliosis of the spine. Her examination is otherwise unremarkable. Blood work reveals normal electrolytes, renal function, blood count, calcium, and thyroid-stimulating hormone (TSH) levels. You order a bone density test, which shows a significant reduction of density in the spine and hips. You diagnose her with osteoporosis and start her on alendronate sodium.

◆ **What is the mechanism of action of parathyroid hormone (PTH) on the bone and in the kidney?**

◆ **What is the mechanism of action of alendronate sodium?**

ANSWERS TO CASE 44: AGENTS AFFECTING CALCIUM HOMEOSTASIS

Summary: A 66-year-old woman with osteoporosis is prescribed alendronate.

◆ **Mechanism of action of PTH on the bone:** Pulsatile administration, the normal physiologic mode, enhances bone formation. Continuous delivery, for example, as a consequence of a parathyroid tumor, results in bone resorption.

◆ **Mechanism of action of PTH in the kidney:** Increases reabsorption of Ca^{2+} and Mg^{2+} and increases production of calcitriol and dihydrotachysterol; decreases reabsorption of phosphate, bicarbonate, amino acids, sulfate, sodium, and chloride.

◆ **Mechanism of action of alendronate sodium:** Inhibition of osteoclastic activity in bone, which reduces bone reabsorption.

CLINICAL CORRELATION

PTH has multiple actions on bone. Chronic elevations in PTH, for example, from a tumor, stimulate the resorption of bone via its stimulation of the number and activity of osteoclasts. This is mediated by specific PTH receptors in the bone, coupled to an increase in cyclic adenosine monophosphate (cAMP). Intermittent administration of PTH stimulates bone growth. Estrogen is an indirect inhibitor of PTH activity in the bone. This effect allows premenopausal women to maintain higher levels of bone density. Following menopause, and the resultant decrease in circulating estrogen levels, there is a relative increase in osteoclastic activity and resorption of bone, with a net loss of bone mineral density. Alendronate sodium is an analog of pyrophosphate that directly binds to bone. It inhibits osteoclastic activity, reducing the resorption of bone. This retards the progression of bone density loss and may allow for increases in density, because osteoblastic activity is not affected. It is administered orally, and its most common adverse effects are gastrointestinal (GI). It may produce esophagitis, and even esophageal perforation, if the pill were to get caught in the esophagus while swallowing. For that reason, patients taking alendronate are instructed to take it on an empty stomach with a full glass of water and to remain upright for at least 30 minutes after ingesting the medication.

APPROACH TO PHARMACOLOGY OF AGENTS REGULATING CALCIUM HOMEOSTATIS

Objectives

1. Know the structure, actions, and uses of PTH.
2. Describe the structure, actions, and uses of calcitonin (CT).

3. Describe the structure, synthesis, actions, and uses of vitamin D and its metabolites.
4. Know the secondary agents that affect calcium homeostasis and their characteristics.

Definitions

Osteocyte: A bone-maintaining cell, an embedded osteoblast.
Osteoblast: Bone-forming cells derived from the stroma of bone.
Osteoclast: Bone-resorptive cell derived from myeloid lineages.
OPG (osteoprotegerin): A member of the OPG, OPGL (osteoprotegerin ligand), RANK (receptor activator of nuclear factor-κB) signal transduction cascade that is central to bone metabolism.

DISCUSSION

Pharmacology of Class

Calcium is the major extracellular divalent ion. It has diverse roles—including enzyme activation, secretion, excitation-contraction coupling in all muscle types, and neuronal function—and is a critical structural element in bone and teeth.

Approximately **40–50 percent of serum calcium exists as free, ionized** Ca^{2+}. This is **the biologically active fraction,** and it is maintained at approximately 2.5 mM in the serum. An additional **40 percent is bound to serum proteins** and the remainder is complexed to ions such as phosphate, citrate, and bicarbonate. The serum concentration of Ca^{2+} is tightly regulated by several endocrine systems and three major tissues: the **gut, kidney, and bone.**

Bone is the **storage depot** for over **99 percent of calcium in the body,** and most of the calcium is in the form of **hydroxyapatite:** $[Ca_{10}(PO_4)_6(OH)_2]$. Bone is a remarkably dynamic tissue and bone remodeling is a continuous process. Normal bone is continuously **reabsorbed by the action of osteoclasts,** and **new bone is formed by the action of osteoblasts;** if these two processes are not equal in magnitude, excess bone can be lost, as in osteoporosis, or too much bone can be formed. **Coupling of the actions of osteoblasts and osteoclasts is largely under the control of the OPG/OPGL signaling system** (Figures 44-1A and 44-1B).

Osteoblasts produce **OPGL,** a polypeptide that binds to receptors on osteoclasts termed **RANK-R. Stimulation of RANK-R** leads to increased **proliferation, maturation, and activation** of osteoclasts. Osteoblasts also elaborate **osteoprotegerin,** which is a **molecular antagonist of OPGL.** OPG can bind OPGL before it can activate the RANK receptor on osteoclasts. Osteoclast activation is thus controlled by the ratio of OPG/OPGL that is secreted by osteoblasts. Most drugs that act to alter calcium homeostasis in bone do so by altering OPG/OPGL.

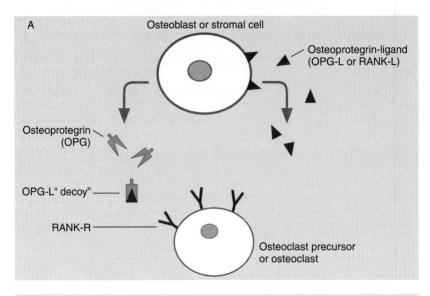

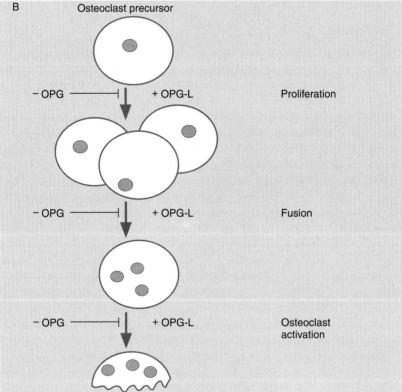

Figure 44-1. Osteoblast (A) and osteoclast (B). The OPG/OPGL-signaling system controls the number and activity of osteoclasts. Osteoblasts secrete both OPG and OPGL. PGL stimulates proliferation and activation of osteoclasts. OPG is a "decoy" that binds OPGL in the interstitial space and prevents its association with its receptor (RANK-R).

PTH is an 84-amino acid peptide synthesized in the **parathyroid glands** and is **secreted in response to low serum-ionized Ca^{2+}.** PTH 1–34 has full biologic activity. In the **kidney it acts to increase Ca^{2+} reabsorption** and **promotes phosphate (PO_4^{2-}) excretion.** It has indirect effects on the **GI** system to **increase Ca^{2+} absorption.** The effects of PTH on bone are complex and dependent on the temporal nature of its release or administration. **Continuously elevated PTH, as in hyper-parathyroidism, increases osteoclast activity via increased OPGL and results in increased bone resorption. Pulsatile release of PTH** activates **osteoblasts** and increases bone formation.

CT is a 32-amino acid polypeptide produced in the **parafollicular cells** of the **thyroid.** It is secreted in response to elevated serum Ca^{2+} levels. **CT increases OPG and decreases OPG-L release** from **osteoblasts,** and its action on bone is to **reduce bone turnover.** In response to CT, osteoclasts withdraw reabsorptive processes, shrink in size, and retract the ruffled border from the surface of bone; CT effectively prevents all stages of osteoclastic bone resorption. It **increases renal excretion of Ca^{2+}, PO_4^{2-}, Mg^{2+}, Cl^-, and K^+ by decreasing reabsorption of these ions.**

The **third endocrine system** that has effects on **bone** is **vitamin D_3** and its **metabolites.** Vitamin D_3 (not a true vitamin in a nutritional sense) is a **prehormone** that undergoes a series of metabolic alterations to the final agonist in the pathway, 1,25-$(OH)_2$ vitamin D_3. **Vitamin D_3 is synthesized from cholesterol** in the skin in a **two-step photo-dependent reaction.** Vitamin D_3 is converted by the **liver enzyme 25-hydroxylase to 25-$(OH)D_3$;** in the **kidney** the enzyme **1-hydroxylase metabolizes 25-(OH) D_3 to 1,25-$(OH)_2$ D_3. 1,25-$(OH)_2$ D_3** acts on the intestine to **increase intestinal absorption of Ca^{2+}.** In the **kidney,** 1,25-$(OH)_2$ D_3 acts to **increase the absorption** of both Ca^{2+} and PO_4^{2-}. 1,25-$(OH)_2$ D_3 stimulates Ca^{2+} mobilization from bone and enhances the resorptive action of PTH on bone. However, **1,25-$(OH)_2$ D_3** also induces **osteocalcin and osteopontin, two matrix proteins** important in bone formation.

Treatment of Hypocalcemia

Calcium Salts

A wide variety of preparations are available for both IV and oral administration for treating **acute hypocalcemic tetany.** These include **calcium gluconate, calcium lactate, calcium carbonate, and calcium citrate.** They vary in the percentage of calcium by weight from a low of 9 percent for calcium gluconate to a high of 40 percent for calcium carbonate.

Vitamin D

Several vitamin D or vitamin D-related agents are available for use for hypocalcemia and osteoporosis (Table 44-1). Selection of which agent to use depends on the desired onset of action, duration of effect, and the presence of

Table 44-1

VITAMIN D-RELATED AGENTS

AGENT	CHEMICAL NATURE	TIME TO MAXIMUM EFFECT	DURATION OF ACTION	REQUIRE- MENT FOR METABOLISM
Cholecalciferol	Vitamin D_3	4 weeks	8 weeks	Liver, kidney
Ergocalciferol	Vitamin D_2	4 weeks	8 weeks	Liver, kidney
Dihydrotachysterol	1-(OH) D_3	1–2 weeks	1–2 weeks	Liver
Doxercalciferol	1-(OH) D_2	1–2 weeks	1–2 weeks	Liver
Calcifediol	25-(OH) D_3	2–3 weeks	2–3 weeks	Kidney
Paricalcitol	25-(OH) D_2	2–3 weeks	2–3 weeks	Kidney
Calcitriol	1,25-(OH)$_2$ D_3	24 hours	3–5 days	None

underlying liver or kidney disease. Thiazide diuretics act on the kidney to increase Ca^{2+} reabsorption in the distal convoluted tubule and can be used in the treatment of hypocalcemia.

Treatment of Hypercalcemia

Hypercalcemia has a number of pathophysiologic causes including **hyperparathyroidism, Paget disease, and hypercalcemia of malignancy. CT** is useful for **short-term treatment of hypercalcemia.** Salmon CT is more potent and has a longer half-life than human CT and is the form used therapeutically. CT has few side effects but **refractoriness** frequently develops. CT is available for parenteral and nasal administration. Peak plasma concentration after an inhaled dose is approximately 30 minutes after administration, but normalization of the rate of bone turnover as in Paget disease may take several months.

Bisphosphonates are **analogs of pyrophosphate in which the phosphodiester bond (P-O-P) is replaced by a nonhydrolyzable bisphosphonate (P-C-P) bond.** First-generation bisphosphonates included sodium **etidronate.** Second-generation aminobisphosphonates include **risedronate, alendronate, pamidronate, tiludronate, clodronate, zoledronate, and ibandronate.** The two classes of bisphosphonates have different mechanisms of action and different potencies. For example, **risedronate** is 1000 times more potent as an inhibitor of bone resorption than etidronate. All bisphosphonates bind to and accumulate in bone, and this provides a measure of tissue specificity. The first-generation nonnitrogenous bisphosphonates are converted into an adenosine triphosphate (ATP) analog that cannot be internalized. This metabolite impairs osteoclast function and triggers osteoclast apoptosis. The aminobisphosphonates are not converted into an ATP analog; rather they interfere with mevalonate and ubiquitin metabolism (similar to statins). This leads to impaired posttranslational modification of a number of proteins that are critical to osteoclast function. Ultimately, the aminobisphosphonates lead to osteoclast hypofunction. **Etidronate** is available for oral use; the aminobisphosphonates may be administered orally or by infusion. Administered orally, all the bisphosphonates have **very poor (approximately 5%) bioavailability,** but sufficient drug is absorbed to achieve therapeutic concentrations in bone. All bisphosphonates are approved for treatment of **Paget disease; alendronate,** risendronate, zoledronate, and ibandronate are also approved for **prevention and treatment of osteoporosis** (pamidronate is approved for treatment of osteoporosis). The remaining aminobisphosphonates are used to treat hypercalcemia of malignancy. Adverse effects of bisphosphonates include **GI upset, diarrhea, and nausea.** Bisphosphonates are associated with **lower esophageal erosion,** and the recommendation with alendronate and risedronate is to **avoid lying down for 30 minutes after oral administration to avoid reflux.** There have been reports of bisphosphonate use associated with the osteonecrosis of the jaw. Although rare, this seems to occur most often in cancer patients receiving bisphosphonate therapy.

Loop diuretics increase the amount of Ca^{2+} excreted and can be used in the acute management of hypercalcemia.

Treatment of Osteoporosis

Osteoporosis, loss of bone mass, affects nearly 30 percent of women aged 65 years and older and a smaller percentage of men. Historically, osteoporosis has been divided into **postmenopausal osteoporosis,** which occurs in women and is related to the loss of ovarian hormones after menopause, and **senile osteoporosis,** which is age related and affects both sexes. Histologically and biochemically, they seem indistinguishable disorders of bone metabolism caused by excessive bone reabsorption or inadequate bone formation. Adequate dietary Ca^{2+} and vitamin D (to facilitate Ca^{2+} absorption) is critical in patients at risk for osteoporosis. The recommended daily allowance (RDA) for Ca^{2+} in patients at risk is **1200 mg/day.**

Teriparatide (PTH 1–34) has been approved for the treatment of osteoporosis. Administered intermittently, once a day by injection, teriparatide **increases bone formation in excess of resorption.** This treatment has been shown to increase bone mass and decrease the incidence of fractures. Studies in **rats** receiving very high doses of teriparatide for 2 years demonstrated an **increased frequency of osteosarcoma. It is contraindicated in patients with bone malignancy or in pediatric patients.** Major adverse effects are **hypotension, hypocalcemia, dizziness, and nausea.**

Estrogens (see Case 40) have been shown to reduce the rate of bone loss in the postmenopausal period when the rate of loss can be as high as 10 percent per year. Estrogens increase bone mineral density and decrease the incidence of vertebral and nonvertebral fractures. However, estrogens do not increase net bone formation.

Selective estrogen receptor modifiers (SERMs) are compounds whose estrogenic activities are tissue selective. Three SERMs are currently approved for use: **tamoxifen, raloxifene, and toremifene. Raloxifene** is approved for the prevention and treatment of osteoporosis; tamoxifen and toremifene are used to treat breast cancer. Raloxifene is a polyhydroxylated nonsteroidal compound that binds to the estrogen receptor, but it has estrogen-agonist activity only in bone and the liver; it has no effect on the uterus, and it is an estrogen antagonist in breast tissue and in the brain. It has antiresorptive activity in bone. It increases bone mineral density and has been shown to decrease the incidence of vertebral and nonvertebral fractures. Adverse effects include hot flashes and leg cramps. More serious adverse effects include an approximate threefold increase in deep vein thrombosis and pulmonary embolism.

Sodium fluoride has been examined in a number of clinical trials for the treatment of osteoporosis. Early studies using relatively high doses reported an increase in bone mineral density but no decrease in the incidence of fractures, probably because of the formation of abnormal hydroxylapatite crystals in bone. More recent studies using slow-release monofluoride have suggested a decrease in fracture rates but fluoride is not yet approved for the treatment of osteoporosis.

COMPREHENSION QUESTIONS

[44.1] Which of the following vitamin D preparations would be the most appropriate in a patient with poor renal function?

    A. Calcifediol
    B. Calcitriol
    C. Cholecalciferol
    D. Ergocalciferol

[44.2] Intermittent administration of PTH produces which of the following?

    A. Impaired Ca^{2+} absorption in the gut
    B. Inhibition of 1-hydroxylase
    C. Net increase in bone formation
    D. Net increase in bone resorption

[44.3] A 53-year-old woman who is being treated for metastatic breast cancer is noted to have some lethargy, fatigue, and an elevated serum calcium level. She is brought into the emergency department for near comatose state, thought to be caused by the hypercalcemia. After addressing the ABCs (airway, breathing, circulation), which of the following is the best therapy for this patient?

    A. Bisphosphonates
    B. CT
    C. IV estrogen therapy
    D. Saline infusion and furosemide

Answers

[44.1] **B.** 1-Hydroxylase activity must be adequate to produce $1,25(OH)_2 D_3$. Calcitriol is the only choice that is already 1-hydroxylated.

[44.2] **C.** Intermittent administration of PTH on its analogs will result in bone formation. Continuous dosing or a PTH-secreting tumor will cause bone resorption.

[44.3] **D.** Loop diuretics are the best choice in a patient with acute onset hypercalcemia.

PHARMACOLOGY PEARLS

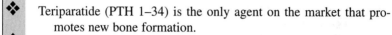 Teriparatide (PTH 1–34) is the only agent on the market that promotes new bone formation.

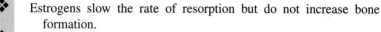 Estrogens slow the rate of resorption but do not increase bone formation.

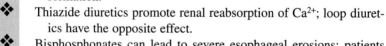 Thiazide diuretics promote renal reabsorption of Ca^{2+}; loop diuretics have the opposite effect.

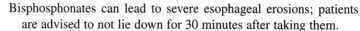 Bisphosphonates can lead to severe esophageal erosions; patients are advised to not lie down for 30 minutes after taking them.

REFERENCES

Ariyan CE, Sosa JA. Assessment and management of patients with abnormal calcium. Crit Care Med 2004;32(4 suppl):S146–54.

Stepan JJ, Alenfeld F, Boivin G, et al. Mechanisms of action of antiresorptive therapies of postmenopausal osteoporosis. Endocr Regul 2003;37:225–38.

Levine JP. Pharmacologic and nonpharmacologic management of osteoporosis. Clin Cornerstone 2006;8:40–53.

A 22-year-old woman enters your clinic with the chief complaint of irregular menstrual periods. She indicates that she was 14 when her periods first started and that they had never really been very regular. On physical examination she is 5'4" and weighs 195 lbs. She has mild acne on her face and shoulders and a more than normal amount of facial hair. There is a darkening of the skin at the base of her neck and across her shoulders. Blood tests reveal an elevated LH and a normal FSH level (LH/FSH 3.2). You suspect she may have polycystic ovary syndrome (PCOS) and start her on metformin.

◆ **What is the effect of insulin on the ovaries?**

◆ **What is the mechanism of action of metformin?**

ANSWERS TO CASE 45: AGENTS FOR THE TREATMENT OF PCOS

Summary: A 22 year old woman with obesity, hirsutism and irregular menstrual cycles, consistent with the diagnosis of PCOS

◆ **Effect of insulin on the ovaries:** Insulin stimulates steroidogenesis, especially androgen production within the ovary.

◆ **Mechanism of action of Metformin:** Metformin activates AMP kinase; this central regulator of metabolism acts to increase glucose uptake and metabolism in skeletal muscle.

CLINICAL CORRELATIONS

PCOS is a very common cause of irregular menstrual periods and infertility. It is frequently associated with obesity and the concomitant insulin resistance and hyperinsulinemia. The excessive insulin increases production of ovarian androgens such as androstenedione and dehydroepiandrosterone, which can act peripherally and increase both sebum production and hair growth. Tunica albicans (darkened shoulders) is a manifestation of hyperinsulinemia. Metformin is a relatively new oral antidiabetic agent that causes metabolic changes that decreases serum glucose and insulin levels.

APPROACH TO PCOS

Objectives

1. Know the agents for the treatment of PCOS.
2. know the mechanism of action, uses, and adverse effects of the agents

Definitions

PCOS: Polycystic ovary syndrome (also known as Stein-Leventhal syndrome or Polycystic Ovary Disease [PCOD]) is one of the leading causes of infertility in women

Acanthosis nigricans: A velvety darkening of the skin commonly seen at the nape of the neck, elbows, axilla, and knuckles.

DISCUSSION

PCOS is characterized by a lack of regular ovulation and excessive amounts or effects of androgenic (masculinizing) hormones. The ovaries accumulate benign cysts produced by abnormal follicular development and lack of ovulation due to endocrine dysfunction. Patients with PCOS tend to have high body mass index (BMI), glucose intolerance, and insulin resistance. The elevated insulin level due to the insulin resistance is a potent stimulator of steroidogenesis, especially of androgens, in the ovary. The androgens cause acne and hirsutism, both frequently associated with PCOS. Hyperinsulinemia increases GnRH pulse frequency, LH over FSH dominance, decreased follicular maturation, and decreased sex hormone–binding globulin; all these steps contribute to the development of PCOS.

Metformin is a biguanine oral antihyperglycemic agent. It appears to act by activating AMP kinase, an important metabolic integrator with effect on adipose tissue, skeletal muscle, cardiac muscle, liver, and hypothalamus. Activation of AMP kinase reduces glycogen production, reduces fatty acid oxidation, and facilitates glucose uptake.

In PCOS patients, metformin reduces insulin resistance and lowers insulin levels, which lowers serum androgen concentrations, restores normal menstrual cycles and ovulation, and may help to resolve PCOS-associated infertility. Metformin, when administered to lean, overweight, and moderately obese women with PCOS, has been found to significantly reduce serum luteinizing hormone (LH) and increase FSH and sex hormone–binding globulin (SHBG). Serum testosterone concentrations were also found to decrease by approximately 50%

GI adverse effects are seen in approximately 30% of patients taking metformin. GI effects include anorexia, nausea/vomiting, abdominal discomfort, dyspepsia, flatulence, diarrhea, and dysgeusia (metallic taste). These side effects tend to decline with continued use and can be minimized by initiating therapy with low doses of metformin. Asymptomatic vitamin B_{12} deficiency was reported with metformin monotherapy in 9% of patients during clinical trials. The risk of hypoglycemia is much less common with metformin than with the sulfonylureas.

Other agents that are used to treat PCOS include oral contraceptives which reduce LH and ovarian androgen production and finasteride, a potent 5α-reductase inhibitor (see Case 40). In PCOS patients desiring to become pregnant, the combination of metformin and clomiphene significantly increase the ovulation and conception rates compared to clomiphene alone.

COMPREHENSION QUESTIONS

[45.1] Which of the following would be the best agent to use in a patient with PCOS?

    A. Pioglitazone
    B. Metformin
    C. Regular insulin
    D. Repaglinide

[45.2] Which of the following is the most common adverse effect of metformin?

    A. Hypoglycemia
    B. Hyperinsulinemia
    C. GI effects
    D. Pruritis

[45.3] Which of the following is the mechanism of action of metformin?

    A. Increase insulin secretion by the pancreas
    B. Increase hepatic sensitivity to insulin
    C. Reduction in DHT production
    D. Increased muscle uptake of glucose

Answers

[45.1] **B.** Pioglitozone, as an insulin sensitizer, might be efficacious in the treatment of PCOS but metformin has fewer and less severe side effects. Repaglinide stimulates insulin secretion which would be detrimental in PCOS.

[45.2] **C.** Metformin infrequently causes hypoglycemia and hypersensitivity reactions, for instance in the skin, are rare.

[45.3] **D.** Metformin does not increase insulin production; it appears to act by decreasing plasma glucose by affecting metabolism rather than altering the sensitivity of tissues to insulin.

PHARMACOLOGY PEARLS

 Metformin reduces insulin levels and can improve insulin sensitivity without weight gain.
 Metformin rarely causes hypoglycemia.

REFERENCES

    Bhathena RK. Therapeutic options in the polycyctic ovary syndrome. J Obstet Gynaecol 2007;27:123–9.
    Reitman ML, Schadt EE. Pharmacogenetics of metformin response: a step in the path toward personalized medicine. J Clin Invest 2007;117:1266–9.

A 48-year-old man comes to your office with a 6-day history of worsening cough productive of green sputum. He has had fever and chills. He complains of pain in the right midback with deep breathing or coughing. Further history reveals that he has smoked one pack of cigarettes a day for 30 years. He has no other significant medical history. On examination, his temperature is 38.1°C (100.5°F); his respiratory rate is 24 breaths per minute; pulse, 98 beats per minute; blood pressure, 120/75 mm Hg; and saturation of oxygen, 96 percent on room air by pulse oximetry. Auscultation of his lungs reveals rales in the right lower-posterior lung field. The remainder of his examination is within normal limits. A posterior-to-anterior (PA) and lateral chest x-ray show a right lower-lobe infiltrate. A sputum Gram-stain reveals gram-positive cocci, and subsequent sputum and blood culture results confirm the diagnosis of pneumonia caused by *Streptococcus pneumoniae* (pneumococcus). You treat him with a combination of amoxicillin and clavulanic acid.

◆ **What is the mechanism of action of amoxicillin?**

◆ **What is the mechanism of action of clavulanic acid?**

ANSWERS TO CASE 46: ANTIBACTERIAL AGENTS

Summary: A 48-year-old man with pneumococcal pneumonia is being treated with amoxicillin and clavulanic acid.

◆ **Mechanism of action of amoxicillin:** Inactivation of bacterial transpeptidases and prevention of cross-linking of peptidoglycan polymers necessary for cell-wall integrity, resulting in loss of cell-wall rigidity and cell rupture; also inhibition of cell-wall synthesis.

◆ **Mechanism of action of clavulanic acid:** Irreversible inhibition of β-lactamase.

CLINICAL CORRELATION

Penicillin is the prototype antibiotic in the β-lactam class. **β-Lactam antibiotics interfere with bacterial transpeptidases** and thereby **prevent the cross-linking of peptidoglycan** polymers essential for **cell-wall integrity.** They do this by binding to the active site of the penicillin-binding protein (an enzyme) that is involved in maintaining cell-wall stability. β-Lactam antibiotics are **bactericidal** in growing cells, with gram-positive bacteria being particularly susceptible. Penicillin has activity against many gram-positive aerobic organisms, some gram-negative aerobes and anaerobic organisms. It does not have significant activity against gram-negative rods. Amoxicillin is an extended-spectrum penicillin with better activity against gram-negative rods and similar activity against other organisms. **Both penicillin and amoxicillin are susceptible to β-lactamases,** which cleave the β-lactam ring required for antibacterial action. Clavulanic acid (and sulbactam and tazobactam) is structurally similar to penicillin. It has no antimicrobial activity of its own but it irreversibly inhibits certain β-lactamases. It frequently is given in fixed combination with amoxicillin, thus allowing it to be used to treat β-lactamase-producing organisms. Penicillins can cause hypersensitivity reactions in susceptible persons. Approximately 5–10 percent of penicillin-allergic persons will have a cross-sensitivity to cephalosporin drugs as well. Penicillins also have gastrointestinal (GI) side effects, and the addition of clavulanic acid significantly increases the incidence of diarrhea.

APPROACH TO PHARMACOLOGY OF ANTIBACTERIAL AGENTS

Objectives

1. Describe the factors in choosing appropriate antibiotic agents.
2. List the classes of antibiotics, and describe their mechanisms of action, therapeutic uses, and adverse effects.
3. Outline mechanism of development of bacterial drug resistance.

Definitions

Chemotherapy: Therapeutic use of chemical agents that selectively act on microbes and cancer.

Plasmids: Extrachromosomal genetic elements that may be transferred between bacteria.

DISCUSSION

Class

The basic principles for the selection of **antibacterial therapy** include consideration of factors such as the **likelihood that the infection is bacterial** and the identification of the **likely infecting organism** to support a rational selection of an antibiotic. Consideration of host and drug factors that could influence antibiotic selection include identification of the site of infection, which will influence the selection of the antibiotic and its route of administration; recognition of concomitant diseases such as AIDS; recognition of the likelihood of drug allergies; recognition of hepatic or renal dysfunction that could alter antibiotic clearance; and recognition of drug toxicity, drug-drug interactions, drug resistance, the patient's age or pregnancy or maternal status; and drug cost.

Antibacterial agents, which target specific components of microorganisms that are unique or more essential to their function than they are to humans, are classified according to their mechanisms of action. The component targets include **enzymes necessary for bacterial cell-wall synthesis, the bacterial ribosome, and enzymes necessary for nucleotide synthesis and deoxyribonucleic acid (DNA) replication.**

Resistance of pathogens to antibacterial and other chemotherapeutic agents may be the result of a natural resistance or may be acquired. In either case, it occurs through mutation, adaptation, or gene transfer. The mechanism of resistance for any antibacterial agent varies, but is a result of either changes in uptake of drug into, or its removal from, the bacterial cell, or to changes in the bacterial cell target site of the drug from a gene mutation. **Multiple drug resistance** is also a major impediment to antibacterial therapy and may be **chromosomal or plasmid mediated,** where genetic elements from resistant bacteria that code for enzymes that inactivate antibacterial agents are transferred to nonresistant bacteria. The emergence of drug resistance is to a large degree the result of the widespread and often unnecessary or inappropriate use of antibiotics in humans.

The **penicillins** (see above) include natural penicillins, penicillins that are resistant to staphylococcal β-lactamase, and extended-spectrum penicillins (Table 46-1).

The **cephalosporins** are classified as first to fourth generation, according to their antibacterial spectrum (Table 46-2).

Table 46-3 lists these and other selected antimicrobial agents. **Aztreonam,** which is relatively β-lactamase resistant, is the only available monobactam.

Table 46-1
PARTIAL LISTING OF PENICILLINS

Natural Penicillin G (prototype) Penicillin V	*Extended-Spectrum* *Aminopenicillins* Ampicillin Amoxicillin
β-Lactamase Resistant Nafcillin Oxacillin Cloxacillin Dicloxacillin	*Ureidopenicillins* Mezlocillin Piperacillin *Carboxypenicillin* Ticarcillin

Table 46-2
SELECTED LISTING OF CEPHALOSPORINS

REPRESENTATIVE CEPHALOSPORINS (route)	NOTES
First generation • Cefazolin (IV) • Cephalexin (PO) • Cefadroxil (PO)	Active against gram-positive cocci, including staphylococci, pneumococci, and streptococci. They are particularly good for soft tissue and skin infection
Second generation • Cefuroxime (IV) oral form is cefuroxime axetil • Cefotoxin (IV) • Cefotetan (IV)	These agents have marked differences in their spectrum of activity. In general, they are active against certain aerobic gram-negative bacteria in addition to activity against many gram-positive organisms sensitive to first-generation cephalosporins. Certain agents are active against *Haemophilus influenza* (e.g., cefuroxime), whereas others are active against *Bacteroides fragilis* (e.g., cefotoxin)
Third generation • Cefotaxime (IV) • Ceftazidime (IV) • Ceftriaxone (IV)	Expanded aerobic gram-negative spectrum. Cross the blood-brain barrier. Useful to treat bacterial strains resistant to other drugs
Fourth generation • Cefepime (IV)	Generally similar activity to third-generation cephalosporins but more resistance to β-lactamases

Table 46-3
PARTIAL LISTING OF ANTIMICROBIAL AGENTS

ANTIBACTERIAL AGENTS	MECHANISM OF ACTION	ADVERSE EFFECTS
β-Lactam antibiotics Penicillins Cephalosporins Monobactams • Aztreonam (p) *Carbapenems* • Imipenem (p) • Meropenem (p) • Ertapenem (p) *Vancomycin* (o,p)	Inhibit synthesis of the bacterial cell wall	*β-Lactam antibiotics:* hypersensitivity with rare potential for anaphylactic shock *Cephalosporins:* may cause local irritation and pain from IM injection. Those with a methylthiotetrazole group, e.g., cefotetan, may cause hypoprothrombinemia and bleeding disorders *Aztreonam:* occasionally may cause skin rashes *Carbapenems:* may cause GI discomfort and skin rashes and seizures in patients with renal dysfunction (particularly imipenem) *Vancomycin:* relatively nontoxic. Fever, chills, and infusion-related flushing ("red-man" syndrome) are encountered. Ototoxicity is a rare effect
Chloramphenicol *Tetracyclines* • Tetracycline (o,p) • Oxytetracycline (o,p) • Doxycycline (o,p) • Methacycline (o) • Minocycline (o,p) *Macrolides* • Erythromycin (o,p) • Clarithromycin (o) • Azithromycin (o) *Ketolides* • Telithromycin (o) *Oxazolidinones* • Linezolid (o,p) *Aminoglycosides* • Streptomycin (p) • Neomycin (o) • Amikacin (p)	Bind to bacterial ribosomes to inhibit protein synthesis	*Chloramphenicol:* GI disturbances, reversible suppression of bone marrow, rarely aplastic anemia *Tetracyclines:* GI disturbances and bacterial overgrowth, teeth and bone deformation in children *Erythromycin and clarithromycin:* severe GI disturbances, hypersensitivity, hepatic P450 inhibition. *Telithromycin:* hepatic P450 inhibition *Linezolid:* reversible thrombocytopenia *Aminoglycosides:* ototoxicity and nephrotoxicity

(Continued)

Table 46-3
PARTIAL LISTING OF ANTIMICROBIAL AGENTS (*continued*)

ANTIBACTERIAL AGENTS	MECHANISM OF ACTION	ADVERSE EFFECTS
• Gentamicin (p) • Tobramycin (p,i) *Spectinomycin (p)* *Lincomycins* • Clindamycin (o,p)		*Clindamycin:* GI disturbances, hepatic dysfunction, potentially fatal colitis
Sulfonamides • Sulfadiazine (o) • Sulfamethizole (o) • Sulfamethoxazole (o) • Sulfanilamide (t) • Sulfisoxazole (t,o) *Trimethoprim*	*Sulfonamides:* structural analogs of p-aminobenzoic acid that inhibit bacterial dihydropteroate synthase to block folic acid synthesis and cell growth *Trimethoprim:* selectively inhibits dihydrofolic acid reductase to block folic acid synthesis and cell growth. Acts synergistically with sulfamethoxazole with which it is often coadministered	*Sulfonamides:* hypersensitivity urinary tract dysfunction, hemolytic or aplastic anemia, potentially fatal Stevens-Johnson syndrome *Trimethoprim:* blood dyscrasias
Fluoroquinolones (selected) • Ciprofloxacin (t,o,p) • Levofloxacin (t,o,p) • Ofloxacin (t,o,p) • Gatifloxacin (o,p) • Moxifloxacin (o,p)	Inhibit activity of bacterial topoisomerase (DNA gyrase) that is necessary for replication	GI disturbances, reversible arthropathy, arrhythmias

t = topical, o = oral, p = parenteral, i = inhalation.

It is nonallergenic and is active only against aerobic gram-negative bacilli (e.g., pseudomonas, serratia). The **carbapenems** (imipenem, meropenem, and ertapenem), which are resistant to most β-lactamases, have a wide spectrum of activity against gram-positive and gram-negative rods and anaerobes. To **prevent its metabolism, imipenem** is administered with an **inhibitor of renal tubule dehydropeptidase, cilastatin.**

Vancomycin, which is unaffected by β-lactamases, **inhibits bacterial cell-wall synthesis** by covalent binding to the terminal two D-alanine residues of nascent peptidoglycan pentapeptide to prevent their elongation and cross-linking, thus increasing the susceptibility of the cell to lysis. It is **active against gram-positive bacteria.**

COMPREHENSION QUESTIONS

[46.1] Which of the following is the most likely explanation for multiple drug resistance to antibiotics that spreads from one type of bacteria to another?

A. Adaptation
B. Decreased bioavailability
C. Gene transfer
D. Mutation

[46.2] Penicillins inhibit which of the following bacterial processes/ compounds?

A. Protein synthesis
B. Topoisomerase
C. Dihydropteroate synthase
D. Cell-wall synthesis

[46.3] Ototoxicity and nephrotoxicity are characteristic adverse effects of which of the following?

A. Aminoglycosides
B. β-Lactam antibiotics
C. Chloramphenicol
D. Fluoroquinolones

Answers

[46.1]   **C.** Antibiotic drug resistance can occur through bacterial cell mutation, adaptation, or gene transfer. The best route for multiple drug resistance that spreads from one type of bacteria to another is via plasmid or chromosomal gene transfer.

[46.2]   **D.** Penicillins inhibit synthesis of the bacterial cell wall. Chloramphenicol, tetracyclines, macrolides, ketolides, oxazolidinones, aminoglycosides, spectinomycin, and the lincomycin bind to bacterial ribosomes to inhibit protein synthesis. The fluoroquinolones inhibit activity of bacterial topoisomerase to inhibit protein synthesis, and the sulfonamides inhibit bacterial dihydropteroate synthase to block folic acid synthesis and cell growth.

[46.3]   **A.** Ototoxicity and nephrotoxicity are characteristic adverse effects of aminoglycosides. Chloramphenicol can cause GI disturbances, reversible suppression of bone marrow, and rarely aplastic anemia. As a group, the β-lactam antibiotics can cause hypersensitivity and have the potential to cause anaphylactic shock. The fluoroquinolones can cause GI disturbances, reversible arthropathy, and arrhythmias.

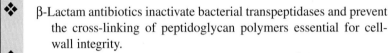

PHARMACOLOGY PEARLS

❖ β-Lactam antibiotics inactivate bacterial transpeptidases and prevent the cross-linking of peptidoglycan polymers essential for cell-wall integrity.
❖ Both penicillin and amoxicillin are susceptible to β-lactamases.
❖ To prevent its metabolism, imipenem is administered with an inhibitor of renal tubule dehydropeptidase, cilastatin.
❖ Vancomycin, which is unaffected by β-lactamases, is active against gram-positive bacteria.
❖ Chloramphenicol can cause GI disturbances, reversible suppression of bone marrow, and rarely aplastic anemia
❖ Aminoglycosides may cause ototoxicity or nephrotoxicity and should be used with caution in those patients who have renal insufficiency or who are elderly.

REFERENCES

Conte JE. Manual of Antibiotics and Infectious Diseases. Philadelphia (PA): Lippincott Williams & Wilkins, 2001.
Tenover FC. Mechanisms of antimicrobial resistance in bacteria. Am J Med 2006;119(6 suppl 1):S3–10; discussion S62–70.
Wright AJ. The penicillins. Mayo Clin Proc 1999;74(3):290–307.

A 58-year-old man presents for the evaluation of a painful rash. He says that for 3 or 4 days he had a sharp, burning pain radiating from his midback around to his left side. He thought that he was having a kidney stone. Yesterday he noticed a rash which spread in a distribution "like a line" in the same area in which he had the pain. He is on glyburide for type II diabetes, simvastatin for high cholesterol, and lisinopril for hypertension, all of which he has been on for several years. He does have a history of having chickenpox as a child. On examination he has a low-grade fever and otherwise normal vital signs. His skin examination is remarkable for a rash in a belt-like distribution from his spine around his left flank to the midline of the abdomen. The rash consists of erythematous patches with clusters of vesicles. The remainder of his examination is normal. You make the diagnosis of herpes zoster and prescribe a course of acyclovir (ACV).

◆ **What is the mechanism of action of ACV?**

◆ **How is ACV eliminated from the body?**

ANSWERS TO CASE 47: ANTIVIRAL AGENTS

Summary: A 58-year-old man with herpes zoster is prescribed ACV.

◆ **Mechanism of action of ACV:** Purine analog that is converted to a nucleoside triphosphate that competes with the natural triphosphate substrate to inhibit the activity of viral DNA polymerase. It is also incorporated into the growing viral DNA where it acts as a chain terminator.

◆ **Elimination of ACV:** Excreted unmetabolized via the kidney through glomerular and tubular filtration.

CLINICAL CORRELATION

Herpes zoster, also known as shingles, is caused by a reactivation of dormant varicella-zoster virus (VZV). It causes a rash and frequently a painful neuropathy, usually in the distribution of a single dermatome. ACV can shorten the course of symptoms of herpes zoster, although it cannot eradicate latent virus. ACV is a purine analog that requires viral thymidine kinase to be converted to a monophosphate form, thus assuring that it accumulates selectively in infected cells. Host cellular enzymes then convert the monophosphate to a triphosphate form that competitively inhibits the activity of viral DNA polymerase. The triphosphate form also is incorporated into viral DNA, where it acts as a chain terminator. ACV has a low oral bioavailability. It is excreted, largely unchanged, via the kidney. Valacyclovir (VCV) is a prodrug form of ACV that has a greater oral bioavailability than ACV. It is rapidly and completely converted to ACV after absorption, resulting in higher concentrations of ACV.

APPROACH TO PHARMACOLOGY OF ANTIVIRAL DRUGS

Objectives

1. List the specific drug classes and drugs used to treat viral disease.
2. Describe the mechanisms of action and adverse effects of antiviral drugs used to treat infections by herpes simplex virus (HSV), VZV, and cytomegalovirus (CMV).

DISCUSSION

Class

Viral Biology

Viruses are obligate intracellular parasites that do not have their own metabolic machinery but rather use the host's own metabolic capabilities to replicate.

Antiviral medications usually attack the virus prior to cell penetration, after the virus leaves the host cell, or while the virus is active within the host cell. Nonspecific effects may be harmful to the host. Figure 47-1 shows a schematic of the viral life cycle summarized, and Table 47-1 describes specific antiviral therapies aimed at the various viral maturation steps.

There are three main types of viruses: (1) **DNA viruses** usually enter the host cell nucleus and direct the production of new viruses, (2) ribonucleic acid **(RNA) viruses** direct the production of new viruses, usually without entering the host cell nucleus (an exception is influenza), and (3) **RNA retroviruses,** such as human immunodeficiency virus (HIV). Retroviruses contain an enzyme, reverse transcriptase that makes a DNA copy of the viral RNA; the DNA copy is spliced into the host DNA and directs the production of the new viruses.

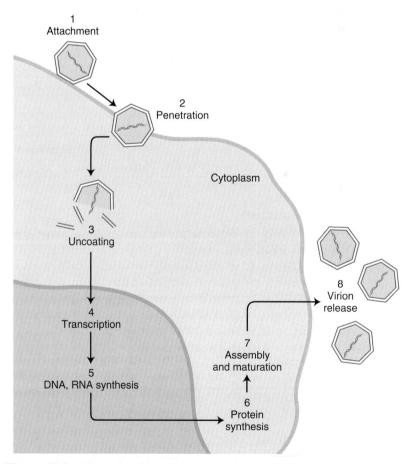

Figure 47-1. Life cycle of the virus.

Table 47-1
EXAMPLES OF ANTIVIRAL MECHANISMS

	VIRAL LIFE CYCLE	ANTIVIRAL THERAPY	EXAMPLES
1.	Virus attaches to the cell	γ-globulin (binds to virus)	Hepatitis A and B
2.	Virus penetrates the cell	γ-globulin	
3.	Virus uncoats its nucleic acid	Influenza A and B	Influenza A
4a.	Synthesis of key viral enzymes such as polymerases (transcription)	ACV, ribavirin (DNA polymerase inhibitor)	Herpes simplex
4b.	Viral nucleic acid is synthesized	Zidovudine (reverse transcriptase inhibitor)	HIV
5.	Late viral structural proteins are synthesized	Indinavir (protease inhibitor)	HIV
6.	Viral proteins and particles are assembled	Influenza A and B	
7.	Viruses are released from the host cell	Influenza A and B	Influenza A and B

Overview of Antiviral Agents

The **four major classes of antiviral agents** are (1) **DNA polymerase inhibitors, (2) reverse transcriptase inhibitors, (3) protease inhibitors, and (4) fusion inhibitors.** It should be noted that HIV treatment usually includes the use of 3–4 antiretroviral agents as standard of care. DNA polymerase inhibitors are categorized as nucleoside or nonnucleoside. Drugs may target viral nucleic acid replication such as DNA polymerase either via nucleoside (purine or pyrimidine analogs) such as ACV or ribavirin, or by attacking a unique viral process needed in nucleic acid synthesis such as viral pyrophosphate (nonnucleoside type).

Antiviral drugs used to treat HSV, VZV, and CMV can be classified as either nucleoside or nonnucleoside, or according to their site of action in the viral replicative cycle or according to their clinical use (see Table 47-1).

Common Antiviral Agents

Influenza. **Amantadine and rimantadine** are primarily used against infections caused by **influenza A.** Their mechanism of action is interfering with **viral uncoating.** Both agents are fairly well absorbed orally and cause some minor central nervous system (CNS) effects (rimantadine less so) and minor GI effects.

Herpes Virus, Varicella-Zoster Virus/Cytomegalovirus

ACV is used against **HSV 1 and HSV 2.** ACV, a **nucleoside DNA polymerase inhibitor,** is a deoxyguanosine triphosphate (**dGTP**) **analog** that is incorporated into the viral DNA and causes DNA chain termination. Its specificity is a result of the presence of **herpes-specific thymidine kinase** in infected cells, which phosphorylates ACV a 100-fold more efficiently than by uninfected cells. The ACV triphosphate is formed in infected cells and incorporated into infected cells' DNA, and not formed in normal cells. ACV can be used topically, orally for recurrent genital herpes, and IV for immunocompromised patients or herpes encephalitis.

Its adverse effects include headache, nausea, and rarely nephrotoxicity with IV use. **VCV** is an analog of ACV and is converted to ACV in the body. Its advantage is better bioavailability.

Penciclovir (PCV) is converted to the triphosphate form and inhibits viral DNA polymerase. **Famciclovir (FCV)** is converted to the active agent PCV in the body. Their main use is to treat **localized herpes zoster in immunocompromised patients.** Headache and GI effects are common. **Ganciclovir (GCV)** is structurally similar to ACV and must be converted to the triphosphate form to be active; it competes with dGTP for incorporation into viral DNA thereby inhibiting DNA polymerase. Its primary role is against **CMV,** and is **far more effective than ACV against CMV.** GCV can induce serious **myelosuppression.**

Foscarnet is a **synthetic nonnucleoside analog of pyrophosphate** and inhibits DNA polymerase or HIV reverse transcriptase by directly binding to the pyrophosphate-binding site. Its use is usually for **ACV-resistant herpes or CMV retinitis.** Significant nephrotoxicity may occur with its use.

Trifluridine is a **fluorinated pyrimidine nucleoside analog.** Its monophosphate form inhibits thymidylate synthetase, and its triphosphate form inhibits DNA polymerase. It is active against HSV 1 and 2 and CMV, and it is used primarily against keratoconjunctivitis and recurrent keratitis.

Structure

VCV, FCV, and valganciclovir: Ester pro-drugs of, respectively, ACV, PCV, and GCV.

Cidofovir (CDV): Phosphonate analog of cytidine.

Idoxuridine (IDU): Analog of thymidine.

Table 47-2 presents a partial listing of antiviral agents and mechanisms of action and Table 47-3 presents the agents used to treat HSV, VZV, and CMV

Table 47-2
PARTIAL LISTING OF ANTIVIRAL AGENTS AND
MECHANISMS OF ACTION

Nucleosides that inhibit RNA or DNA genomic replication: ACV,
cidofovir (CDV), FCV, GCV/valganciclovir, PCV, IDU, trifluridine, VCV

Nonnucleosides that inhibit RNA or DNA genomic replication: foscarnet

Nonnucleosides that inhibit transcription: interferons

Nonnucleosides that inhibit translation: fomivirsen

Nonnucleosides that inhibit uncoating: amantadine, rimantadine

Nonnucleosides that inhibit release and budding: zanamivir, oseltamivir

Other Viral Infections

Hepatitis B and C:
Lamivudine, adefovir, interferon alfa, and ribavirin

Influenza:
Amantadine and rimantadine (nonnucleosides that inhibit uncoating), zanamivir and
oseltamivir (nonnucleosides that inhibit release and budding)

HIV-1:
Nucleoside and nucleotide reverse transcriptase inhibitors (NRTIs; abacavir, didanosine,
lamivudine, stavudine, tenofovir, zalcitabine, zidovudine)

Nonnucleoside reverse transcriptase inhibitors (NNRTIs; delavirdine, efavirenz,
nevirapine)

Protease inhibitors (amprenavir, atazanavir, fosamprenavir, indinavir, lopinavir/
ritinovir, nelfinavir, ritonavir, saquinavir, tipranavir)

Fusion inhibitors (enfuvirtide)

Mechanism of Action

VCV, GCV, and valganciclovir act like ACV.

IDU and FCV and the prodrug FCV, which is converted to the active agent
PCV, also act like ACV except that they do not cause DNA chain termination.

Trifluridine (activated by host cell phosphorylation) and foscarnet (acts
directly to inhibit viral DNA polymerase and RNA polymerase) do not require
activation by viral thymidine kinase for their activity and therefore can be used
to treat ACV-resistant viral infections.

CDV is phosphorylated to mono- and diphosphate nucleotides by cellular
kinases and, therefore, accumulates in both infected and uninfected cells. As a

Table 47-3
AGENTS USED TO TREAT HSV, VZV, AND CMV
(ROUTE OF ADMINISTRATION)

AGENTS	VIRAL INFECTIONS	ADVERSE EFFECTS
ACV (t,o,p)	HSV, VSV	Nausea, vomiting, diarrhea, headache; parenteral administration may cause reversible neuropathy and nephropathy
Cidofovir CDV (p)	HSV, CMV	Nephrotoxicity
Docosanol (t)	HSV, VSV	Well tolerated
Famciclovir FCV (o)	HSV, VSV	Nausea, vomiting, diarrhea, headache, confusion in elderly
Ganciclovir (GCV) (intraocular implant, o,p)	CMV	Generally reversible myelosuppression with neutropenia and thrombocytopenia
Valganciclovir (o)		
Penciclovir (PCV) (t)	HSV, VSV	Well tolerated
Idoxuridine (IDU) (o)	HSV	Edema and burning and stinging of the eye
Valacyclovir (VCV) (o)	HSV, VSV	Nausea, vomiting, diarrhea, headache
Trifluridine (t)	HSV	Edema and burning and stinging of the eye
Foscarnet (p)	HSV, VSV, CMV	Reversible nephrotoxicity, hypo- or hypercalcemia and phosphatemia that may lead to neural and cardiac dysfunction; hallucinations, genital ulceration, and anemia are not uncommon
Fomivirsen (p)	CMV	Iritis, vitreitis, increased ocular pressure

t = topical, o = oral, p = parenteral.

diphosphate, CDV inhibits and serves as an alternative dCTP substrate for viral DNA polymerase, resulting in inhibition of viral DNA synthesis and termination of chain elongation.

Fomivirsen is an antisense oligonucleotide that binds to the major immediate early region 2 (IE2) of CMV mRNA to prevent its translation to protein and therefore to block viral replication.

Administration

ACV: Administered IV and orally and is used as a topical agent.

Foscarnet: Reserved to treat ACV-resistant viral infections and can only be administered IV.

VCV, FCV: Available only for oral use.

GCV: Administered orally; parenterally (IV); and as an intraocular, slow-release implant.

PCV, trifluridine, IDU: Available only for topical use.

Cidofovir: Administered parenterally with probenecid to block its active tubular secretion.

Fomivirsen: Administered by intravitreal injection.

Pharmacokinetics

ACV: Low oral bioavailability.

VCV: An ester prodrug with greater oral bioavailability than ACV that is rapidly and completely converted to ACV after absorption.

FCV, valganciclovir: Ester prodrugs that are rapidly converted by first-pass metabolism to their respective active agents, PCV and GCV.

NNRTI and PI agents are metabolized by and induce the cypP450 enzyme system (3A4) resulting in numerous drug-drug interactions.

COMPREHENSION QUESTIONS

[47.1] Which of the following drugs is most likely to cause myelosuppression?

    A. FCV

    B. Fomivirsen

    C. GCV

    D. PCV

[47.2] Which of the following drugs is a prodrug that after oral administration is converted to an active agent, PCV?

    A. ACV

    B. FCV

    C. Fomivirsen

    D. GCV

[47.3] The high levels of ACV obtained in target viruses such as HSV is a result of which of its properties?

    A. Binding to the major immediate early region 2 (IE_2) of CMV mRNA

    B. Direct inhibition of viral DNA polymerase and RNA polymerase

    C. Host cell enzyme conversion to triphosphate compounds

    D. Monophosphorylation by viral thymidine kinase

Answers

[47.1] **C.** GCV can cause a generally reversible myelosuppression. FCV can cause nausea, vomiting, diarrhea, and headache. PCV is generally well tolerated. Fomivirsen causes ocular problems, including iritis, vitreitis, and increased ocular pressure.

[47.2] **B.** FCV is a diacetyl ester prodrug that after oral administration is converted to PCV by first-pass metabolism. Fomivirsen is administered by intravitreal injection. ACV and GCV act directly and can be administered orally and parenterally. ACV can also be administered topically. GCV can also be administered as an intraocular implant.

[47.3] **A.** The high levels of ACV obtained in target viruses such as HSV result from its monophosphorylation by viral thymidine kinase. Antiviral drugs that are activated only by host cell kinases, for example, cidofovir (CDV), will accumulate in host cells with or without viral infection. Fomivirsen is an antisense oligonucleotide that binds to the major immediate early region 2 (IE_2) of CMV mRNA to prevent its translation to protein and therefore to block viral replication. Foscarnet acts directly to inhibit viral DNA polymerase and RNA polymerase.

PHARMACOLOGY PEARLS

❖ The primary strategy of antiviral agents is to attack a unique but vital viral enzyme or process.

❖ The three major types of antiviral agents include DNA polymerase inhibitors, reverse transcriptase inhibitors, and protease inhibitors.

❖ HIV therapy generally uses at least two reverse transcriptase inhibitors and one protease inhibitor.

❖ Didanosine is also a nucleoside reverse transcriptase inhibitor for HIV infections and is associated with peripheral neuropathy and pancreatic damage.

❖ Foscarnet is a synthetic nonnucleoside analog of pyrophosphate and is associated with reversible nephrotoxicity, and hypo- or hyper-calcemia and phosphatemia that may lead to neural and cardiac dysfunction. Also, hallucinations, genital ulceration, and anemia may occur.

❖ Implantable GCV and oral valganciclovir are more widely used for CMV disease than the IV agents foscarnet, cidofovir, and GCV.

REFERENCES

Coen DM, Richmann DD. Antiviral agents. In: Knipe DM, Howley PN, Griffin DE, et al., eds. Fields Virology, 5th ed. Philadelphia (PA): Lippincott, Williams & Wilkins, 2006.

Drugs for non-HIV viral infections. Med Lett Drugs Therapy. 2007;5(59):59–70.

AIDS info: U.S. Department of Health and Human Services. www.aidsinfo.nih.gov

A 4-year-old boy is brought in by his mother because he keeps scratching a spot on his arm. His mother says that this has been going on for several days, and it appears that the spot is growing larger. No one else at home has anything similar. He has not had a fever or any systemic signs of illness. There have been no recent exposures to new foods, medications, lotions, or soaps. He attends preschool during the day. On examination of his skin you see a circular, nickel-sized ring on his right forearm. It has a red, raised border and central clearing. The remainder of his skin examination and his general physical examination are normal. You diagnose him with tinea corporis (ringworm) and prescribe topical nystatin.

◆ **What is the mechanism of action of nystatin?**

◆ **Nystatin is similar in structure and function to which other antifungal medication?**

ANSWERS TO CASE 48: ANTIFUNGAL

Summary: A 4-year-old boy with tinea corporis is prescribed topical nystatin.

◆ **Mechanism of action of nystatin:** Creates pores in fungal membranes by binding ergosterol.

◆ **Nystatin is similar in structure and action to:** Amphotericin B.

CLINICAL CORRELATION

Superficial fungal infections of the skin are very common, particularly in the pediatric population. There are many topical preparations available that are effective against this problem. Nystatin is a polyene antifungal agent with similarities in structure and function to the systemic antifungal agent amphotericin B. Nystatin, which is too toxic for parenteral use, is administered topically for skin infections. It is not absorbed through the GI tract; therefore, oral preparations are used only to treat fungal infections of the mucous membranes of the mouth or intestinal tract. Amphotericin B is given IV and is only used for severe, systemic fungal infections. It has significant toxicities and adverse effects. It frequently causes fever, chills, and impaired renal function. Less often it will cause anaphylactic reactions, pain, thrombocytopenia, and seizures.

APPROACH TO PHARMACOLOGY OF ANTIFUNGAL DRUGS

Objectives

1. List the antifungal drugs and describe their mechanisms of action, therapeutic uses, routes of administration, and adverse effects.

DISCUSSION

Class

In addition to the pyrimidine analog, flucytosine, and the *Penicillium*-derived antifungal agent, griseofulvin, the three major classes of antifungal agents are the polyene macrolides, azoles, and allylamines (Table 48-1).

Of all the available antifungal agents, **amphotericin B** has the **broadest spectrum of activity,** including **activity against yeast, mycoses, and molds.** It is the **drug of choice for disseminated or invasive fungal infections in immunocompromised** patients. The **major adverse effect** resulting from amphotericin B administration is the almost invariable **renal toxicity** that results from decreased renal blood flow and from tubular and basement membrane

Table 48-1
SELECTED ANTIFUNGAL DRUGS (ROUTE)

Polyene Macrolides	*Allylamines*
Nystatin (t,o for GI tract)	Naftifine (t)
Natamycin (t)	Terbinafine (o,t)
Amphotericin B (t,o for GI tract, p)	
Azoles	*Other Antifungal Agents*
Miconazole (t)	Flucytosine (o)
Clotrimazole (t)	Griseofulvin (o)
Itraconazole (o,p)	
Fluconazole (o,p)	
Voriconazole (o,p)	

t = topical, o = oral, p = parenteral.

destruction that may be irreversible and may require dialysis. Therefore, it is often given acutely to patients with severe infections followed soon after by a less toxic agent such as an azole. Other adverse effects of amphotericin B relate to its IV infusion and include fever, chills, vomiting, hypotension, and headache, which can be ameliorated somewhat by careful monitoring and slow infusion.

The **azole antifungal agents** have a **broad spectrum of activity,** including activity against **candidiasis, mycoses, and dermatophytes,** among many others. As topical agents the azoles are relatively safe. Administered orally, their **most common adverse effect is GI dysfunction.** Hepatic dysfunction may rarely occur. **Itraconazole** interaction with quinidine can result in cardiac arrhythmias. Monitoring patients who receive itraconazole for potential **hepatic toxicity** is also highly recommended. **Voriconazole** frequently causes an **acute blurring of vision** with changes in color perception that resolves quickly.

The **allylamine antifungal agents, naftifine and terbinafine,** are used **topically** to treat dermatophytes. Contact with mucous membranes may lead to local irritation and erythema and should be avoided. **Terbinafine** administered orally is effective against the **onychomycosis. Monitoring for potential hepatic toxicity is highly recommended.**

Flucytosine is active against only a **relatively restricted range of fungal infections.** Because of rapid development of resistance, it is used concomitantly for its synergistic effects with other antifungal agents. The most commonly reported adverse effect is **bone marrow suppression,** probably as a result of the **toxicity of the metabolite fluorouracil,** which should be continuously monitored. Other reported but less common adverse effects include reversible hepatotoxicity, enterocolitis, and hair loss.

Griseofulvin, the use of which is declining relative to the azoles terbinafine and itraconazole, is an effective antifungal agent that is used only **systemically** to treat a very **limited range of dermatophyte infections.** The most common adverse effects include **hypersensitivity** (fever, skin rash, serum sickness-like syndrome) and **headache.** It is **teratogenic.**

Structure

Depending on whether there are two or three nitrogen atoms in the azole ring, azole antifungal agents are subclassified, respectively, as either imidazoles (ketoconazole, clotrimazole, miconazole) or triazoles (itraconazole, fluconazole, voriconazole).

Mechanism of Action

Nystatin and amphotericin B bind to ergosterol, a major component of **fungal cell membranes.** This disrupts the stability of the cell by forming pores in the cell membrane that result in leakage of intracellular constituents. Bacteria are not susceptible to this because they lack ergosterol.

Azoles (imidazoles less so) have a greater affinity for fungal than human cytochrome P450 enzymes and therefore more effectively reduce the synthesis of fungal cell ergosterol than human cell cholesterol. The allylamine antifungal agents, naftifine and terbinafine, decrease ergosterol synthesis and increase fungal membrane disruption by inhibiting the enzyme squalene epoxidase.

Flucytosine must first be transported into fungal cells via a cytosine permease and converted to 5-fluorouracil (5-FU) and then sequentially converted to 5-fluorodeoxyuridylic acid, which disrupts DNA synthesis by inhibiting thymidylate synthetase. Human cells are unable to synthesize the active flucytosine metabolites.

The mechanism of antifungal action of griseofulvin is not clearly known. It acts only on growing skin cells and has been reported to inhibit cell-wall synthesis, interfere with nucleic acid synthesis, and disrupt microtubule function, among other activities.

Administration

Amphotericin B is insoluble in water and, therefore, is generally administered as a colloidal suspension with sodium deoxycholate. Because of its poor absorption from the GI tract, amphotericin B must be given IV to treat systemic disease, although it is effective orally for fungal infections within the GI lumen. Likewise, nystatin is poorly absorbed but may also be used for fungal infection of the GI tract. It is too toxic for systemic use and therefore is mostly used topically to treat fungal infections of the skin and mucous membranes (e.g., oropharyngeal thrush, vaginal candidiasis). Costly lipid formulations of amphotericin B are available for IV use, which reduce its nonspecific binding to cholesterol of human cell membranes and therefore lessens its potential to cause renal damage. Griseofulvin is administered in a microparticulate form to improve absorption.

Pharmacokinetics

Amphotericin B and nystatin are poorly absorbed from the GI tract. The absorption of the azole antifungal agent, itraconazole, is reduced by antacids that block acid secretion. Through their actions on hepatic microsomal enzymes, itraconazole and voriconazole significantly decrease the metabolism of numerous other drugs (e.g., the rifamycins, phenytoin, carbamazepine, digoxin, cyclosporine). In the presence of a number of these other drugs, the metabolism of itraconazole and voriconazole may be increased.

COMPREHENSION QUESTIONS

[48.1] Which of the following antifungal agents binds to ergosterol?

    A. Amphotericin B
    B. Fluconazole
    C. Flucytosine
    D. Terbinafine

[48.2] Bone marrow suppression is a common adverse effect of which of the following drugs?

    A. Fluconazole
    B. Flucytosine
    C. Griseofulvin
    D. Terbinafine

[48.3] Which of the following is the drug of choice for disseminated or invasive fungal infections in immunocompromised patients?

    A. Amphotericin B
    B. Flucytosine
    C. Griseofulvin
    D. Terbinafine

Answers

[48.1]   **A.** Amphotericin B, like nystatin, binds to ergosterol to create pores in fungal membranes. Flucytosine must first be transported into fungal cells via a cytosine permease and converted to 5-FU and then sequentially converted to 5-fluorodeoxyuridylic acid, which disrupts DNA synthesis by inhibiting thymidylate synthetase. Fluconazole binds fungal cell cytochrome P450 enzymes to reduce the synthesis of ergosterol. Terbinafine decrease ergosterol synthesis by inhibiting the enzyme squalene epoxidase.

[48.2] **B.** Bone marrow suppression is a common adverse effect of flucytosine. A common adverse effect of griseofulvin is hypersensitivity
(fever, skin rash, serum sickness-like syndrome). Terbinafine may
cause hepatic toxicity. Fluconazole causes GI dysfunction.

[48.3] **A.** Amphotericin B is the drug of choice for at least the initial treatment of disseminated or invasive fungal infections in immunocompromised patients.

PHARMACOLOGY PEARLS

 Itraconazole has been associated with heart failure when used to
treat onychomycosis and therefore should not be used in patients
with ventricular abnormalities.

 A common side effect of griseofulvin is hypersensitivity.

❖ Because of renal toxicity, amphotericin B is often used to initiate a
clinical response before substituting a continuing maintenance
dose of an azole.

REFERENCES

Groll AH, Gea-Banacloche JC, Glasmacher A, et al. Clinical pharmacology of anti-
fungal compounds. Infection Dis Clin North Am 2003;17(1):159–91.
Rex JH, Stevens DA. Systemic antifungal agents. In: Mandell GL, Bennett JE,
Dolin R, eds. Principles and Practice of Infectious Diseases, 6th ed. New York:
Elsevier, Vol.1; 2005:502.

A 66-year-old man presents for evaluation of skin growths on his face. For several years he has had scaly, rough growths on his face, forehead, and scalp. He has had individual lesions frozen off by previous physicians, but keeps getting more and more. He has never been diagnosed with skin cancer. He has a long history of sun exposure and multiple sunburns, primarily as a consequence of working outdoors and playing golf. He takes an aspirin a day and pravastatin for high cholesterol. He has no other significant medical history. On examination of his skin, you note multiple 4- to 7-mm lesions on the face and scalp that are flat, pink, and scaly. They feel rough on palpation. They are all in areas that would be sun exposed. He has several on the dorsal surfaces of his hands and forearms. You diagnose him as having multiple actinic keratoses. Along with recommending skin protection from the sun, you prescribe topical 5-fluorouracil (5-FU).

◆ **What is the mechanism of action of 5-FU?**

◆ **What are the adverse effects of 5-FU when given systemically?**

ANSWERS TO CASE 49: ALKYLATING AND ANTIMETABOLITE AGENTS

Summary: A 66-year-old man with multiple actinic keratoses is prescribed 5-FU.

◆ **Mechanism of action of 5-FU:** Pyrimidine antagonist that, after a complex conversion to 5-fluoro-2'-deoxyuridine-5'-monophosphate (FdUMP), covalently inhibits thymidylate synthetase and thus impairs DNA synthesis.

◆ **Adverse effects of systemic 5-FU:** Myelosuppression, nausea, vomiting, and hair loss.

CLINICAL CORRELATION

Actinic keratoses are premalignant skin lesions that frequently occur as a result of excessive sun exposure. Untreated, actinic keratoses may progress to become squamous cell carcinomas of the skin. Persons with multiple lesions are often treated with topical 5-FU. Systemic 5-FU is given parenterally primarily for the treatment of certain solid tumors. Systemic 5-FU is myelosuppressive and causes frequent GI disturbances and hair loss. Topical 5-FU does not have the systemic side effects but can cause significant local redness, itching, and burning of the skin.

APPROACH TO PHARMACOLOGY OF ALKYLATING AND ANTIMETABOLITE AGENTS

Objectives

1. Outline the principles of cancer chemotherapy and the development of resistance to chemotherapeutic agents.
2. List the antimetabolite and alkylating chemotherapeutic agents and describe their mechanisms of action, therapeutic uses, and adverse effects.

DISCUSSION

Class

Appropriate **cancer chemotherapy** demands a thorough understanding of the kinetics of **tumor cell growth,** including its **control and regulation,** a thorough understanding of the **pharmacologic properties of available anticancer agents,** and an appreciation of the interactions between them.

    Combination chemotherapy early in therapy increases the likelihood of destroying drug-resistant populations of cells that are refractory to treatment and therefore is **generally more effective than monotherapy.** To be most effective, the drugs used in combination chemotherapy should each have **therapeutic activity with different dose-limiting toxicities** and should be **administered during several cycles** of treatment **to allow recovery from acute adverse effects.**

The drugs used to treat cancer are **classified** as **alkylating agents, antimetabolites, cytotoxic antibiotics, plant alkaloids, hormonal agents, and miscellaneous agents** (Table 49-1). Depending on the tumor type, they are often used in combinations or as adjunct therapy to surgical and radiation procedures.

Table 49-1

SELECTED ANTICANCER DRUGS
(MAY BE COMBINED WITH OTHER ANTICANCER AGENTS)

SELECTED ANTICANCER DRUGS	TOXICITY—ACUTE AND DELAYED	SELECTED INDICATIONS
Alkylating agents Cyclophosphamide Melphalan Chlorambucil Busulfan Thiotepa Carmustine Lomustine Mechlorethamine	Nausea and vomiting, GI ulceration, alopecia, myelosuppression, bone marrow depression (thrombocytopenia, leucopenia) with bleeding	*Cyclophosphamide:* acute lymphocytic leukemia, non-Hodgkin lymphomas *Melphalan:* multiple myeloma *Chlorambucil:* chronic lymphocytic leukemia *Busulfan:* chronic myelogenous leukemia *Thiotepa*: ovarian cancer *Carmustin, Lomustin:* brain tumors *Mechlorethamine:* Hodgkin's disease (advanced stage III and IV)
Antimetabolites Methotrexate 5-Fluorouracil 6-Mercaptopurine	*Methotrexate:* diarrhea, mucositis, myelosuppression *5-Fluorouracil:* nausea, vomiting, diarrhea, myelosuppression, neurotoxicity, head and foot syndrome *6-Mercaptopurine:* myelosuppression, hepatotoxicity	*Methotrexate:* acute lymphocytic leukemia *5-Fluorouracil:* colorectal cancer, solid tumors of the breast, pancreas, liver, etc. *6-Mercaptopurine:* acute lymphocytic leukemia

Primary resistance to anticancer drugs is thought to occur because of some **inherent genetic characteristics of tumor cells. Acquired resistance** of tumor cells to a specific anticancer drug may occur via several different mechanisms that usually involve either **amplification or overexpression of one or more genes.** For example, resistance to methotrexate is caused by either decreased drug transport into tumor cells, a modification of the target enzyme dihydrofolate reductase (DHFR) that results in a decreased affinity for methotrexate, or an increased level of DHFR in tumor cells. Resistance to the chemotherapeutic effects of alkylating agents may develop because of decreased cell permeability, increased cell thiol content that serves as a "decoy" target for alkylation, increased activity of glutathione transferases, and modification of DNA repair mechanisms. Alternatively, after exposure of a tumor cell to a number of structurally different agents, a so-called multidrug, or pleiotropic, resistance may develop to chemotherapeutic agents because of decreased uptake or retention of the drugs. This is a result of either increased expression of the constitutively expressed multidrug resistance gene (MDR-1), which codes for a surface cell membrane P-glycoprotein involved in drug efflux, or by overproduction of one of a number of other multidrug resistance proteins, for example, MRP-1, that are involved in the transmembrane export of drugs. Multidrug resistance is the major form of resistance to vinca alkaloids, etoposide, paclitaxel, anthracyclines, and dactinomycin.

Other Classes of Selected Anticancer Drugs

Cytotoxic antibiotics: Dactinomycin (actinomycin D), bleomycin, doxorubicin

Plant alkaloids: Vinblastine, vincristine, vinorelbine, etoposide, paclitaxel, topotecan

Hormonal agents: Steroid hormones: megestrol acetate, hydrocortisone, prednisone

Antiandrogens: Flutamide

Antiestrogens: Tamoxifen

Gonadotropic-releasing hormone (GRH) agonists: Goserelin acetate, leuprolide

Aromatase inhibitors: Aminoglutethimide, anastrozole, exemestane, letrozole

Growth factor receptor inhibitors: Cetuximab, gefitinib, erlotinib, bevacizumab

Miscellaneous agents: Cisplatin, imatinib, hydroxyurea, mitotane, arsenic trioxide, procarbazine

Mechanism of Action

Alkylating Agents

The cytotoxic effects of alkylating agents result from the transfer of their alkyl groups to numerous cellular components, most notably the bases of

DNA, particularly the N7 position of guanine, which in replicating cells (G_1 and S phase) results in either miscoding or strand breakage.

Antimetabolites

Methotrexate (MTX): Folic acid antagonist that binds the catalytic site of DHFR to reduce the synthesis of tetrahydrofolate that results in downstream reduction of thymidylate and an indirect inhibition of DNA synthesis as well as RNA and protein synthesis.

Fluorouracil (5-FU): A prodrug that is converted to FdUMP by a multistep process. FdUMP covalently forms an inhibitory ternary complex with the enzyme thymidylate synthetase and reduced folate N5,10-methylene tetrahydrofolate, which are essential to the synthesis of thymidylate and the production of DNA. Through other metabolic conversions, 5-FU is also incorporated into DNA as 5-fluorodeoxyuridine-5'-triphosphate (FdUTP) and into RNA as 5-fluorouridine-5'-triphosphate (FUTP), which results in further inhibition of DNA function as well as inhibition of RNA processing and mRNA activity.

Mercaptopurine (6-MP): The precise mechanism of action of mercaptopurine, a modified purine, is unknown. Like the natural purines, hypoxanthine and guanine, it is converted to a nucleotide by hypoxanthine guanine phosphoribosyltransferase (HGPRT). The product, in this case 6-thioinosinic acid, inhibits purine nucleotide interconversion.

Pharmacokinetics

Cyclophosphamide is not itself cytotoxic but must first be converted by hepatic microsomal enzymes to form the cytotoxic agents, phosphoramide mustard and acrolein.

COMPREHENSION QUESTIONS

[49.1] Resistance to methotrexate is a result of which of the following?

    A. Increased activity of glutathione transferases
    B. Increased cell thiol content
    C. Modification of DNA repair mechanisms
    D. Modification of the target enzyme DHFR

[49.2] Which of the following agent forms an inhibitory ternary complex with the enzyme thymidylate synthetase?

    A. Cyclophosphamide
    B. Fluorouracil (5-FU)
    C. Mercaptopurine (6-MP)
    D. Methotrexate (MTX)

[49.3] Which of the following is true in general of combination cancer chemotherapy?

    A. It is administered during several cycles of treatment.
    B. It is less effective than monotherapy.
    C. It includes at least two drugs with similar dose-limiting toxicities.
    D. It includes one drug that has no inherent therapeutic activity.

Answers

[49.1]   **D.** Resistance to methotrexate may be a result of a modification of the target enzyme DHFR. It may also be a consequence of decreased drug transport into tumor cells or an increased level of DHFR in tumor cells. Resistance to the chemotherapeutic effects of alkylating agents may develop because of decreased cell permeability; increased cell thiol content, which serves as a "decoy" target for alkylation; increased activity of glutathione transferases; and modification of DNA repair mechanisms.

[49.2]   **B.** Fluorouracil (5-FU) is a prodrug that is converted to FdUMP, which covalently forms an inhibitory ternary complex with the enzyme thymidylate synthetase and reduced folate $N5,10$-methylene tetrahydrofolate, both of which are essential to the synthesis of thymidylate and the production of DNA. Mercaptopurine (6-MP) is thought to inhibit purine nucleotide interconversion. Methotrexate (MTX) is a folic acid antagonist that binds the catalytic site of DHFR to reduce the synthesis of tetrahydrofolate that results in downstream reduction of thymidylate and an indirect inhibition of DNA synthesis as well as RNA and protein synthesis. The cytotoxic effects of alkylating agents like cyclophosphamide are a result of the transfer of their alkyl groups to numerous cellular components, most notably the bases of DNA that in replicating cells (G_1 and S phase) results in either miscoding or strand breakage.

[49.3]   **A.** Combination chemotherapy early in therapy increases the likelihood of destroying drug-resistant populations of cells that are refractory to treatment and therefore is generally more effective than monotherapy. To be most effective, the drugs used in combination chemotherapy should each have therapeutic activity with different dose-limiting toxicities and should be administered during several cycles of treatment to allow recovery from acute adverse effect.

PHARMACOLOGY PEARLS

 Smaller tumors are generally more responsive to chemotherapy than larger tumors because of the increased probability of drug-resistant mutations in the larger tumors.

 Development of a mild leukopenia is evidence of the adequate absorption of orally administered alkylating agents.

 Leucovorin (citrovorum factor), a folic acid analog that does not require reduction by DHFR, can be used to "rescue" patients from MTX overdose or high-dose MTX therapy.

REFERENCES

Chabner BA, Longo DL. Cancer Chemotherapy and Biotherapy, 4th ed. Philadelphia (PA): Lippincott Williams and Wilkins, 2005.

DeVita VT Jr, Hellman S, Rosenberg SA. Cancer: Principles and Practices of Oncology, 7th ed. Philadelphia (PA): Lippincott Williams and Wilkins, 2004.

Perry MD. The Chemotherapy Source Book, 3rd ed. Baltimore (MD): Lippincott Williams and Wilkins, 2001.

A 60-year-old woman presents to her oncologist for follow-up of her metastatic ovarian cancer. She was diagnosed approximately a year ago. Initial treatment included surgery and a cisplatin-based chemotherapy regimen. Unfortunately, she was recently diagnosed with recurrent disease. She currently takes only promethazine as needed for nausea and a combination of hydrocodone and acetaminophen as needed for pain. On examination she appears comfortable. She has a thin growth of hair on her scalp. Her abdomen has a well-healed surgical scar but is otherwise unremarkable. The remainder of her examination is normal. She is diagnosed with recurrent metastatic ovarian cancer and placed on a chemotherapeutic regimen that includes paclitaxel.

◆ **What is the mechanism of action of paclitaxel?**

◆ **What are the common adverse reactions seen with paclitaxel?**

ANSWERS TO CASE 50: PLANT ANTICANCER ALKALOIDS

Summary: A 60-year-old woman with recurrent metastatic ovarian cancer is being treated with combination chemotherapy including paclitaxel.

◆ **Mechanism of action of paclitaxel:** Promotes formation and inhibits disassembly of stable microtubules, resulting in inhibition of mitosis.

◆ **Adverse effects of paclitaxel:** Myelosuppression, peripheral neuropathy, GI side effects.

CLINICAL CORRELATION

Paclitaxel is a chemical derived from bark of the Pacific yew tree. Its chemotherapeutic effect is based on its ability to inhibit mitosis. Its mechanism of action is to promote the formation of and inhibit the disassembly of stable microtubules in the M phase of cell division. Paclitaxel is used for the treatment of metastatic ovarian, breast, and small cell lung cancers. It is metabolized in the liver and excreted in the bile. Myelosuppression and peripheral neuropathy are often dose-limiting toxicities, and hypersensitivity reaction, GI side effects, and hair loss are common.

APPROACH TO PHARMACOLOGY OF PLANT ANTICANCER ALKALOIDS

Objectives

1. List the plant alkaloids used as cancer chemotherapeutic agents and describe their mechanisms of action, therapeutic uses, and adverse effects.

Definitions

Microtubules: Structures composed of tubulin polymers that are critical components of the cell cytoskeleton and the mitotic spindle.
Topoisomerases (I and II): Nuclear enzymes that cleave and unwind DNA to relieve torsional stress. They are necessary for DNA replication and RNA transcription. Topoisomerase II is also necessary for mitosis.

DISCUSSION

Class

Table 50-1 describes selected anticancer drugs. See also Case 49.

Table 50-1
SELECTED ANTICANCER DRUGS
(MAY BE COMBINED WITH OTHER ANTICANCER AGENTS)

AGENT	SELECTED INDICATIONS	SELECTED TOXICITY (ACUTE AND DELAYED)
Vinblastine	Non-Hodgkin lymphomas, Hodgkin disease, breast cancer	Nausea and vomiting, myelosuppression, neurotoxicity, alopecia
Vincristine	Acute lymphocytic leukemia, non-Hodgkin lymphomas, Hodgkin disease, multiple myeloma	Neurotoxicity is dose limiting. GI dysfunction, myelo-suppression, muscular-skeletal disorders, aberrant antidiuretic hormone secretion (SIADH)
Vinorelbine	Non-small cell lung cancer, breast cancer	Myelosuppression is dose limiting. Nausea and vomiting, GI dysfunction, neurotoxicity, SIADH
Paclitaxel	Breast cancer and a wide variety of other solid tumors	Myelosuppression is dose-limiting. Nausea and vomiting, hypotension, arrhythmias, neurotoxicity
Etoposide	Testicular and ovarian germ cell cancers, lung cancers, acute lymphoblastic leukemia	Myelosuppression is dose-limiting. Nausea and vomiting, mucositis, hypotension

Structure

Vinblastine and vincristine are derived from the periwinkle plant (*Vinca rosea*). Vinorelbine is a semisynthetic vinca alkaloid.

Paclitaxel is a complex diterpene derived from the Western and European yew (*Taxus brevifolia* and *Taxus baccata*).

Etoposide is a semisynthetic podophyllotoxin, an extract from the Mandrake root (*Mandragora officinarum*) or May apple root (*Podophyllum peltatum*).

Mechanism of Action

Vinca alkaloids (vinblastine, vincristine, vinorelbine): Bind tubulin to terminate microtubule assembly and cause cell arrest in metaphase (M) by blocking mitosis and chromosomal aggregation and causing mitotic spindle dissolution.

Taxanes (paclitaxel): Bind to microtubules resulting in their stabilization and in an enhancement of aberrant tubulin polymerization that result in cytotoxicity, including mitotic arrest.

Epipodophyllotoxins (etoposide): Reversibly complex with the enzyme topoisomerase II that results in double-stranded DNA strand breakage.

Administration

Hypersensitivity to paclitaxel can be reduced by premedication with dexamethasone and histamine H_1- and H_2-receptor blockers.

Pharmacokinetics

Abraxane is a formulation of paclitaxel bound to albumin, approved for treatment of breast cancer, that does not cause hypersensitivity reactions, and is less likely to result in severe neurotoxicity or myelosuppression.

Vinca alkaloid hepatic metabolism is decreased by L-asparaginase.

Paclitaxel is metabolized extensively by hepatic P450 enzymes (CYP450 3A4) with potential, therefore, of drug-drug interactions. Dose reduction is necessary for patients with liver dysfunction.

Etoposide is 95 percent plasma protein bound. Dose reduction is necessary for patients with renal dysfunction.

COMPREHENSION QUESTIONS

[50.1] Which of the following classes of cancer chemotherapeutic agents bind tubulin and cause arrest of cells in metaphase?

    A. Alkylating agents
    B. Antimetabolites
    C. Taxanes
    D. Vinca alkaloids

[50.2] Abraxane is often used to reduce hypersensitivity to which of the following drugs?

    A. Etoposide
    B. Paclitaxel
    C. Vinblastine
    D. Vincristine

[50.3] Neurotoxicity is dose-limiting for which of the following drugs?

    A. Etoposide
    B. Methotrexate
    C. Paclitaxel
    D. Vincristine

Answers

[50.1]   **D.** Vinca alkaloids (vinblastine, vincristine, vinorelbine) bind tubulin to terminate microtubule assembly and cause cell arrest in metaphase (M) by blocking mitosis and chromosomal aggregation and causing mitotic spindle dissolution. Alkylating agents form covalent bonds with adjacent guanine residues and inhibit DNA replication and transcription. Antimetabolites compete with naturally occurring compounds for binding sites on enzymes or else become incorporated into DNA or RNA to interfere with cell growth and division. Taxane (paclitaxel) binds to microtubules resulting in their stabilization and in an enhancement of aberrant tubulin polymerization that result in cytotoxicity, including mitotic arrest.

[50.2]   **B.** Hypersensitivity to paclitaxel can be reduced by abraxane, a formulation of paclitaxel bound to albumin.

[50.3]   **D.** Neurotoxicity is dose-limiting for vincristine. Myelosuppression is dose-limiting for paclitaxel, etoposide, and methotrexate.

PHARMACOLOGY PEARLS

 The plant anticancer alkaloids act on the microtubules, during the mitosis (M) phase of the cell cycle.

 The vinca alkaloids cause sensory and motor toxicities with the following order of activity: vincristine is greater than vinblastine is greater than vinorelbine.

 Neurotoxicity is dose limiting for vincristine, whereas myelosuppression is dose limiting for paclitaxel, etoposide, and methotrexate.

REFERENCES

Abal M, Andreu JM, Barasoain I. Taxanes: microtubules and centrosome targets, and cell cycle dependent mechanism of action. Curr Cancer Drug Targets 2003;3(3):193–203.

Gradishar WJ. Albumin-bound paclitaxel: a next-generation taxane. Expert Opin Pharmacother 2006;7(8):1041–53.

A 62-year-old woman presents for the evaluation of a breast lump. She noticed the lump in her left breast approximately 3 months ago but didn't come in because she "hates doctors." She denies pain, nipple discharge, or weight loss. Her last mammogram was 3 years ago. She stopped having menstrual periods at the age of 50. She is on no medications and has no significant medical history. On examination she is anxious, but her general examination is normal. Breast examination reveals a hard, 2-cm mass in the upper, outer quadrant of her left breast and several small lymph nodes in the left axilla. A fine needle aspiration of the mass confirms the diagnosis of breast carcinoma. Further workup does not reveal distant metastases. She subsequently undergoes a modified radical mastectomy and lymph node dissection. Pathology studies of the tumor reveal it to be estrogen- and progesterone-receptor positive, and she has microscopic metastases in the lymph nodes. She is started on tamoxifen.

◆ **What is the mechanism of action of tamoxifen?**

◆ **What are the side effects commonly associated with tamoxifen?**

ANSWERS TO CASE 51: STEROID HORMONES AND ANTAGONISTS

Summary: A 62-year-old woman with estrogen-receptor-positive breast cancer is begun on tamoxifen therapy.

◆ **Mechanism of action of tamoxifen:** Competitive inhibitor of estrogen receptors.

◆ **Common adverse effects:** Nausea, vomiting, hot flashes.

CLINICAL CORRELATION

Tamoxifen is a competitive inhibitor of estrogen binding to both isoforms of the estrogen receptor. This inhibits estrogen-dependent synthesis and autocrine growth-promoting actions of estrogen within the breast. Its primary use is as a chemotherapeutic agent in women with metastatic, estrogen-receptor positive breast cancer. It is also used to reduce the incidence of breast cancer development in women who are at high risk for developing breast cancer as a consequence of genetic factors and family history. As an antiestrogen, tamoxifen causes menopausal side effects, predominantly hot flashes and vaginal dryness. It can cause menstrual irregularities in premenopausal women. Tamoxifen has an estrogen agonistic effect on other parts of the body. It may simulate the effect of unopposed estrogen on the endometrium, resulting in an increased risk of endometrial carcinoma. Similarly, tamoxifen, like estrogen, increases the risk of thromboembolic disease.

APPROACH TO PHARMACOLOGY OF ANTIESTROGENS

Objective

1. Know the steroid hormone antagonists used in chemotherapy, their mechanisms of action, therapeutic uses, and adverse effects.

Definitions

Selective estrogen receptor modulators (SERMs): These are compounds that display a range of agonist-to-antagonist actions in a tissue-selective manner.

DISCUSSION

Class

Many breast cancers depend on the **proproliferative signals** produced by **estrogens** to support their growth. Similarly, the vast majority of **prostate**

cancers depend on the effects of **androgens** to support their growth. This has given rise to a class of anticancer agents that interfere with the action of estrogens or androgens in particular tissues. The **SERMs** are a relatively new class of compounds that have been developed in large part because of the understanding of the details of the molecular functioning of the estrogen receptor. There are **two forms of the estrogen receptor** (ER; see also Case 40) ERα and ERβ, which are derived from separate genes and have overlapping but distinct functions in a cell and promoter-dependent manner. Both ERs are weakly bound to the promoter/regulatory regions of genes that contain a particular DNA sequence, the estrogen response element (ERE). Binding of agonist, for example, 17β-estradiol, causes a significant and important change in the conformation of ER. This concept of ligand-mediated changes in receptor conformation is the key to the mechanism of action of the SERMs. The change in ER conformation causes ER to dimerize (ERα/ERα, ERβ/ERβ, or heterodimers of ERα/ERβ) and to bind more strongly to the ERE. One particular portion of the receptor, helix 12, is positioned and available to interact with other proteins called coactivators. Coactivators recruit other proteins of the RNA polymerase complex to the target gene(s) and produce the increase in transcription. Ligands that are not pure agonists cause a different conformation of ER and these different conformations can interact with different coactivators. Estrogen antagonists cause a conformational shift in ER that facilitates the interaction with corepressors, proteins that reduce transcriptional activity from target genes. The effect of a given drug will depend on the nature of the compound, the ratio of ERα/ERβ, and the particular repertoire of coactivators and corepressors present in any given cell.

The **pharmacologic goal in the development of SERMs is to produce estrogenic actions in those tissues where it would be beneficial** (e.g., bone, brain, liver) and to have either **no activity or antagonist activity in tissues, such as the endometrium or the breast, where estrogenic activity** (e.g., proproliferative signals and increased risk of cancer) **might be deleterious.**

There are **three SERMs approved for use, tamoxifen, toremifene, and raloxifene;** several more SERMs are in various stages of clinical trials. **Tamoxifen is a triphenylethylene** derived from the estrogen agonist **diethylstilbestrol.** It binds to both ERα and ERβ. Tamoxifen has antiestrogenic, estrogenic, or mixed activity depending on the tissue and the target gene. Tamoxifen is an estrogen **antagonist in human breast** and ER-positive breast cancer cells. However, it has **agonist activity in the uterus** and stimulates proliferation in the endometrium. It has **estrogen agonist activity in the liver** where it causes a **decrease in total cholesterol and low-density lipoprotein (LDL) but does not increase triglycerides or high-density lipoprotein (HDL).** Tamoxifen is **antiresorptive in bone and** is very useful in the treatment of breast cancer. It is used alone or in combination with other agents for treatment of advanced breast cancer in ER-positive tumors and is indicated for both early and advanced cancer in women of all ages. Response rates are approximately 50 percent in tumors that are ER positive and nearly 70 percent in ER and progestin-receptor-positive (PR positive) tumors; response in ER-negative tumors is less than 10 percent. Tamoxifen reduces the risk of recurrence by approximately 50 percent. It is also approved for primary prevention in women at high risk of breast cancer; in clinical trials it caused a 50 percent reduction in invasive breast cancer and a 47 percent reduction in noninvasive cancers. **Treatment should be discontinued after 5 years because of the development of drug-resistant tumors.** The adverse effects of tamoxifen include hot flashes, nausea, and vaginal bleeding; more serious adverse effects include a two- to threefold increase in the risk of endometrial cancer and a twofold increase in the risk if thromboembolic disease. It may cause GI disturbances.

Tamoxifen is administered orally and a major metabolite produced in the liver is 4-OH tamoxifen which has a 25- to 50-fold higher affinity for ERα and ERβ. Peak blood levels are attained 4–7 hours after administration. Tamoxifen is metabolized by the hepatic cytochrome P450 **system and excreted in the feces. Toremifene** is similar structurally to tamoxifen, with a chlorine substitution in one-ring structure. It has the same indications and effects as tamoxifen.

Raloxifene (see Case 40) is a benzothiophene that has been polyhydroxylated. Raloxifene has estrogen agonist activity in bone and inhibits resorption. It is indicated for the **treatment and prevention of osteoporosis.**

Like SERMs, **progestin receptor modulators (PRMs)** and **androgen receptor modulators (ARMs),** which would have tissue-selective hormonal actions, are in clinical development.

Aromatase Inhibitors

Estrogens produced locally, that is, within a tissue, may play a significant role in breast cancer. This has greatly stimulated interest in the use of aromatase inhibitors to selectively block the production of estrogens. Current agents include both **steroidal** (e.g., **formestane** and **exemestane**) and **nonsteroidal agents** (e.g., anastrozole, letrozole, and vorozole). The **steroidal, or type 1 agents,** are **substrate analogs** that act as **inhibitors and irreversibly inactivate the enzyme,** while the nonsteroidal, or type 2 agents, interact reversibly with the heme group in the cytochrome P450 **moiety. Exemestane, letrozole, and anastrozole** are currently indicated for the treatment of breast cancer.

These agents may be used as first-line treatment of breast cancer or as second-line drugs after tamoxifen. They are **highly efficacious,** but unlike tamoxifen they **do not increase the risk of uterine cancer or venous thromboembolism.** Because they dramatically reduce circulating as well as local levels of estrogens, they **do produce hot flashes,** and there is concern about their long-term effects on bone and plasma lipid profiles. **Aromatase inhibitors are under investigation for the prevention of breast cancer.**

COMPREHENSION QUESTIONS

[51.1] A woman entering your cancer clinic is concerned about her chance of developing breast cancer. Her mother died of the disease, and her sister has been diagnosed with the disease. A breast examination is negative. Which of the following might be used prophylactically in this woman?

A. Clomiphene
B. Leuprolide
C. Progesterone
D. Tamoxifen

[51.2] As compared to 17β-estradiol, SERMs have which of the following properties?

A. They are active orally.
B. They are antagonists in all tissues.
C. They have tissue-specific effects.
D. They are more potent than 17β-estradiol.

[51.3] A 44-year-old woman has developed breast cancer and is asked to participate in a clinical trial. She will be given formestane for 3 years. Which of the following are accurate statements about this medication?

A. It reversibly antagonizes the enzyme responsible for estrogen production.
B. It is a SERM similar to tamoxifen.
C. It is a nonsteroidal medication.
D. The patient will likely experience significant hot flashes.

Answers

[51.1]   **D.** Tamoxifen may be used in woman at high risk to develop breast cancer. Leuprolide and clomiphene have antiestrogenic activities but are not used prophylactically in women at high risk of breast cancer. Progesterone may cause proliferation and cancer in the breast.

[51.2]   **C.** SERMs are agonists at estrogen receptors in some but not all tissues.

[51.3]   **D.** Formestane is a steroidal aromatase inhibitor that irreversibly inactivates the aromatase. Patients generally have significant hot flashes because of the low estrogen levels.

PHARMACOLOGY PEARLS

 Tamoxifen reduces the risk of hormonally responsive breast cancer recurrence by approximately 50 percent.

 Tamoxifen treatment should be discontinued after 5 years to avoid the development of drug-resistant breast tumors or uterine cancer.

 Aromatase inhibitors are highly efficacious, and unlike tamoxifen they do not increase the risk of uterine cancer or venous thromboembolism.

REFERENCES

Rutqvist LE. Adjuvant endocrine therapy. Best Pract Res Clin Endocrinol Metab 2004;18:81–95.

Wickerham DL. Tamoxifen's impact as a preventive agent in clinical practice and an update on the STAR trial. Recent Results Cancer Res 2003;163:87–95.

Hind D, De Negris E, Ward S, et al. Hormonal therapies for early breast cancer: systematic review and economic evaluation. Health Technol Assess 2007;11:1–152.

A 22-year-old man is brought to the emergency room unresponsive and in respiratory distress. He was found unconscious at home next to a suicide note and an empty bottle of methanol. A brief history from an accompanying family member is significant for the patient having depression, but he is not currently on any medications. On examination he is not responsive to verbal stimuli but has pupillary and pain responses, and he is tachypneic and tachycardic (rapid respiratory and heart rates). His lungs are clear. You quickly institute supportive measures, intubate the patient, and send blood tests that confirm a profound anion-gap metabolic acidosis. No other drugs are found in his system. You diagnose him with an acute methanol overdose, start him on IV fluids, sodium bicarbonate, and an IV infusion of ethanol.

◆ **What enzyme metabolizes methanol?**

◆ **Why is ethanol used to treat methanol toxicity?**

ANSWERS TO CASE 52: SOLVENT TOXICITIES

Summary: A 22-year-old man with methanol poisoning is being treated with IV ethanol.

◆ **Enzyme that metabolizes methanol:** Alcohol dehydrogenase.

◆ **Reason for use of ethanol in methanol poisoning:** Competes for metabolism by alcohol dehydrogenase to reduce the production of toxic metabolites of methanol.

CLINICAL CORRELATION

The toxicity of methanol is primarily mediated by its metabolites. Methanol is metabolized by alcohol dehydrogenase to formaldehyde and subsequently to formic acid, the most likely cause of major organ toxicity. Formic acid inhibits cytochrome oxidase activity, resulting in tissue hypoxia and lactic acid production. The metabolic acidosis that occurs in methanol overdose is a result of the combination of formic acid and lactic acid that is produced. The most characteristic symptom in methanol poisoning is visual disturbances with blurred vision and a sense of "being in a snowstorm." Isopropyl alcohol and ethylene glycol similarly are metabolized by alcohol dehydrogenase to toxic metabolites. Unfortunately, the toxic metabolites of all of these solvents can cause permanent neurologic damage, blindness, coma, and death. In these clinical settings ethanol can be used therapeutically. It is given by continuous IV infusion to compete for metabolism by alcohol dehydrogenase. With hemodialysis, this can help to reduce the ongoing production of toxins. Sodium bicarbonate can be given to help correct the metabolic acidosis. Fomepizole, another available, very costly (~$4000 per patient) inhibitor of alcohol dehydrogenase is also available.

APPROACH TO PHARMACOLOGY OF SOLVENT TOXICITY

Objectives

1. Outline the basic principles of toxicology, including the dose-response relationship and risk and duration of exposure to toxins.
2. List the classes of solvent toxins and describe how exposure occurs and the effects of exposure.

Definitions

Toxicology: Study of the deleterious effects of chemical, biological, and physical substances, including their deleterious effects on the human body.

Xenobiotics: Deleterious foreign substances.

Toxicokinetics: Study of the absorption, distribution, metabolism, and elimination of xenobiotics.

DISCUSSION

Class

In considering the human toxicity of xenobiotics, it is important to keep in mind the following general principles:

The **toxicokinetics of xenobiotics** is equivalent to the pharmacokinetics described for drugs used as therapeutic agents.

Exposure to toxic substances is generally either **occupational** or **environmental** (air, soil, water, etc.).

Certain xenobiotics (e.g., acids, alkali, strong reducing and oxidizing agents, detergents) **cause nonspecific damage** to tissues by altering proteins, nucleic acids, lipids, and other macromolecules that are integral to cell structure and integrity.

Biotransformation of **chemical toxicants** may result in formation of **reactive metabolites** or the production of **free radicals and reactive oxygen** that form covalent bonds with proteins, nucleic acids, and lipids to disrupt cell function.

For many xenobiotics, a **dose-response relationship** for toxicity cannot be directly determined from human data but rather must be based on data derived strictly from **animal studies.**

In addition to decreasing or eliminating exposure, management of the poisoned patient is supportive and depends on the specific tissue or organ or tissue involved (Table 52-1).

Table 52-1
SOLVENT CLASSIFICATION AND TOXICITY

SELECTED SOLVENT CLASSES*	SELECTED TOXICITY
Aliphatic alcohols (e.g., methanol)	See clinical correlation
Aliphatic hydrocarbons (e.g., hexane)	CNS depression, sensorimotor disturbances
Glycols and glycol ethers (ethylene glycol, propylene glycol, etc.)	CNS depression, renal and hepatic toxicity
Halogenated aliphatic hydrocarbons (e.g., chloroform, carbon tetrachloride, trichloroethylene, tetrachloroethylene, 1,1,1-trichloroethane)	CNS depression, impaired memory, *Tetrachloroethylene:* peripheral neuropathy *Carbon tetrachloride* (acute or chronic exposure): hepatic injury *Chloroform, carbon tetrachloride, trichloroethylene:* renal injury carcinogenicity in animals (certain halogenated hydrocarbons)
Aromatic hydrocarbons (e.g., benzene, toluene)	*Benzene:* CNS depression that may result in ataxia, vertigo, and coma. Chronic exposure can result in severe bone marrow depression and possibly leukemia *Toluene:* CNS depressant that acutely can cause ataxia at low exposure and at high exposure lead rapidly to loss of consciousness. The effects of chronic exposure are uncertain

*These agents are used as industrial solvents, as cleaning agents, in synthesis of other chemicals, or as components of personal and household products.

COMPREHENSION QUESTIONS

[52.1] Which of the following is the most characteristic symptom in methanol poisoning?

    A. Carcinogenicity
    B. Hepatic injury
    C. Renal injury
    D. Visual disturbances

[52.2] Which of the following compounds is the most likely cause of organ toxicity from methanol?

    A. Formaldehyde
    B. Formic acid
    C. Lactic acid
    D. Methanol

[52.3] Severe bone marrow depression is most likely to result from exposure to which of the following solvents?

A. Benzene
B. Ethylene glycol
C. Hexane
D. Toluene

Answers

[52.1] **D.** The most characteristic symptom in methanol poisoning is visual disturbances. Hepatic injury, renal injury, and potential carcinogenicity are more characteristic of the halogenated aliphatic hydrocarbons.

[52.2] **B.** Methanol is metabolized by alcohol dehydrogenase to formaldehyde, which is then metabolized to formic acid, the most likely cause of methanol's organ toxicity. Formic acid inhibition of cytochrome oxidase activity results in tissue hypoxia with the production of lactic acid, which with formic acid, can result in metabolic acidosis.

[52.3] **A.** Chronic exposure to benzene can result in bone marrow depression. Exposure to toluene results in CNS depression. The effects of chronic exposure to toluene are uncertain. Hexane is more likely to cause CNS depression and sensorimotor disturbances. Ethylene glycol is likely to cause CNS disturbances and renal disturbances.

PHARMACOLOGY PEARLS

 Toxicity from the solvents commonly affect the CNS, causing sedation or CNS depression.

 Exposure to carbon tetrachloride can lead to hepatic toxicity.

Chronic exposure to benzene may lead to bone marrow depression and possibly leukemia.

REFERENCES

Klassen CD, ed. Casarett and Doull's Toxicology, the Basic Science of Poisons, 7th ed. New York: McGraw-Hill, 2007.

Rom WM, Markopwitz S, ed. Environmental and Occupational Medicine, 4th ed. Philadelphia (PA): Lippincott Williams and Wilkins, 2007.

U.S. National Library of Medicine. Toxnet: http://toxnet.nlm.nih.gov, 2007.

A woman brings her 5-year-old son in for evaluation. He has had progressive difficulty walking in the past few months and has seemed irritable. He has also seemed quite tired. He has vomited on one or two occasions. His past medical history is unremarkable. He was born after an uncomplicated, full-term pregnancy. He has had all of his vaccines and had achieved all of his developmental milestones for his age. He lives with his parents in a home that was built in the 1920s, which they have been renovating. On examination, he is somewhat restless but cooperative. His conjunctiva and mucous membranes are pale. Neurologic examination is significant for an ataxic gait (clumsiness). His general examination is otherwise unremarkable. A complete blood count (CBC) shows him to be anemic. A serum lead level is markedly elevated. You admit him to the hospital and start him on succimer.

◆ **How does chronic lead exposure cause anemia?**

◆ **What is the mechanism of action of succimer?**

ANSWERS TO CASE 53: HEAVY METAL POISONING

Summary: A 5-year-old boy with lead toxicity is admitted to the hospital and started on succimer.

◆ **Mechanism of lead-induced anemia:** Inhibition of δ-aminolevulinic acid dehydratase, which blocks the conversion of δ-aminolevulinic acid to porphobilinogen, disrupting hemoglobin synthesis.

◆ **Mechanism of action of succimer:** Chelates lead to increase lead excretion in the urine.

CLINICAL CORRELATION

Most lead toxicity in children is a result of GI ingestion. Children absorb a greater portion of ingested lead than adults do. The source of this lead is often from lead-based paint that was widely used before the 1970s. Inorganic lead binds to hemoglobin and distributes to soft tissues, including the brain. It later accumulates in the bone, from which it eliminated very slowly. Lead produces anemia via the inhibition of the enzyme δ-aminolevulinic acid dehydratase, which converts δ-aminolevulinic acid to porphobilinogen. This interrupts the pathway of synthesis of hemoglobin. Lead can also cause CNS effects, especially in children. Common signs include vertigo, ataxia, headache, restlessness, and irritability. Vomiting, delirium, and seizures may occur. Lowered IQ and behavioral disturbances may be the result of childhood exposure. Peripheral neuropathy is another possible outcome of chronic lead poisoning. Treatment of lead toxicity requires cessation of exposure and, in severe cases, chelation therapy. In children, succimer is frequently used. It can be administered orally. It binds to lead and increases the excretion of lead in the urine. Other drugs used for chelation include calcium disodium ethylenediaminetetraacetic acid (EDTA), dimercaprol, and penicillamine.

APPROACH TO PHARMACOLOGY OF HEAVY METAL POISONING

Objectives

1. Discuss the general principles related to heavy metal poisoning.
2. List the common sources of heavy metal exposure and describe their mechanisms of action and their toxicities (Table 53-1).
3. List agents used for the management of heavy metal poisoning and describe their mechanisms of action.

Table 53-1
HEAVY METALS AND TOXIC EFFECTS

HEAVY METAL	TOXICITY	NOTES
Iron (Fe)	GI mucosa destruction, with severe gastroenteritis, abdominal pain, and bloody diarrhea, that lead to systemic absorption as transferrin with subsequent endothelial damage in the liver and kidney that can result in metabolic acidosis, coma, shock, cardiovascular collapse, and death	Exposure in children is generally by accidental ingestion of iron supplements. In adults toxicity is generally the result of repeated transfusions, inherited disorders, or intentional overdosing
Mercury (Hg)	Neurologic and behavioral changes, including visual deficits, because of neuronal injury and encephalopathy are among the most common adverse effects of mercury. Excitability, tremors, and gingivitis are hallmarks of mercury toxicity. GI and renal injury are common with exposure to mercury salts, which can also cause severe pain and vomiting because of its corrosive action on the mucosa of the mouth, pharynx, and intestine. Mercury vapor can result in severe respiratory difficulty with residual fibrosis	Elemental mercury vapor is well absorbed from the lungs. Elemental mercury in liquid form is relatively nontoxic. Inorganic mercury salts are generally ingested and when absorbed concentrate in the kidney. They have a long half-life Organomercury compounds are absorbed readily from the GI tract. They undergo enterohepatic recycling with long half-lives. The developing nervous system is especially vulnerable to mercury exposure in utero
Arsenic (As)	Nonspecific GI, CNS, and cardiovascular toxicity. Arsine gas can cause severe abdominal pain and, rarely, extensive hemolysis with renal damage from degraded hemoglobin	Exposure can be through ingestion or inhalation

(Continued)

Table 53-1
HEAVY METALS AND TOXIC EFFECTS (*continued*)

HEAVY METAL	TOXICITY	NOTES
Lead (Pb)	Acute: uncommon; includes paresthesia, muscle weakness, hemolysis, renal damage Chronic: see Clinical Correlation; most serious toxicity is encephalopathy that can lead to impaired learning and mental retardation, especially in children	See Clinical Correlation. Crosses placental barrier and can cause in utero damage leading to impaired CNS development

DISCUSSION

Class

The general principles related to heavy metal toxicity are the following:

Exposure to heavy metals may be **acute or chronic,** generally through accidental occupational or environmental exposure.

Most, if not all, heavy metals **interact with SH groups** and perhaps other functional groups of cell proteins to cause their toxicity.

Multiple organ systems may be affected but particularly the **CNS, liver, kidney, and respiratory and immune systems.**

Management of metal poisoning involves **removal of the source, decontamination,** and **supportive treatment for symptoms.** In addition, **metal chelators** can be used to remove or prevent metal binding to important cell constituents (Table 53-2). The major chelators interact with the same functional groups as the heavy metals to form complexes which can then be eliminated from the body. With the exception of **deferoxamine,** their selectivity is relatively poor in that they **also bind important endogenous divalent cations, notably Ca^{2+}.**

Table 53-2
HEAVY METAL CHELATORS

HEAVY METAL CHELATORS	PRIMARY METALS CHELATED	NOTES
Dimercaprol	Mercury (Hg), Arsenic (As)	Administered parenterally; avoid in iron or cadmium poisoning because complex is extremely hepatotoxic; avoid with methylmercury poisoning because it facilitates entry into the CNS
EDTA	Lead (Pb)	Administered parenterally; chronic treatment requires "off" periods to allow redistribution out of bone
Deferoxamine	Iron (Fe), Aluminum (Al)	Administered parenterally
Penicillamine trientine	Copper (Cu), adjunct for Pb, Hg	Administered orally; used to chelate excess copper in Wilson disease; may result in allergic reaction
Succimer	Lead (Pb), adjunct for Hg, As	Administered orally; causes GI disturbances and rash

COMPREHENSION QUESTIONS

[53.1] Which of the following heavy metal chelators is used as a primary treatment for mercury poisoning?

   A. Dimercaprol
   B. EDTA
   C. Penicillamine
   D. Succimer

[53.2] GI mucosa destruction, with severe gastroenteritis, abdominal pain, and bloody diarrhea are characteristic symptoms of poisoning from which of the following heavy metals?

   A. Arsenic
   B. Elemental liquid mercury
   C. Iron
   D. Lead

[53.3] Lead-induced anemia is a result of inhibition of which of the following
        enzymes?

    A. Aldehyde dehydrogenase
    B. Cytochrome oxidase
    C. δ-Aminolevulinic acid dehydratase
    D. Monoamine oxidase

Answers

[53.1] **A.** Dimercaprol is used as a primary heavy metal chelator for treat-
        ment of mercury poisoning. EDTA and succimer are used for lead
        poisoning. Penicillamine is used to treat copper poisoning. EDTA and
        penicillamine are used as adjuncts to treat mercury poisoning.

[53.2] **C.** Iron poisoning causes characteristic GI mucosa destruction, with
        severe gastroenteritis, abdominal pain, and bloody diarrhea.
        Elemental liquid mercury is relatively nontoxic. A nonspecific GI,
        CNS, and cardiovascular toxicity is caused by arsenic. The most seri-
        ous (chronic) toxicity from lead poisoning is encephalopathy.

[53.3] **C.** Lead produces anemia via the inhibition of the enzyme δ-
        aminolevulinic acid dehydratase, which converts δ-aminolevulinic
        acid to porphobilinogen. This interrupts the pathway of synthesis of
        hemoglobin.

PHARMACOLOGY PEARLS

 Iron toxicity can lead to gastroenteritis, liver, and kidney damage
and, if severe enough, death.

 The most common manifestations of mercury poisoning are the neuronal toxicity such as visual deficits.

 Lead poisoning can lead to mental retardation in the developing
fetus or children.

REFERENCES

Klassen CD, ed. Casarett and Doull's Toxicology, the Basic Science of Poisons, 7th
    ed. New York: McGraw-Hill, 2007.
Rom WM, Markopwitz S, ed. Environmental and Occupational Medicine, 4th ed.
    Philadelphia (PA): Lippincott Williams and Wilkins, 2007.
U.S. National Library of Medicine. Toxnet: http://toxnet.nlm.nih.gov, 2007.

Listing of Cases

Listing by Case Number

Listing by Disorder (Alphabetical)

LISTING BY CASE NUMBER

LISTING BY DISORDER (ALPHABETICAL)

❖ INDEX